I0884975

Building a Patient-Centered Interprofessional Education Program

Steven D. Waldman
University of Missouri-Kansas City School of Medicine, USA

Stephanie Bowlin
Western University of Health Sciences, USA

A volume in the Advances in Medical Education, Research, and Ethics (AMERE) Book Series

IGI Global
PUBLISHER of TIMELY KNOWLEDGE

Published in the United States of America by
IGI Global
Medical Information Science Reference (an imprint of IGI Global)
701 E. Chocolate Avenue
Hershey PA, USA 17033
Tel: 717-533-8845
Fax: 717-533-8661
E-mail: cust@igi-global.com
Web site: http://www.igi-global.com

Library of Congress Cataloging-in-Publication Data

Names: Waldman, Steven D., editor. | Bowlin, Stephanie, editor.
Title: Building a patient-centered interprofessional education program / Steven D. Waldman, Stephanie Bowlin, editors.
Description: Hershey, PA : Medical Information Science Reference, [2020] | Includes bibliographical references and index. | Summary: "This book explores how to facilitate patient-centered interprofessional education programs"--Provided by publisher.
Identifiers: LCCN 2019047157 (print) | LCCN 2019047158 (ebook) | ISBN 9781799830665 (hardcover) | ISBN 9781799830672 (ebook)
Subjects: MESH: Education, Medical, Continuing | Patient-Centered Care | Interprofessional Relations
Classification: LCC R834 (print) | LCC R834 (ebook) | NLM W 20 | DDC 610.71--dc23
LC record available at https://lccn.loc.gov/2019047157
LC ebook record available at https://lccn.loc.gov/2019047158

This book is published in the IGI Global book series Advances in Medical Education, Research, and Ethics (AMERE) (ISSN: 2475-6601; eISSN: 2475-661X)

British Cataloguing in Publication Data
A Cataloguing in Publication record for this book is available from the British Library.

All work contributed to this book is new, previously-unpublished material.
The views expressed in this book are those of the authors, but not necessarily of the publisher.

For electronic access to this publication, please contact: eresources@igi-global.com.

Advances in Medical Education, Research, and Ethics (AMERE) Book Series

ISSN:2475-6601
EISSN:2475-661X

Editor-in-Chief: Steven D. Waldman, University of Missouri-Kansas City School of Medicine, USA & Stephanie Bowlin, Western University of Health Sciences, USA)

MISSION

Humans are living longer now than ever as a result of advances in the medical field. Having the tools available to train knowledgeable and ethical future generations of doctors and medical researchers is essential to continuing to advance our understanding of the human body and develop new ways of treating and curing sickness and disease.

The **Advances in Medical Education, Research, and Ethics (AMERE)** book series highlights publications pertaining to advancements in pedagogical practice for developing future healthcare professionals, research methods, and advancements in the medical field, as well as moral behavior and practice of healthcare professionals, students, and researchers. Featuring research-based book publications that are highly relevant to the healthcare community, this series is ideally designed for library inclusion at medical universities and research institutions as well as personal use by medical professionals, researchers, and upper-level students entering the field.

COVERAGE

- Clinical Research
- Conflicts of Interest
- Ethics in Medicine
- Healthcare Pedagogy
- Medical Curricula
- Medical Simulation
- Patient Data
- Professional Development
- Research Methods
- Scientific Misconduct

IGI Global is currently accepting manuscripts for publication within this series. To submit a proposal for a volume in this series, please contact our Acquisition Editors at Acquisitions@igi-global.com or visit: http://www.igi-global.com/publish/.

The Advances in Medical Education, Research, and Ethics (AMERE) Book Series (ISSN 2475-6601) is published by IGI Global, 701 E. Chocolate Avenue, Hershey, PA 17033-1240, USA, www.igi-global.com. This series is composed of titles available for purchase individually; each title is edited to be contextually exclusive from any other title within the series. For pricing and ordering information please visit http://www.igi-global.com/book-series/advances-medical-education-research-ethics/132365. Postmaster: Send all address changes to above address.

Titles in this Series

For a list of additional titles in this series, please visit:
http://www.igi-global.com/book-series/advances-medical-education-research-ethics/132365

Exploring Best Child Development Practices in Contemporary Society
Nava R. Silton (Marymount Manhattan College, USA)
Medical Information Science Reference • © 2020 • 305pp • H/C (ISBN: 9781799829409) • US $245.00

Handbook of Research on the Efficacy of Training Programs and Systems in Medical Education
Ruth Gotian (Weill Cornell Medicine, USA) Yoon Kang (Weill Cornell Medicine, USA) and Joseph Safdieh (Weill Cornell Medicine, USA)
Medical Information Science Reference • © 2020 • 566pp • H/C (ISBN: 9781799814689) • US $365.00

Gender Equity in the Medical Profession
Maria Irene Bellini (Belfast Health and Social Care Trust, UK) and Vassilios E. Papalois (Imperial College London, UK)
Medical Information Science Reference • © 2020 • 339pp • H/C (ISBN: 9781522595991) • US $265.00

Preparing Physicians to Lead in the 21st Century
Valerie Anne Storey (University of Central Florida, USA) and Thomas Edward Beeman (University of Pennsylvania Health System, USA)
Medical Information Science Reference • © 2019 • 245pp • H/C (ISBN: 9781522575764) • US $245.00

Optimizing Medical Education With Instructional Technology
Erdem Demiroz (Trakya University, Turkey) and Steven D. Waldman (University of Missouri-Kansas City School of Medicine, USA)
Medical Information Science Reference • © 2019 • 291pp • H/C (ISBN: 9781522562894) • US $215.00

For an entire list of titles in this series, please visit:
http://www.igi-global.com/book-series/advances-medical-education-research-ethics/132365

IGI Global
PUBLISHER of TIMELY KNOWLEDGE

701 East Chocolate Avenue, Hershey, PA 17033, USA
Tel: 717-533-8845 x100 • Fax: 717-533-8661
E-Mail: cust@igi-global.com • www.igi-global.com

Editorial Advisory Board

Table of Contents

Detailed Table of Contents

Interprofessional education has been gaining traction in the educational and professional climate today. As a shift has been made to incorporate the collaboration of health professionals into education, benefits in overall quality of education and patient care have been observed. Students who are involved in IPE are able to learn about other careers, learn the limitations of their own career, cement existing knowledge, develop relationships with members of various fields, improve teamwork skills, and enhance their job satisfaction. Patients have also benefited from the new IPE implementation. As a result of increased collaboration, there has been a reduction in patient errors and overall improved quality of care among programs who participate in IPE.

The goal of allopathic and osteopathic medical education is to develop the medical student into a competent and caring physician. As the evolving healthcare system continues to evolve and intersect with an increased breadth and depth of medical knowledge and an aging and more complex patient population, the emerging physician must now rely more on a team-based approach to patient-centered healthcare. Integrating interprofessional competencies into the span of the medical education and assessment process via the core competencies and the Entrustable Professional Activities has the potential to help instill not only the knowledge and skills required to practice as a member of an interprofessional healthcare team, but can also help to normalize the culture and thus the expectation of practicing collaboratively with all members of the health team toward the goal of improved patient outcome.

The widespread availability and use of digital technology including the internet, cell phones, remote electrocardiogram, PACS (picture archiving and communication) systems, and video chat platforms such as Facetime and Zoom have fueled the growth of telehealth. In 2013, only about 350,000 Americans utilized telehealth technology as part of their care plan, and most of these patient interactions involved the use of telephone consults. By the end of 2018, that number had jumped to over 7,000,000. Coupled with the exponential increase in the use of telehealth technology has been a rapid decrease in the cost of telehealth technology and HIPAA compliant telehealth platforms. The ease of use and relative affordability of these technologic advances make telehealth technology an ideal tool to enhance the interprofessional community of practice.

Older persons commonly experience complex health needs that are best met by a multifaceted healthcare team. Most healthcare disciplines provide geriatric competencies specific to their professions which support the development of IPE curricula. The American Geriatric Society provided a list of formal geriatric competencies that are useful to curriculum designers and health professions educators. The chapter provides ideas for imbedding commonly occurring geriatric concepts and clinical assessment tools that are relevant to all disciplines for the creation of interprofessional learning activities.

Teaching in the 21st century requires universities to offer educational programs based on skill development, student-centered settings, focus on the needs of the community, and context-rich experiences that prepare graduates for both local and international practice. Several educational strategies and trends have been designed and implemented to incorporate rapid sociocultural and care model transitions. This chapter focuses on the challenge-based learning (CBL) strategy application in medical education to foster a transformative learning experience in which the patient is the center of the educational process. Several examples of CBL are presented, and an analysis is performed of the benefits and difficulties for its implementation in medical education. In the end, there is a discussion about enabling resources and dynamics for excellence in medical education.

Diabetes is a growing public health epidemic in the U.S. African Americans are particularly at-risk for diabetes with rates twice as high as whites. Health professionals are recommended to encourage their at-risk patients to participate in evidence-based lifestyle change programs, such as CDC's National Diabetes Prevention Program (DPP) and support their weight loss efforts. This chapter describes feasibility/outcomes of a community-based collaborative care model used to implement a weekly-group DPP facilitated by interprofessional teams of medical school students with three African American churches (N=72 participants; 93% overweight/obese). At 12-weeks, 30% of participants had lost at least 5 lbs.; among those attending at least nine sessions, 55% achieved at least 3% weight loss. Findings suggest interprofessional student teams can feasibly partner with churches to deliver the DPP and achieve weight-loss outcomes associated with reducing diabetes risk. Future research is needed to determine scalability/costs of using community-based collaborative care student models to address diabetes.

In the United States, quality healthcare is an expectation. The accepted healthcare delivery approach relies on interprofessional, collaborative, and person-centered teams. As a result, health professions education must implement education and training to graduate a healthcare workforce that is competent in interprofessional collaboration. Physician assistants (PA) have an important role in the healthcare team. The purpose of this chapter is to provide a historical background to the interprofessional collaborative healthcare team, the formation of interprofessional

Foreword

As an emergency room nurse who has recently had the privilege of caring for patients during the recent pandemic, I can tell you unequivocally that the interprofessional care team has never been more important. In regular times, some healthcare professionals may view interprofessionalism as something of a value-added proposition, a nicety, or something that might make you a little happier at work. During a pandemic, I have found that interprofessional care is the element that can make the difference between life and death for our patients. I suspect that some of you that are reading this that have not been involved in the care of sick Covid-19 patients are thinking that this is an overstatement. Let me assure you that this is not the case.

What we learned early on in the care of patients who were critically ill with Covid-19 is that minutes mattered and our safety as well as the safety of the patient depended on facilitated communication and flawless teamwork. It was not unusual to see a sick Covid patient present to the emergency department with a high fever and cough, but with an initial oxygen saturation determination of 96…only for that initially acceptable O2 sat to drop precipitously over a very short period of time while IV's were getting started, labs drawn, insurance cards copied. etc. What we also learned is that if we wanted to optimize the patient's chance of survival, all members of the interprofessional care team needed to work together like a well-oiled machine. Waiting for a blood gas from respiratory therapy, an IV start from nursing, an EKG from the patient care associate, getting an ICU bed cleaned and ready to go, receiving crucial medications from the pharmacy was simply not an option. We knew that if we all didn't pull together as a team, it was the patient who would ultimately suffer. Dramatic words for dramatic times, but they are true.

This text is worth reading because if provides healthcare educators a clear, how-to-do-it roadmap for embedding interprofessionalism into the healthcare curriculum. The authors all have hands-on experience in building successful interprofessional practice and education programs. Unlike many works on interprofessional practice and education, which spend much effort on telling anyone who will listen what is wrong with the current healthcare delivery system, this text actually tells you how to do something about it. I wholeheartedly recommend this text as a "must-have" for anyone who is committed to improving the care of our patients.

Kelley Sharp
Department of Emergency Medicine, Hartford Hospital, Hartford, USA
May 1, 2020

Preface

Patient-Centered Interprofessional Education: The Time Is Now

Time has shown that the first goal of every healthcare professional has always been to provide the highest quality care to their patients. One could argue that this care has always been, for better or worse, provided in some form of team environment. So, you might ask, why is there such a sudden interest in building the interprofessional care team? One answer might be that medicine has never been more specialized and it is unreasonable to expect one person to know everything about everything. Another answer might be that medicine has become depersonalized with the replacement of the family physician who has known the patient for years by the anonymous hospitalist. Another answer might be that the electronic medical record has destroyed the art of patient communication and we all need to band together to prevent patient care Armageddon. I am sure that you can think of many more answers, each more plausible that the next.

Regardless of the answer, the goal of each dedicated health care professional has remained constant……quality care for our patients……and it has become increasingly clear that the best way to attain that goal is to harness the unique perspectives, insights, and talents of each member of the interprofessional team. While we are still in the process of discovering the best ways to facilitate interprofessional collaboration for the benefit of the patient, we know that the following is true:

1. Interprofessional patient-centric care improves outcomes by utilizing the unique perspectives that each professional brings to the bedside to optimize patient care.
2. Interprofessional patient-centric care helps bridge myriad barriers to communication by allowing for the right information to get to the right team members in the most efficient manner possible.
3. Interprofessional patient-centric care helps reduce errors by involving the entire team in clinical decision making. Everyone caring for the patient knows the "why".

4. Interprofessional patient-centric care makes care? saves healthcare dollars by reducing operational inefficiencies and redundancies, e.g. duplicate lab tests, medical imaging, etc.
5. Interprofessional patient-centric care makes care? improves the culture of care by making all team members feel valued not just for their unique knowledge base, but as an active and vital member of the patient care team.

If we accept that the above is true, then it is incumbent on all health care educators to equip our students to flourish in an interprofessional team environment. As many of us who have embraced the concept of interprofessional patient-centered care have discovered, this is something that is easier said than done.....hence our desire to draw upon experts with practical experience in this endeavor to help us identify the best ways to teach ourselves and our students.

Building A Patient-Centered Interprofessional Education Program has brought together a group of authors who not only believe in the promise of interprofessional patient-centered care, but have the hands-on practical experience and smarts to help us achieve our goal.

We hope you will enjoy reading *Building A Patient-Centered Interprofessional Education Program* as much as we did writing it and hope you will find it a valuable resource as you train your students.

Steven D. Waldman
University of Missouri-Kansas City School of Medicine, USA

Stephanie Bowlin
Western University of Health Sciences, USA

Chapter 1
How to Build Effective Interprofessional Healthcare Teams

Stefanie R. Ellison
University of Missouri-Kansas City School of Medicine, USA

Christi L. Bartlett
University of Kansas Medical Center, USA

Valerie L. Ruehter
University of Missouri-Kansas City School of Pharmacy, USA

ABSTRACT

Building effective interprofessional (IP) teams is an important process for healthcare systems across the world. In order to be truly effective, professional degree programs must teach our future health professionals to learn and collaborate on teams during their education. The goal of building effective IP healthcare teams will be achieved when each healthcare system effectively supports IP collaboration, the development of dynamic teams, and the appropriate use of resources. Advancing the effort to build effective IP healthcare teams will take an investment from key stakeholders such as educators, faculty and students, leaders and researchers in academic medicine, hospital and system administrators, policymakers, as well as patients and their families to create a culture of IP collaboration and provide the resources necessary to be sustainable and successful. This chapter will serve to show that effective IP healthcare teams can successfully improve patient outcomes, provide quality care, improve the healthcare team's experience, and reduce costs.

DOI: 10.4018/978-1-7998-3066-5.ch001

INTRODUCTION

Interprofessional teams are an imperative for all health systems in the current healthcare work force in the United States. These teams are what patients and their families, as well as the healthcare providers, deserve and need to provide compassionate, high quality, state-of-the-art care. Defining effective and efficient care is difficult but included in this book chapter are definitions of effective interprofessional teams, examples of published standards for interprofessional care that improve patient outcomes, and examples of interprofessional teams that function to support the Quadruple Aim. This is the foundation to help healthcare organizations and health professions programs to educate and build effective IP teams for healthcare.

Health professions education in the United States and Canada now incorporates interprofessional education (IPE) in the curricula for most if not all health professional degree programs because there are existing accreditation criteria for degrees in dentistry, medicine, nursing and pharmacy. In order to construct IP teams, it is important to know and understand key definitions and terms for Interprofessional Education (IPE), Interprofessional Collaborative Practice (ICPT), Interprofessional Teamwork (IPT), and Interprofessional Team-Based Care (IPTBC) (Table 1).

Over the past decade, health professions learners in the United States and Canada have completed their degrees educated and trained to provide patient-centered care on IP teams, however the team structures in most healthcare systems are not adequately developed to accommodate the skill set of these graduates. Health professionals are finding that while they are practice ready for IP care, the teams they are joining do not reflect the care they have practiced during clinical training. Healthcare systems are growing in complexity and technology but oftentimes lack the efficiency and effectiveness described in training. Healthcare systems, to be effective, must be more patient-driven and centered, recognizing the importance of teams, and optimizing the healthcare workforce to increase the value and quality of the care that IP teams provide.

BACKGROUND

Recommendations for education in all health professions has been explored extensively through the Interprofessional Education Collaborative (IPEC). In 2009, six national representatives formed this collaborative to promote interprofessional education and to provide guidelines to advance the ability for professional programs to promote learning and interprofessional practice (IPEC, 2016). In 2016-2017, additional members and supporting organizations joined and now include representatives from academic health sciences libraries, allied health, dentistry, dietetics, dental hygiene,

Table 1. Consensus terminology in the published literature

Term	Definition	Organization
Interprofessional Education (IPE)	"When students from two or more professions learn about, from and with each other to enable effective collaboration and improve health outcomes."	WHO*
Interprofessional Collaborative Practice (IPCP)	"When multiple health workers from different professional backgrounds work together with patients, families, careers†, and communities to deliver the highest quality of care."	WHO*
Interprofessional Teamwork (IPT)	"The levels of cooperation, coordination and collaboration characterizing the relationships between professions in delivering patient-centered care."	IPEC‡
Interprofessional Team-Based Care (IPTBC)	"Care delivered by intentionally created, usually relatively small work groups in health care who are recognized by others as well as by themselves as having a collective identity and shared responsibility for a patient or group of patients (e.g., rapid response team, palliative care team, primary care team, and operating room team)."	IPEC‡

* World Health Organization (2010). *Framework for action on interprofessional education & collaborative practice.* Retrieved January 8, 2019, from http://whqlibdoc.who.int/hq/2010/WHO_HRH_HPN_10.3_eng.pdf.

†The term "caregivers" is more commonly used in the United States.

‡Interprofessional Education Collaborative (2016). *Core competencies for interprofessional collaborative practice: 2016 update.* Retrieved January 8, 2019, from https://nebula.wsimg.com/2f68a39520b03336b41038c370497473?AccessKeyId= DC06780E69ED19E2B3A5&disposition=0&alloworigin=1.

medicine, nursing, occupational and physical therapy, optometry, osteopathic health, pharmacy, physician assistant, podiatry, programs of public health, psychology, respiratory therapy, simulation in healthcare, social work, speech language and hearing, and veterinary programs. Although the original 2011 panel focused its recommendations on the professions of medicine, nursing, pharmacy, dentistry, and public health, IPEC continues to engage multiple health professions in its efforts to guide curriculum development across health professions schools.

In 2019, the Health Professions Accreditors Collaborative (HPAC) and the National Center for Interprofessional Practice and Education developed a guide to improve the quality of IPE for the health professions. (HPAC, 2019) This guiding document was developed through a multi-year, multi-phase consensus aimed at supporting the implementation of excellent IPE and to advise health professions educators on quality IPE while meeting accreditation standards. In this document, the societal importance of IPE is recognized in educating our future health professionals. This body also recognizes the current redesign of the United States health care system to become more patient-driven and the pivotal role that teams will play in this effort. The HPAC also emphasizes the need to optimize the healthcare workforce, increase the value of the care provided, and combine these with the use of technology. Health professions education now, more than ever, will have a key role in ensuring health professions' educational commitment to provide and achieve high quality IPE and improve IP collaboration for quality care.

MAIN FOCUS: ISSUES, CONTROVERSIES, PROBLEMS

The main issues of building and establishing IP care are inconsistencies in the education and training of our professionals, the changing needs of healthcare systems, the ability of the system to adapt to IP teams, and the unique needs of today's patients. As a result of increased professional accreditation standards, IPE efforts are growing across healthcare professions programs but silos of education still exist. To support the effort to establishing more consistent IPE for our graduates, there are more resources in the public domain to prepare educators and academic programs as well as graduate healthcare professionals to be practice ready to join IP teams. There are now IPE models and tool kits to assist health professions educators in designing effective educational programs to prepare professional learners to join IP teams ready to collaborate and provide team-based care upon entering practice. These resources are working to establish common definitions and shared language along with curriculum and assessments to guide consistent IP learning. Health professions learners also need adequate context to apply what they are learning in real, clinical environments in order to establish the clinical practice skills necessary for the healthcare systems they are going to enter. Community-oriented learning environments and realistic clinical experiences are necessary to prepare our learners.

IPE is growing in programs in the United States, Canada and worldwide. Research shows that IPE courses are offered in 92% of United States medical schools with 89% providing clinical IPE training in academic health centers. (Gilbert, Yan & Hoffman, 2010). In Canada, IPE is provided in 12 out of 17 medical schools (You, Malik, Scott & Fung, 2017). In Japan, a 2016 survey of all 81 of Japan's medical schools demonstrated that IPE courses were provided in only 46 medical schools in the early years of medical school and less frequently in later years (Maeno et al., 2019). Successful IPE shows that it is preferable for medical students to receive IPE continuously throughout all years of medical school (Reeves, 2016, 185-197). To enhance readiness for interprofessional collaboration, clinical encounters are favorable to classroom activities. (Reeves, Perrier, Goldman, Freeth & Zarenstein, 2013). To train learners to be ready to collaborate, health professions educational programs will need to implement IPE across all years in school in authentic clinical contexts to achieve the experience necessary to participate in effective, team-based IP care.

The remaining problem is that graduates are going into practice in healthcare systems that do not reflect the IP teams and collaboration that graduates are prepared to join. The training and patient care in academic centers does not always reflect the ideal IP teams and collaborations that are taught. Further, academic centers must commit to faculty development in IPE and community engagement with stakeholders to meet the needs of healthcare systems and the needs of patient communities and community centers. To remedy this, IPE and IPC must share a common set of definitions and language to further the consistency of our health professions education programs.

INTERPROFESSIONAL DEFINITIONS AND COMMON TERMS

1. Interprofessional Team-Based Care
2. Interprofessional Education Collaborative Domains
3. Patient-Centered Care
4. Goals: Quadruple Aim in Healthcare

Interprofessional team-based care can and should be the standard of care for all health systems. It embodies the vision of Flexner:

"Once students understand how to work interprofessionally, they are ready to enter the workplace as a member of the collaborative practice team. This is a key step in moving health systems from fragmentation to a position of strength." -- Abraham Flexner

Another tenet of Abraham Flexner was the need for educational programs of both the undergraduate and graduate education programs to consider the needs of society when designing their programs. Clinical medical education cannot just stop at meeting the acute care needs of the sick patient in the hospital and emergency setting. Understanding the health care needs of our patients must expand and include acute, urgent and emergent care needs; chronic care needs, particularly in the outpatient setting; critical and palliative care; population and community-based care; and preventive and wellness care (Flexner, 1910). Organizing medical education as a continuum so that all of these unique health care needs are taught and practiced in a clinical environment can prepare professionals to be more successful at meeting the needs of a population of patients. Truly effective IP teams that serve the patient within the health care system are essential to meeting the clinical needs of a population of patients. (Whitcomb, 2009; Flexner, 1910).

The final challenge for building effective interprofessional teams are the unique needs of modern-day patients. Patients are more complex with acute and chronic medical conditions. Social determinants of health and layers of complexity must also be addressed and overcome to meet the health and preventive needs of patients in any nation. Healthcare system leaders and stakeholders must research, know and understand the health priorities for the patients within their region and community and work to design systems to treat medical conditions as well as promote health and wellness. Further, to improve population health outcomes, systems need to focus on the Quadruple Aim: improve patient satisfaction, improve patient outcomes, do it in a cost-effective way all while evaluating the system to improve the IP team experience to avoid burnout and encourage the providers to find joy in practice,

- Improve patient satisfaction
- Improve patient outcomes
- Ensure cost-effective care
- Evaluate the system to improve the IP experience, avoid burnout and increase joy in practice.

Interprofessional Education, Team-Based Care and Competencies

When students are educated using IPE, they are ready to provide collaborative care on teams in the workforce. The definition of interprofessional team-based care:

"Care delivered by intentionally created, usually relatively small, work groups in health care who are recognized by others as well as by themselves as having a collective identity and shared responsibility for a patient or groups of patients (e.g. rapid response team, palliative care team, primary care team, and operating room team)." (IPEC 2016)

When students understand and learn how to work interprofessionally, they are ready to enter the workplace as a member of the collaborative practice team. According to the World Health Organization, this is a key step in moving health systems forward (WHO, 2010). It is important to have a shared set of competencies when developing any healthcare system or team. IPEC has defined interprofessional competencies and competency domains that serve as the foundation for the education of professionals and include learning objectives and performance standards for individuals and teams. The interprofessional competencies in healthcare are defined by IPEC as: "integrated enactment of knowledge, skills, values, and attitudes that define working together across the professions, with other health care workers, and with patients, along with families and communities, as appropriate to improve health outcomes in specific care contexts." (IPEC 2016)

Interprofessional Education Collaborative Competency Domains

IPEC 2011 established interprofessional identity domains to guide educators in establishing IP curricula and assessments. These are essential competencies for members of IP teams and serve as the foundation of educational programs in constructing and teaching team-based IP care. These competencies are also essential for effective IP healthcare teams in practice and were updated in 2016. The IPEC Competency Domains are:

"Competency 1, **Ethics and Values***: work with individuals of other professions to maintain a climate of mutual respect and shared values.*

Competency 2, **Roles and Responsibilities***: Use the knowledge of one's own role and those of other professions to appropriately assess and address the health care needs of patients and to promote and advance the health of populations.*

Competency 3, **Interprofessional Communication***: Communicate with patients, families, communities, and professionals in health and other fields in a responsive and responsible manner that supports a team approach to the promotion and maintenance of health and the prevention and treatment of disease.*

Competency 4, **Teams and Teamwork***: Apply relationship-building values and principles of team dynamics to perform effectively in different team roles to plan, deliver, and evaluate patient/population-centered care and population health programs and policies that are safe, timely, efficient, effective, and equitable. "*

When building an interprofessional healthcare team, the educational system and the healthcare system that health professionals will enter need to align to meet the needs of that community of patients.

Patient-Centered Care

Patient-centered care is embedded and essential in effective IP care. Interprofessional teams should consider the patient as part of the team and should include the patient in shared decision-making. It is important to understand the definition of patient-centered care in order to effectively include patients on the IP team. The Institute of Medicine (IOM) defines patient-centered care as: "Providing care that is respectful of, and responsive to, individual patient preferences, needs and values, and ensuring that patient values guide all clinical decisions." (IOM, 2001).

The Josiah Macy Foundation recognized the need to link reforms in health professions education to the reforms that are necessary in clinical practice which focus on team-based, patient-centered care and population health. Because there has been too little connection between interprofessional education and clinical practice redesign, they convened a conference called Partnering with Patients, Families and Communities to Link Interprofessional Practice and Education in April 2013. Educators, healthcare delivery experts, patients, and patient advocates came together to align goals and develop recommendations to engage patients and families to link interprofessional education and practice redesign. The proceedings from this group made the following recommendations (Fulmer & Gaines, 2014):

1. Make changes in the content and conduct of health professions education necessary to graduate practitioners who partner with patients, families and communities.
2. Make changes in health professions education organizations and healthcare organizations necessary to facilitate durable partnerships, both new and existing, with patients, families, and communities.
3. Build the capacity for partnerships among patients, families and communities and health professions education and healthcare organizations.
4. Make regulatory and payment reforms that require, support, and sustain partnerships among patients, families, and communities and health professions education and healthcare organizations.

This important document provides recommendations that guide leaders in health professions education and the healthcare system on ways to partner with patients and families to create an effective care system that meets the needs of the public. There was consensus that this partnership creates a "sweet spot" in order to improve population health. (Figure 1)

The National Center for Interprofessional Practice and Education supports the patient-centered approach of the Picker Institute that defines eight principles for patient-centered care which provide a more thorough approach to accomplish patient-

Figure 1.
(https://www.nhpf.org/uploads/Handouts/Thibault-slides_05-15-15.pdf)

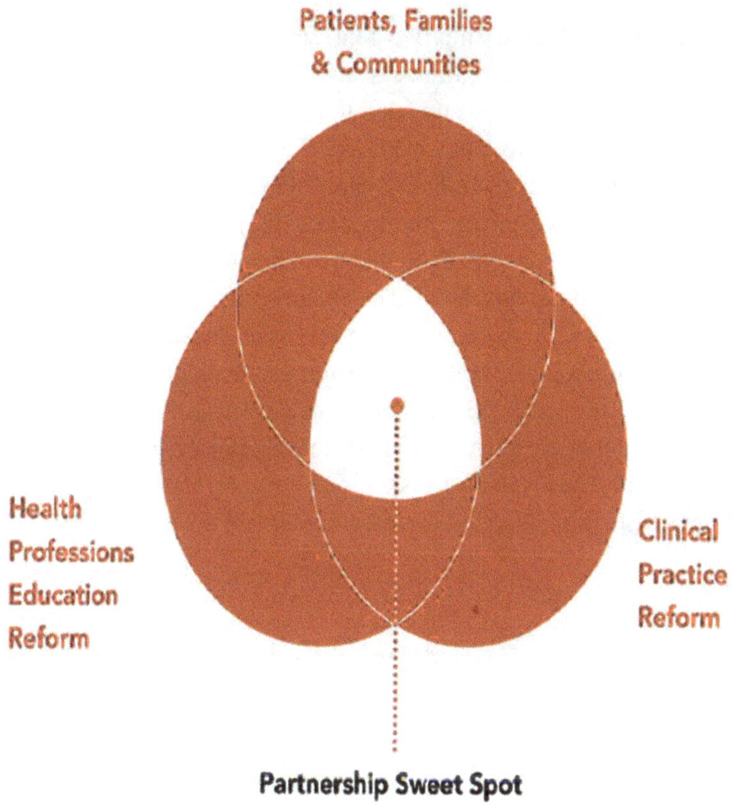

centered care for teams. It includes respect for patient preferences, coordination and integration of care, information and education, physical comfort, emotional support, involvement of family and friends, continuity and transition, and access to care (figure 2). Each of these eight principles are fundamental responsibilities of effective IP teams and can be broken down further into two sets of responsibilities; those of the individuals and those of the team. Individuals demonstrate respect, inform and educate, ensure physical comfort, provide emotional support, and involve family and friends. Coordination and integration of care, continuity and transition of care and access to care are considered to be examples of team efforts. Coordination and integration of care requires effective IP teams of nurses, physicians, and patient care technicians to communicate well, to work between professionals and disciplines in healthcare to ensure continuity and accuracy in diagnosis and treatment of the patient. (NexusIPE, 2015)

The Institute for Healthcare Improvement Quadruple Aim for Effective IP Teams

The Institute for Healthcare Improvement first developed the Triple Aim for healthcare in 2008 in order to optimize healthcare system performance to improve population health. In 2017 it was updated to become the Quadruple Aim and now includes improving the care team experience to improve care team well-being. Similarly, interprofessional team-based care endeavors to improve the quality of safe patient care, to avoid errors, and to place the patient at the center of care. With any educational enhancement or change to healthcare systems and teams, the Quadruple Aim should be considered. The Quadruple Aim changed from the Triple Aim in healthcare to create more opportunities for our healthcare team members to be included in the outcome of how their system and team provides care for patients (Berwick & Finkelstein, 2010; Bodenheimer & Sinsky, 2014). Working to improve outcomes and patient safety has resulted in system changes that have inadvertently led to provider burnout, stress, and dissatisfaction with care. Burnout has been shown to lower patient satisfaction, increase errors, and increase costs (Patel, Bachu, Adikey,

Figure 2.
https://www.oneviewhealthcare.com/the-eight-principles-of-patient-centered-care/ accessed on August 30, 2019

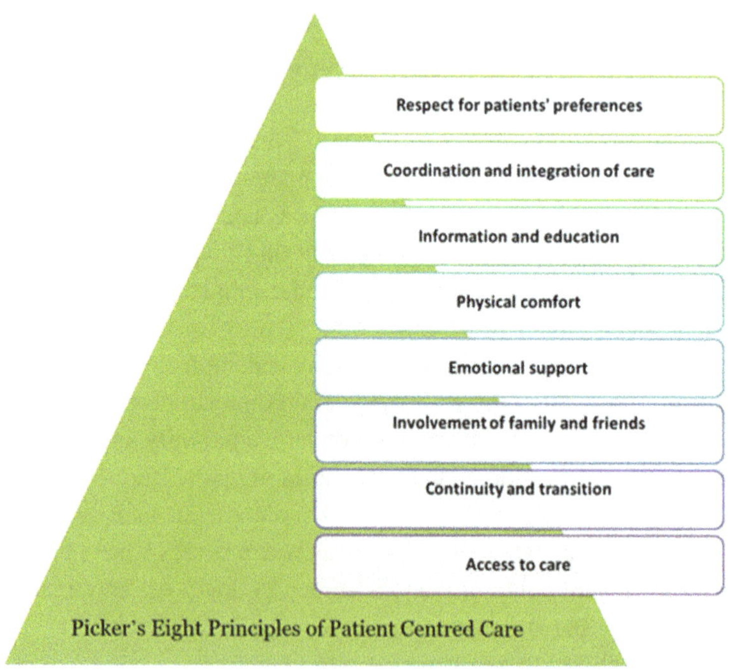

Malik & Shah 2018; Moss, Good, Gozal, Kleinpell & Sessler, 2016; Wright & Katz, 2018). Adding this fourth element, care team well-being, was an important step to help the workforce achieve an acceptable work life balance (Figure 3). Positive buy-in and engagement of the healthcare team is necessary to accomplish the primary goal of the Quadruple Aim to improve population health.

Figure 3.
https://www.google.com/search?q=quadruple+aim&client=safari&rls=en&tbm=isch&source=iu&ictx=1&fir=RbADvyHlghLk-M%253A%252C_4xIL2MyljJDoM%252C_&vet=1&usg=AI4_-kSkQRulvRzzKjb8vjDJS0Z3MMv6sA&sa=X&ved=2ahUKEwj7w920vaPlAhUCUa0KHeIqBiwQ9QEwAHoECAMQKw#imgrc=RprB7rrjqGKU9M:&vet=1 Accessed September 1, 2019

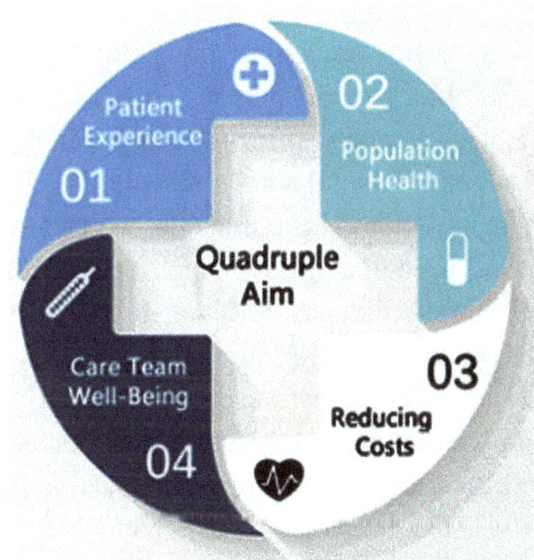

Teaching our healthcare workforce about real and applicable methods to provide safe patient care is imperative to the care and wellness of our patients and promotes the goals of the Quadruple Aim. Creating healthcare providers that function interdependently,-to develop effective communication and teamwork skills, and defining roles and responsibilities and the interplay of collaborative care are essential to building functional healthcare teams today.

Interprofessional Teams and Best Practice

The Institute of Medicine report, *Crossing the Quality Chasm*, states that effective teams are a means to improve quality of care. (IOM, 2001; Fernandopulle, p. 178-190, 2003; Strasser et al., 2008). Observational studies in chronic disease management have shown the effectiveness of the IP team approach in chronic disease management especially in the areas of self-care tasks, high risk patients, complex health systems, elderly patients and heart failure patients. (Von Korff, Gruman, Schaefer, Curry, & Wagner, 1997; Boult, Kane, Pacala & Wagner. 1999; Rich et al., 1995). In acute hospital settings, recent clinical trials provide evidence for enhanced patient outcomes in the areas of surgical outcomes, Alzheimer's care, cancer treatment and pediatric asthma when care is delivered by an IP team when compared with a nonteam approach. (IOM, 1999; Young, et al., 1998; Langhorne & Dennis 2004; Callahan, et al., 2006; Rummans, Clark & Sloan, 2006; Walders et al., 2006).

A white paper published by the Institute of Medicine provides a core set of principles in team-based care to assist in creating effective healthcare teams (Mitchell et al., 2012):

- **Shared goals:** The team—including the patient and, when appropriate, family members or other support persons—works to establish shared goals that reflect patient and family priorities, and can be clearly articulated, understood, and supported by all team members.
- **Clear roles:** There are clear expectations for each team member's functions, responsibilities, and accountabilities, which optimize the team's efficiency and facilitate appropriate division of labor, thereby allowing the team as a whole to accomplish more than the sum of its parts.
- **Mutual trust:** Team members earn each other's trust, creating strong norms of reciprocity and greater opportunities for shared achievement.
- **Effective communication:** The team prioritizes and continuously refines its communication skills. It has consistent channels for candid and complete communication, which are accessed and used by all team members across all settings.
- **Measurable processes and outcomes:** The team agrees on and implements reliable and timely feedback on successes and failures in both the functioning of the team and achievement of the team's goals. These are used to track and improve performance immediately and over time. SOURCE: Mitchell et al., 2012.

Conceptual Framework of Interprofessional Teams

Effective IP healthcare teams must also function well in the system and culture in which they practice. There are factors that occur within the team, between team members and the system itself. Team members come from many different educational and training backgrounds and have different experiences and cultural influences that become part of the team dynamic. Team members must demonstrate a respect for one another and leadership doesn't always come from a single professional on the team. Effective professionals must understand the unique roles that each plays on the IP team and the competencies and strengths that will best serve the patient and their needs. Teams that function well will also allow for leadership to be determined by the person, not the profession, to best serve the patient. All members must be prepared to learn with and from one another in their respective roles.

The UK Center for the Advancement of Interprofessional Care and Education (CAIPE) defines an IP framework designed to apply IP teamwork across different national and clinical contexts of care. The CAIPE framework identifies three important areas, each contributing to IP teamwork and recommends building and educating team members to be successful at working together utilizing this model (Figure 4):

1. Relational Factors
2. Processual Factors
3. Organizational and Contextual Factors

Relational factors describe the mindset and what affects the relationship between health professionals. The relationships are determined by the interplay of power, hierarchy, roles, and the composition of the team. Processual factors define the processes involved in teamwork and the learning process for teams to function effectively and competently. Learning must continue in health care systems which are based on highly complex activities so it must teach individuals to establish routines to reinforce safe care, and develop roles that adapt and respond to unpredictable and urgent patient care needs. Examples include managing unpredictability and urgency and task shifting to meet patient care needs. Relational and processual factors interplay in defining roles between team members. Contextual factors and organizational factors create the culture of teams and how they function within the system. Relational factors coincide with organizational factors as do processual factors and contextual factors.

Working competently as a team doesn't just happen, it is a process that occurs within systems and should include learning on collaboration and the team process. (Lingard & Hodges, 2013, pp. 14–41; Singer, Falwell & Gaba, 2009). An increasing volume of literature reports that deficiencies in collaboration and communication between healthcare professionals have a negative impact on the provision of healthcare and on patient outcomes (Fagin, 1992; Makary et al., 2006; Rosenstein & O'Daniel, 2005). In particular, new models of care emphasizing the need for close IP collaboration and a focus on the use of technology to provide continuous and coordinated care to the aging and chronically ill population are needed in Western countries. (Sommers, Marton, Barbaccia & Randolph, 2000; Krein et al., 2004; Callahan et al., 2006). Review of the literature demonstrates, that the vast majority of the systems that implemented IP teams have shown at least one improved outcome

Figure 4. Conceptual framework of interprofessional teamwork.
Note: *Reproduced from Reeves S, Lewin S, Espin S, Zwarenstein M. A Conceptual Framework for Interprofessional Teamwork. Chichester, West Sussex; Ames, IA: John Wiley and Sons; 2010.9 With permission from John Wiley and Sons, Copyright © 2010.*

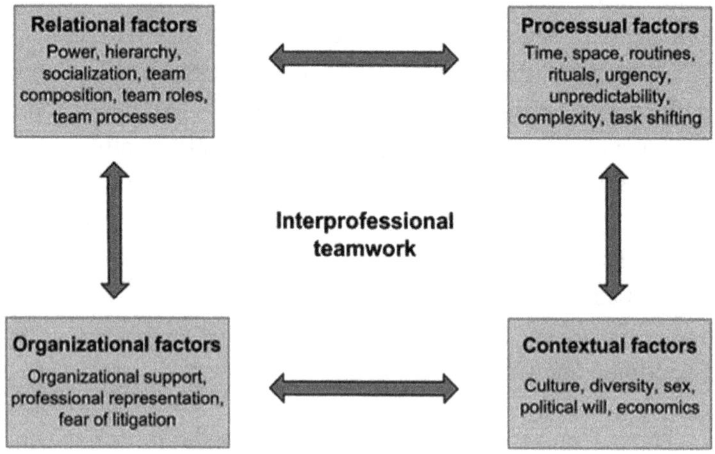

following interventions based on IP collaboration. (Martin, Ummenhofer, Manser & Spirig, 2010).

Examples of Effective Interprofessional Teams

The medical literature is now robust with examples and evidence of effective interprofessional healthcare teams. This section serves to provide examples of effective healthcare IP teams that are working to accomplish the Quadruple Aim through modeling of interprofessional teams and collaboration. These examples provide effective team structure with two or more healthcare professionals as part of the team construct and are examples that show improvements based on patient satisfaction or patient outcomes, and include IP teams as core to the intervention within systems.

1. Emergency Medicine
2. Elder Care
3. Physical Medicine & Rehabilitation
4. Cancer Care
5. Palliative Care
6. Behavioral Health

Emergency Medicine Teams

Emergency Medicine (EM) is provided by an IP team and is delivered by multiple professions and specialties to treat acute, undifferentiated, and sometimes critical patients. EM consists of a team of professionals that includes but is not limited to emergency medicine trained physicians, physician assistants, nurse practitioners, nurses and other allied health professionals. Providers in the emergency department often receive specialized training in advanced cardiac life support ACLS™, advanced trauma life support ATLS™, and training in various areas such as pediatrics, emergency medical services and toxicology, to name a few. Ideally these professionals collaborate on a daily basis with other professionals such as social workers, nurse case managers, patient care assistants, radiology technicians, respiratory therapists, emergency medical responders, pastoral care, and administrative assistants and clerks who help with the clerical registration of patients. EM providers will consult and communicate regularly with other specialists who meet the specialized needs of the acute patient. These specialists include but are not limited to trauma surgeons, radiologists, urologists, neurologists, obstetrician and gynecologists, internal medicine physicians, pulmonary/critical care specialists and cardiologists. Every health system may differ in the specialties and professions available but in busy urban emergency departments there is a need for each of the afore mentioned professionals working interdependently to meet the needs of a patient.

The literature shows growing evidence that acute care and critical care patient populations can and do benefit from interprofessional practice and team-based care in the emergency department setting. Campbell et al. demonstrated that the interprofessional approach and training from the Pennsylvania Family Violence Prevention Fund improves the effectiveness of the emergency department (ED) response to intimate partner violence. Control groups of emergency department teams of physicians, nurses and social workers were educated in protocols for intimate partner violence screening and response. Staff knowledge and attitudes about battered women improved as did their ability to provide patient pertinent information and measures of patient satisfaction also improved. Overall, the culture and knowledge about the protocols improved as an IP system-change indicator. (Campbell et al., 2001)

There is growing evidence that when acute care teams are constructed modeling aviation crew resource management there are improved patient outcomes. (more on aviation crews) In a randomized, controlled trial by Morey et al. of emergency department staff organized into caregiver teams of physicians, nurses and patient care technicians who received an Emergency Team Coordination Course™ (ETCC) showed improvements in team behavior, ED performance, attitudes and opinions toward teamwork. Teams were created of physician and nurse instructor pairs that educated teams of physicians, nurses, medical technicians and unit clerks who completed eight hours of instruction on five team dimensions: 1) maintain team structure and climate, 2) apply problem-solving strategies, 3) communication with the team, 4) execute plans and manage workload, and 5) improve team skills. Trained observers rated ED staff teams on team behaviors and observations of clinical errors. Patients in the ED completed surveys measuring their attitudes and opinions. There was a statistically significant improvement in quality of team behaviors in the experimental and control groups following training. Subjective workload was not affected by the intervention. The clinical error rate significantly decreased from 30.9% to 4.4% in the experimental group. The ED staff's attitudes toward teamwork also improved in the experimental group and staff assessments of institutional support showed a significant increase. Team behavior, ED performance, attitudes and opinions all qualitatively improved through this interprofessional, ETCC-training in the emergency department (Morey et al., 2002).

Interprofessional teamwork has been proposed and shown to improve trauma care in the ED. Trauma care is complex, critically important, and expensive, as traumatic injuries continue to be a significant public health problem. In the U.S. and worldwide, trauma remains the leading cause of death and disability in young adults and children (Stewart et al., 2003). During trauma resuscitation, potentially life-threatening injuries must be identified and treated rapidly, and coordinated decisions must occur between team members and disciplines present in the trauma bay. Studies have shown that time in patient care is saved and error reductions occur with team training for the ED (Steineman et al., 2011, Capella, et al. 2010, Morey, et al. 2002; Patel & Vinson, 2005). Team assignment system: expediting emergency department care. *Ann Emerg Med.* 46:499-506. 2005). Team error analysis in trauma patient care has demonstrated four error types including interpretation, communication, management and concurrency errors (Sarcevic, 2011). Teamwork behaviors shown to reduce errors in intensive care units were identified as team communication, coordination, leadership and decision-making (Reader, et al. 2009).

Workplace violence is a growing problem in emergency departments worldwide. Patients present to EDs with intoxication from alcohol and drugs, with acute mental health issues and with organic causes such as brain injury or stroke. Studies have shown that emergency nurses are at greatest risk of verbal and physical assault when compared to physicians and nurses in other specialty settings (Hodge & Marshal, 2007; Wolf, Delao & Perhats, 2014). Implementation of a structured IP team response to manage patients with behavioral emergencies has shown a significant impact, resulting in diminishing patient aggression (Rintoul, Wynaden & McGowan, 2009; Downes, Healy, Page, Bryant &Isbister. 2009). Wong and colleagues showed that an IP curriculum in coordinating a team response to behavioral issues in the ED improved ED staff attitudes. The IP curriculum included formal lectures and training in de-escalation techniques, role clarification, IP communication and teamwork skills for teams of EM residents, nurses and hospital police officers with standardized patients portraying aggressive patients. Attitudes were measured pre and post intervention and showed the constructs for internal factors, external factors and situational interactional perspectives on patient aggression significantly improved with the intervention. In fact, as a result of this curriculum the department developed an ED-based IP crisis management alert and response protocol (Wong, Wing, Weiss & Gang, 2015).

Geriatrics and Elder Care

Interprofessional team collaboration is improving outcomes for elderly individuals with chronic conditions. It has been shown that care of the elderly, especially those with disabilities, can be fragmented and lead to hospitalization and institutionalization. Integrated models of care that improve health, decrease hospitalization, improve satisfaction and decrease injuries are of special interest for this patient population. Among community-dwelling older adults, Trivedi and colleagues conducted a systematic review of 37 randomized controlled trials of the Interprofessional Patient Collaborative Teams (IPCT) models of care. Effective IPCT care teams most often included teams of nurses, medical assistants or patient care technicians, physical therapists and a form of supervisor rounds that worked to reduce poor outcomes such as falls, injuries, missed medications or relapse of chronic medical conditions. The goals of most studies were to show an increase or decrease in direct patient care processes impacting health, such as improved cost-effectiveness, and indirect outcomes such as patient satisfaction, empowerment or reduced caregiver burden. Their findings demonstrated that models that had a well-integrated and shared-care design, showed improved processes of care. There was also greater potential to reduce indirect measures of health, such as hospital or nursing home use. The authors argued, however, that currently, the evidence of overall effectiveness and cost-effectiveness of the IPCT models is rather weak. (Trivedi, Goodman & Gage, 2013). Other studies highlighted many positive impacts such as improvement in elder satisfaction (Beland et al., 2006; Eng, Pedulla, Eleazer, McCann & Fox, 1997; Hebert et al., 2010; and Challis, Darton, Johnson, Stone & Traske, 1991), improvement in elder empowerment (Hebert et al., 2010), reduction of caregiver burden (Tourigny, Durand, Bonin, Hébert & Rochette, 2004), decrease in functional decline (Hebert et al., 2010, Tourigny et al, 2004, Bernabei et al, 1998), reduction in hospital use, reduction in emergency- department visits (Hebert, et al. 2010), reduction in nursing home utilization (Béland, et al., 2006; Eng, et al., 1997; Tourigny et al., 2004; Bernabei et al., 1998; Landi et al., 1999), and reduction in costs (Eng, et al. 1997, Dubuc, Dubois, Raîche, Gueye & Hébert R, 2011).

In a study of nursing homes in Georgia, a falls management program (FMP) was implemented in response to the Centers for Medicare and Medicaid Services quality initiatives. An IP team including a facility-based falls coordinator, an advanced practice nurse (APP), nursing staff and patient care assistants in nineteen nursing homes conducted training to reduce falls and the use of restraints for elder care. All team members underwent extensive training and were led by the APP with expertise in falls management. Restraint use decreased substantially by 44% when compared to the nursing homes without the intervention during the study period. Fall rates remained stable in the intervention nursing homes while they increased in nursing homes without the intervention. This study showed that IPCT implementation of the FMP significantly improved care process documentation, stabilized the fall rate and reduced the use of restraints substantially.

The medical literature also shows that IP teams can make an impact on elder abuse. In an article written by Lachs & Pillemer it is estimated that the incidence of elder abuse is likely higher than previously thought and is a virtual epidemic. Elderly patients with one or more chronic illnesses are more likely to be abused financially, emotionally and/or physically. Studies show that elder abuse occurs more often among residents of nursing home facilities (Lachs & Pillemer, 2015). Interprofessional teams combating elder abuse have proven to be a successful intervention strategy to assist physicians in identifying and protecting victims of elder abuse and in referring them for further care. (Blowers, et al. 2012, Navarro, Gassoumis &Wilber, 2013). Evidence shows that IP teams of physicians, nurses, social workers, law-enforcement personnel, lawyers and other community advocates can work in a coordinated fashion to successfully assist victims of elder abuse. (Teaster, Nerenberg & Stansbury, 2003; Rizzo, Burnes & Chalfy, 2015).

Physical Medicine and Rehabilitation

Physical Medicine and Rehabilitation (PM&R) is another specialty area where there is evidence to show that IPCTs improve outcomes and patient care. Patients that require the care of PM&R specialists and facilities are complex with multiple chronic medical conditions and physical needs. The complex nature of these patients and their conditions often requires professionals such as physical and occupational therapists, speech therapists, nurses, physicians and long-term care facilities for their rehabilitation. In fact, Medicare requires that care be interdisciplinary, team-based care for inpatient rehabilitation reimbursement (Centers for Medicare and Medicaid Reimbursement, 2019). As with the care of elderly patients, falls are a risk for this group of patients. Strasser et al. showed positive outcomes in a cluster, randomized trial of stroke victims when the Falls Management Program (FMP) was implemented on IPCTs. Teams included a physical or occupational therapist, two to four certified nursing assistants, a member of maintenance staff that served as a "falls engineer" and the director of nursing. All teams attended a full-day workshop and a one-month follow-up support module to address ongoing issues and concerns. Training regarding living space and strategies to reduce fall risk were included. The workshops were provided by an IP team of two nurse practitioners, a geriatric nurse practitioner, and a nurse educator experienced in long-term care, conducted the education and discussion workshops. As a result of this training, documentation of care processes related to falls prevention and fall risk improved. A reduction in restraint use was also noted. The assessment and management of residents at risk of falls improved through IP team training (Strasser et al., 2008). Similarly, stroke patients treated by staff who participated in an IP team training program were more likely to make functional gains than those treated by staff receiving information only. (Centers for Medicare and Medicaid Reimbursement, 2019).

Cancer Care

Oncology teams and programs are an example of effective IPCTs. Cancer care is complex and requires the coordination of different healthcare professionals to provide the best treatment and patient experience. The IOM provided a report in 1999 on the quality of cancer care which recognized the need for coordinated care to be delivered by experienced professionals. (IOM and NRC, 1999). Cancer care requires specialty disciplines of physicians partnering with one another to determine the optimal plan of care for each individual patient. Tumor conferences are an example of interdisciplinary care in oncology. These are held to allow for collaboration among oncology, radiation oncology, surgery, primary care, palliative care and other physician specialists to determine the best plan of care based on the cancer type and patient needs. Interprofessional Collaborative Team functions in cancer care, as described in the literature, include but are not limited to teamwork, IP collaboration, integrated care delivery, interorganizational collaboration, continuity of care and case management. Gagliardi et al describes effective IP cancer care as collaborative involving two or more health care professionals with shared patient goals and interacting on a continuum from consultation to integration. Professional roles, with varying degrees of interaction with patients, will vary based on different decision-making capacity and the scope of overall patient management. Team structure, traits, and processes may vary by system. Outcomes, systems and organizational support are also variables to consider in establishing and measuring effective IP cancer care teams (Gagliardi, Dobrow & Wright, 2001).

Once the best treatment plan has been determined by an interdisciplinary team, the patient will need to navigate the system to receive chemotherapy, surgery and/or radiation. It is important to recognize and build IPCTs to support patients, to ensure treatment adherence and provide a quality experience for patients receiving complex cancer treatment. IP teams of physicians, pharmacists, advanced practice nurses, physician assistants, psychologists, palliative care and hospice clinicians, spiritual care, rehabilitation clinicians, dieticians and oncology nurses are often necessary to provide for the unique needs of cancer patients. (Committee on Improving the Quality of Cancer Care, 2013). Oncologists develop individualized treatment plans based on the specific patient and these plans are supported by cancer center pharmacies and infusion centers. Each IP provider has a role and responsibility for the care of the patient and the coordination of that care is important in the effectiveness of the treatment and optimization of patient care. It takes access to multiple professional perspectives to address institutional issues and to work together to avoid medical errors, especially in cancer care.

In a review of research on IP cancer care improvements in patient outcomes in cancer care have been demonstrated through the use of IPCTs. Cancer conferences and discussion of cancer care by IPCTs improved the planning of therapy, adherence to recommended preoperative assessment, pain control, and adherence to medications. There was not convincing evidence that IPCTs affect patient survival or cost of care, nor studies suggest how or which processes or structures were associated with success. (Taplin, Weaver & Salas, 2015). In another review of the evidence on multi-disciplinary teams, or the use of teams with varying specialty experience and expertise of physicians, there are measurable positive outcomes for cancer patients with certain types of cancer. Interdisciplinary teams resulted in better clinical approaches and survival outcomes for cancer patients with colorectal, head and neck, breast, esophageal and lung cancers. This review also demonstrated that multi-disciplinary teams are associated with changes in diagnosis and treatment decisions in bladder, breast, colorectal, gastroesophageal, gynecological, head and neck, melanoma, pancreatic, prostate and urological cancers. This resulted in positive consequences for patient management (Prades, Remue, van Hoof & Borras, 2015). However, evidence standardizing structure and standards of such teams is lacking.

There is still more research that needs to be completed to show that IPCTs are effective at improving patient outcomes, cost and quality in cancer care. There is evidence that patient satisfaction is improved during care provided by IPCTs but more research will need to be completed to demonstrate effective team structure and to show positive effects on outcomes, cost, provider and staff satisfaction.

Hospice and Palliative Care

Palliative care teams function interprofessionally and are associated with improved patient outcomes, patient satisfaction and provider satisfaction. Palliative care is a philosophy of care focused on symptom management and quality of life for patients with a life threatening or terminal illness or injury. Palliative care uses an interprofessional approach to help manage pain and other distressing symptoms while also ensuring that a patient's overall goals of care are respected and incorporated into the treatment plan. Patients receiving palliative care are not limited in terms of medical interventions. Hospice is similar to palliative care in terms of focus on quality of life and symptom management, with some notable differences. Hospice services are reserved for patients who have an anticipated prognosis of 6 months or less and are no longer pursuing curative or life prolonging interventions. Hospice provides care that allows for patients to live comfortably and die as naturally and peacefully as possible.

Studies have repeatedly shown that hospice and palliative care services are beneficial to both patients and caregivers. Patients receiving interdisciplinary palliative care report better quality of life, symptom management and spiritual well-being, in addition to lower psychological distress (Ferrell B et al., 2015). Early palliative care has also shown benefit in terms of caregiver satisfaction and psychological well-being. (El-Jawahri A et al., 2017) In a landmark study, Temel et al demonstrated a survival benefit of nearly three months for patients with metastatic non-small cell lung cancer when they received early palliative care (Temel et al., 2010). Incorporating palliative care as part of the overall treatment plan has also shown benefit in terms of reducing aggressive non-beneficial interventions at the end of life and reducing overall cost. Because of these benefits, organizations like the American Society of Clinical Oncology recommend the early integration of palliative care services for oncology patients. (Smith, Phillips & Smith, 2017).

The benefits that have been shown from palliative care interventions are likely due to both the holistic approach applied to patient care as well as the involvement of a skilled interprofessional team. Hospice providers, under Medicare guidelines, are required to involve an interdisciplinary team to provide patients with a comprehensive assessment and an individualized plan of care. As the palliative care movement has grown, it continues to incorporate the interprofessional team as a central component. Most palliative care teams are composed of some combination of physicians, nurses, social workers, chaplains and pharmacists, depending on resources and availability.

While research analyzing the effect of the interprofessional structure of the team on patient outcomes is sparse, it can be extrapolated that the team approach, being an integral tenet of palliative care, is at least to some extent, responsible for the benefits noted above. The interprofessional model allows for multiple patient needs (including symptom management, psychological support, spiritual support and resource referrals) to be assessed and satisfied by one team. Each palliative care team is unique in its structure, and this varies based on the location of service (hospital, clinic, home-based). Most teams operate with the goal of using the unique attributes and skill sets of each member of the team to meet the needs of each patient. For example, inpatient palliative care teams generally start the day by discussing each patient and the individual needs that might arise that day. If the team identifies that the patient will need special attention to pain management as well as counseling to address spiritual distress, the team will structure its visit to ensure that these needs are addressed. A physician or advance practice provider nurse with specialized training in symptom management will be present to evaluate and treat the patient's pain and a chaplain will be present to explore their spiritual concerns.

Because palliative care teams incorporate the expertise of various disciplines, it is critical that the team clarify the role of each member. This is often an ongoing process as the roles of members can be fluid, for example: a social worker may coordinate discharge planning for one patient, and may provide counseling and psychosocial support for another. Growing a healthy interprofessional team also requires strong leadership, to facilitate mutual purpose among team members as well as shared values. The health of the interprofessional team hinges on mutual respect, clear expectations for performance and open lines of communication. Meeting frequently enables teams to discuss not only patient care, but also the team dynamic, efficiency, areas for potential improvement and also the emotional needs of the team members.

Recognizing that burnout is a growing problem in healthcare, particularly in emotionally charged specialties like palliative care, attention to personal and team wellness is paramount. Many teams prioritize scheduled wellness and team building activities as a way to strengthen team dynamics and personal relationships. Setting clear boundaries both personally and professionally and focusing on self-care are important in maintaining job satisfaction, combating burnout and building resiliency. The concept of "collective resilience" has been emphasized as a characteristic that enables stronger individuals and stronger teams (Koh et al., 2019).

Behavioral Health

Effective mental health care requires high performing, interprofessional teams to address the complex needs for patient's physical and mental health as well as their psychosocial needs. The Center for Health Care Strategies advocates for *Advancing Integrated Models* of care including use of interprofessional health care teams for such patients with a focus on improving health outcomes and fostering health equity (Advancing Integrated Models, 2019). Many patients present to their primary care provider for management of behavioral health symptoms. Finley and colleagues describe a collaborative care model in which clinical pharmacists worked under the supervision of psychiatrists to provide drug therapy management and patient education (Finley, Crismon & Rush AJ, 2003). In this study, patients were referred by their primary care provider to participate in the study immediately after starting antidepressant therapy for depressive symptoms. Results of this randomized controlled trial found increased drug adherence rates, enhanced patient satisfaction and decreased number of primary care visits. Additional publications support the integration of psychiatric pharmacists into the patient medical home model. (Gibu, Clark & Gold, 2018; Mishra, Krishna & Alla, 2017; Finley, Rens & Pont, 2003; Locke & Kamo, 2016; Goldstone et al., 2015; Capoccia, Boudreau & Blough, 2004).

Behavioral health patients can be high resource utilizers and face frequent hospitalization. Transitional care strategies are an important factor in reducing re-hospitalization rates among all patients. Many interventions focus on pre-discharge needs but do not emphasize psychosocial stressors such as housing, occupation, economics, and access to health care, which can hinder a patient's recovery and continued engagement in care. Addressing the psychosocial needs are critical as psychiatric diagnoses increase the likelihood of medical readmission. DeCaporale-Ryan et. al. implemented a pilot study of a team-based service delivery model in an effort to decrease 30- and 90-day preventable readmission rates. The integrated care team, consisting of a physician, psychologist, pharmacist, care managers and interprofessional trainees addressed psychosocial needs and comprehensive medication review in a family medicine setting. While the study size was small, they were able to demonstrate feasibility of this care model and a positive impact on readmission rates by addressing psychosocial factors of patients after hospital discharge. (DeCaporale-Ryan, Ahmed-Sarwar, Upham, Mahler & Lashway. (2017).

Addressing behavioral health issues in the pediatric population is a challenging area. Walter and colleagues published impressive five-year outcomes data from integration of behavioral health into pediatric primary care addressing mild and moderate presentations of common psychiatric disorders including anxiety, depression and attention-deficit/hyperactivity disorder (ADHD). Results showed increased patient access to psychotherapy, improved rates of prescription adherence for guideline-congruent medications used to treat anxiety, depression, and ADHD, and a favorable impact on cost, as well as provider satisfaction (Walter, Vernacchio & Trudell, 2019).

As we move toward more integrated, IP team-based care for physical and mental health, it is important to consider staff perceptions on the benefits and challenges of this model of care. Staff within the Veteran's Health Administration increased staff communication, collaboration and shared decision-making through team meetings where members could share perspectives with each other regarding patient care plans. Implementation challenges were identified as well including lack of guidance from leadership, lack of clear roles and expectations for staff, staff shortages and turnover and difficulty finding time to attend team meetings. (Barry, Abraham, Weaver & Bowersox, 2016).

Future Research Directions

More research is needed to show the effect of interprofessional teams to support the Quadruple Aim through the four applications to improve population health: 1) patient experience, 2) population health outcomes, 3) reduced cost, and 4) the care team's well-being. Funding of IPE and IPCT programs with intentional measurements to show improved patient outcomes, patient and family satisfaction and improved provider and staff wellness must increase. Healthcare systems must also evolve to create a patient-centered IP culture of practice that partners with patients and families as well as IP provider and staff teams.

CONCLUSION

The elements to build effective IP teams are many. It begins with educating our healthcare professionals through effective IPE and opportunities for our learners to learn with, from and about one another while placing patients at the center of their care. To advance the quality of care, healthcare systems must also adapt and design systems that support and encourage interprofessional team training and assessment of those delivering care. System administrators must be engaged in the process to build and advance effective teams based on the evidence that IPCTs improve quality of care, patient outcomes, patient and family satisfaction, team satisfaction and lead to a reduction in errors.

REFERENCES

AI Models. (n.d.). Center for Healthcare Strategies Web site: https://www.chcs.org/project/advancing-integrated-models/

Barry, C. N., Abraham, K. M., Weaver, K. R., & Bowersox, N. W. (2016). Innovating Team-Based Outpatient Mental health Care in the Veterans Health Administration: Staff-Perceived Benefits and Challenges to Pilot Implementation of the Behavioral health Interdisciplinary Program (BHIP). *Psychological Services*, *13*(2), 148–155. doi:10.1037er0000072 PMID:27148949

Béland, F., Bergman, H., Lebel, P., Clarfield, A.M., Tousignant, P., Contandriopoulos, A.P., & Dallaire, L. (2006). A System of Integrated Care for Older persons with disabilities in Canada: a randomized, controlled trial. *J Gerontol A Biol Sci Med Sci.*, *61*(4), 367-73.

Bernabei, R., Landi, F., Gambassi, G., Sgadari, A., Zuccala, G., Mor, V., Rubenstein, L. Z., & Carbonin, P. (1998). Randomised trial of impact of model of integrated care and case management for older people living in the community. *BMJ (Clinical Research Ed.)*, *316*(7141), 1348–1351. doi:10.1136/bmj.316.7141.1348 PMID:9563983

Berwick, D., & Finkelstein, J. (2010). Preparing medical students for the continual improvement of health and health care: Abraham Flexner and the New "Public Interest". *Academic Medicine*, *85*, S56–S65. doi:10.1097/ACM.0b013e3181ead779 PMID:20736631

Blowers, A. N., Davis, B., Shenk, D., Kalaw, K., Smith, M., & Jackson, K. (2012). A multidisciplinary approach to detecting and responding to elder mistreatment: Creating a university-community partnership. *American Journal of Criminal Justice*, *37*(2), 276–290. doi:10.100712103-012-9156-4

Bodenheimer, T., & Sinsky, C. (2014). From Tripe to Quadruple Aim: Care of the patient requires care of the provider. *Annal Family Med*, *12*(6), 573-576.

Boult, C., Kane, R. L., Pacala, J. T., & Wagner, E. H. (1999). Innovative healthcare for chronically ill older persons: Results of a national survey. *The American Journal of Managed Care*, *5*, 1162–1172. PMID:10621082

Callahan, C. M., Boustani, M. A., Unverzagt, F. W., Austrom, M. G., Damush, T. M., Perkins, A. J., Fultz, B. A., Hui, S. L., Counsell, S. R., & Hendrie, H. C. (2006). Effectiveness of collaborative care for older adults with Alzheimer disease in primary care: A randomized controlled trial. *Journal of the American Medical Association*, *295*(18), 2148–2157. doi:10.1001/jama.295.18.2148 PMID:16684985

Campbell, J. C., Coben, J. H., McLoughlin, E., Dearwater, S., Nah, G., Glass, N., Lee, D., & Durborow, N. (2001). An Evaluation of a System-change Training Model to Improve Emergency Department Response to Battered Women. *Academic Emergency Medicine*, *8*(2), 131–138. doi:10.1111/j.1553-2712.2001.tb01277.x PMID:11157288

Capella, J., Smith, S., Philp, A., Putnam, T., Gilbert, C., Fry, W., Harvey, E., Wright, A., Henderson, K., Baker, D., Ranson, S., & ReMine, S. (2010). Teamwork training improves the clinical care of trauma patients. *Journal of Surgical Education*, *67*(6), 439–443. doi:10.1016/j.jsurg.2010.06.006 PMID:21156305

Capoccia, K. L., Boudreau, D. M., Blough, D. K., Ellsworth, A. J., Clark, D. R., Stevens, N. G., Katon, W. J., & Sullivan, S. D. (2004). Randomized trial of pharmacist interventions to improve depression care and outcomes in primary care. *American Journal of Health-System Pharmacy*, *61*(4), 364–372. doi:10.1093/ajhp/61.4.364 PMID:15011764

Centers for Medicare & Medicaid Services Documentation requirements for inpatient rehabilitation (A18990). (n.d.). http://www.wvtra.org/conference/2006/Veritus_IRF.doc

Challis, D., Darton, R., Johnson, L., Stone, M., & Traske, K. (1991). An evaluation of an alternative to long-stay hospital care for frail elderly patients: II. Costs and effectiveness. *Age and Ageing*, *20*(4), 245–254. doi:10.1093/ageing/20.4.245 PMID:1656718

Committee on Improving the Quality of Cancer Care. (2013). *Addressing the Challenges of an Aging Population; Board on Health Care Services*. Washington, DC: National Academies Press. Available from: https://www.ncbi.nlm.nih.gov/books/NBK202149/

DeCaporale-Ryan, L. N., Ahmed-Sarwar, N., Upham, R., Mahler, K., & Lashway, K. (2017). Reducing Hospital Readmission Through Team-Based Primary Care: A 7-Week Pilot Study Integrating Behavioral health and Pharmacy. *Families, Systems & Health*, *35*(2), 217–226. doi:10.1037/fsh0000269 PMID:28617022

Downes, M. A., Healy, P., Page, C. B., Bryant, J. L., & Isbister, G. K. (2009). Structured team approach to the agitated patient in the emergency department. *Emergency Medicine Australasia*, *21*, 196–202. PMID:19527279

Dubuc, N., Dubois, M., Raîche, M., Gueye, N. R., & Hébert, R. (2011). Meeting the home-care needs of disabled older persons living in the community: Does integrated services delivery make a difference? *BMC Geriatrics*, *11*(1), 67. doi:10.1186/1471-2318-11-67 PMID:22029878

El-Jawahri, A., Greer, J. A., Pirl, W. F., Park, E. R., Jackson, V. A., Back, A. L., Kamdar, M., Jacobsen, J., Chittenden, E. H., Rinaldi, S. P., Gallagher, E. R., Eusebio, J. R., Fishman, S., VanDusen, H., Li, Z., Muzikansky, A., & Temel, J. S. (2017). Effects of Early Integrated Palliative Care on Caregivers of Patients with Lung and Gastrointestinal Cancer: A Randomized Clinical Trial. *The Oncologist*, *22*(12), 1528–1534. doi:10.1634/theoncologist.2017-0227 PMID:28894017

Eng, C., Pedulla, J., Eleazer, G. P., McCann, R., & Fox, N. (1997). Program of All-inclusive Care for the Elderly (PACE): An innovative model of integrated geriatric care and financing [see comments]. *Journal of the American Geriatrics Society*, *45*(2), 223–232. doi:10.1111/j.1532-5415.1997.tb04513.x PMID:9033525

Fagin, C. M. (1992). Collaboration between nurses and physicians: No longer a choice. *Academic Medicine*, *67*(5), 295–303. doi:10.1097/00001888-199205000-00002 PMID:1575859

Fernandopulle, R., Ferris, T., Epstein, A., McNeil, B., Newhouse, J., Pisano, G., & Blumenthal, D. (2003). A research agenda for bridging the "quality chasm". *Health Affairs (Project Hope)*, *22*(2), 178–190. doi:10.1377/hlthaff.22.2.178 PMID:12674420

Ferrell, B., Sun, V., Hurria, A., Cristea, M., Raz, D. J., Kim, J. Y., Reckamp, K., Williams, A. C., Borneman, T., Uman, G., & Koczywas, M. (2015). Interdisciplinary Palliative Care for Patients With Lung Cancer. *Journal of Pain and Symptom Management*, *50*(6), 758–767. doi:10.1016/j.jpainsymman.2015.07.005 PMID:26296261

Finley, P. R., Crismon, M. L., & Rush, A. J. (2003). Evaluating the Impact of Pharmacists in Mental Health: A Systematic Review. *Pharmacotherapy*, *23*(12), 1634–1644. doi:10.1592/phco.23.15.1634.31952 PMID:14695043

Finley, P. R., Rens, H. R., Pont, J. T., Gess, S. L., Louie, C., Bull, S. A., Lee, J. Y., & Bero, L. A. (2003). Impact of a Collaborative Care Model on Depression in a Primary Care Setting: A Randomized Controlled Trial. *Pharmacotherapy*, *23*(9), 1175–1185. doi:10.1592/phco.23.10.1175.32760 PMID:14524649

Flexner, A. (1910). *Medical Education in the United States and Canada*. A Report to the Carnegie Foundation for the Advancement of Teaching. Bulletin No. 4. Boston: Updyke.

Fulmer, T., & Gaines, M. (2014). Partnering with Patient, Families and Communities to Link Interprofessional Practice and Education. *Proceeding of a conference sponsored by the Josiah Macy Jr. Foundation in April 2014*. New York: Josiah Macy Jr. Foundation.

Gagliardi, A., Dobrow, M., & Wright, F. (2001). How can we improve cancer care? A review of interprofessional collaboration models and their use in clinical management. *Surgical Oncology*, *20*(3), 146–154. doi:10.1016/j.suronc.2011.06.004 PMID:21763127

Gibu, M., Clark, J., & Gold, J. (2018). Mental health pharmacists as interim prescribers. *Ment Health Clin*, *7*(3), 111–115. doi:10.9740/mhc.2017.05.111 PMID:29955508

Gilbert, J. V., Yan, J., & Hoffman, S. J. (2010). A WHO Report: Framework for action on interprofessional education and collaborative practices. *Journal of Allied Health*, *39*, 196–197. PMID:21174039

Goldstone, L. W., DiPaula, B. A., Caballero, J., Park, S., Price, C., & Sister, M. (2015). Improving medication-related outcomes for patients with psychiatric and neurologic disorders: Value of psychiatric pharmacists as part of the health care team. *MHC*, *5*(1), 1–23. doi:10.9740/mhc.2015.01.001

Health Professions Accreditors Collaborative. (2019). *Guidance on developing quality interprofessional education for the health professions*. Health Professions Accreditors Collaborative.

Hébert, R., Raiche, M., Dubois, M. F., Gueye, N. R., Dubuc, N., & Tousignant, M. (2010). Impact of PRISMA, a coordination-type integrated service delivery system for frail older people in Quebec (Canada): A quasi-experimental study. *The Journals of Gerontology. Series B, Psychological Sciences and Social Sciences*, *65B*(1), 107–118. doi:10.1093/geronb/gbp027 PMID:19414866

Hodge, A. N., & Marshal, A. P. (2007). Violence and aggression in the emergency department: A critical care perspective. *Australian Critical Care*, *20*(2), 61–67. doi:10.1016/j.aucc.2007.03.001 PMID:17568534

Institute of Medicine. (2001). Crossing the quality chasm. National Academies Press.

Institute of Medicine and National Research Council. (1999). *Ensuring quality cancer care*. National Academy Press.

Interprofessional Education Collaborative. (2016). *Core competencies for interprofessional collaborative practice: 2016 update*. Washington, DC: Interprofessional Education Collaborative. (https://www.ipecollaborative.org/membership.html

Interprofessional Education Collaborative Mission and Vision. (n.d.). https://www.ipecollaborative.org/vision---mission.html

Koh, M., Hum, A. Y. M., Khoo, H. S., Ho, A. H. Y., Chong, P. H., Ong, J., ... Yong, W. C. (2019). Burnout And Resilience after a Decade in Palliative Care (BARD) (2019). What "Survivors" have to teach us. A Qualitative Study of Palliative Care Clinicians with more than 10 years of experience. *Journal of Pain and Symptom Management*. PMID:31465787

Krein, S. L., Klamerus, M. L., Vijan, S., Lee, J. L., Fitzgerald, J. T., Pawlow, A., Reeves, P., & Hayward, R. A. (2004). Case management for patients with poorly controlled diabetes: A randomized trial. *The American Journal of Medicine*, *116*(11), 732–739. doi:10.1016/j.amjmed.2003.11.028 PMID:15144909

Lachs, M., & Pillemer, K. (2015). Elder Abuse. *The New England Journal of Medicine*, *373*(2), 1947–1955. doi:10.1056/NEJMra1404688 PMID:26559573

Landi, F., Gambassi, G., Pola, R., Tabaccanti, S., Cavinato, T., Carbonin, P., & Bernabei, R. (1999). Impact of integrated home care services on hospital use. *Journal of the American Geriatrics Society*, *47*(12), 1430–1434. doi:10.1111/j.1532-5415.1999.tb01562.x PMID:10591237

Langhorne, P., & Dennis, M. S. (2004). Stroke units: The next 10 years. *Lancet*, *363*(9412), 834–835. doi:10.1016/S0140-6736(04)15771-1 PMID:15031023

Lingard, L. (2013). Rethinking competence in the context of teamwork. In B. D. Hodges & L. Lingard (Eds.), *The Question of Competence: Reconsidering Medical Education in the Twenty-First Century* (pp. 14–41). ILR Press.

Locke, A., & Kamo, N. (2016). Utilizing clinical pharmacists to improve delivery of evidence-based care for depression and anxiety in primary care. *BMJ Quality Improvement Reports*, *5*(1), 1–5. doi:10.1136/bmjquality.u211816.w4748 PMID:27493753

Maeno, T., Haruta, J., Takayashiki, A., Yoshimoto, H., Goto, R., & Maeno, T. (2019). Interprofessional education in medical schools in Japan. *PLoS One*, *14*(1), e0210912. doi:10.1371/journal.pone.0210912 PMID:30653563

Makary, M. A., Sexton, J. B., Freischlag, J. A., Holzmueller, C. G., Millman, E. A., Rowen, L., & Pronovost, P. J. (2006). Operating room teamwork among physicians and nurses: Teamwork in the eye of the beholder. *Journal of the American College of Surgeons*, *202*(5), 746–752. doi:10.1016/j.jamcollsurg.2006.01.017 PMID:16648014

Martin, J. S., Ummenhofer, W., Manser, T., & Spirig, R. (2010). Interprofessional collaboration among nurses and physicians: Making a difference in patient outcome. *Swiss Medical Weekly*, *140*, w13062. doi:10.4414mw.2010.13062 PMID:20458647

Mishra, A., Krishna, G. S., Alla, S., Kurian, T. D., Kurian, J., Ramesh, M., & Kishor, M. (2017). Impact of Pharmacist-Psychiatrist Collaborative Patient Education on Medication Adherence and Quality of Life (QOL) of Bipolar Affective Disorder (BPAD) Patients. *Frontiers in Pharmacology*, *8*(722), 722. doi:10.3389/fphar.2017.00722 PMID:29066976

Mitchell, P., Wynia, M., Golden, R., McNellis, R., Okun, S., Webb, C. E., Rohrbach, V., & Von Korhorn, I. (2012). *Core principles and values of effective team-based health care*. Institute of Medicine. doi:10.31478/201210c

Morey, J. C., Simon, R., Jay, G. D., Wears, R. L., Salisbury, M., Dukes, K. A., & Berns, S. D. (2002). Error reduction and performance improvement in the emergency department through formal teamwork training: Evaluation results of the MedTeams project. *Health Services Research*, *37*(6), 1553–1581. doi:10.1111/1475-6773.01104 PMID:12546286

Moss, M., Good, V. S., Gozal, D., Kleinpell, R., & Sessler, C. N. (2016). An Official Critical Care Societies Collaborative Statement: Burnout Syndrome in Critical Care Health Care Professionals: A Call for Action. *American Journal of Critical Care*, *25*(4), 368–376. doi:10.4037/ajcc2016133 PMID:27369038

Navarro, A. E., Gassoumis, Z. D., & Wilber, K. H. (2013). Holding abusers accountable: An elder abuse forensic center increases criminal prosecution of financial exploitation. *The Gerontologist*, *53*(2), 303–312. doi:10.1093/geront/gns075 PMID:22589024

Nexus, I. P. E. (n.d.). *National Center for Interprofessional Practice and Education. Picker Institutes Eight Principles of Effective Patient Care*. https://nexusipe.org/informing/resource-center/picker-institute's-eight-principles-patient-centered-care

Patel, P. B., & Vinson, D. R. (2005). Team assignment system: Expediting emergency department care. *Annals of Emergency Medicine*, *46*(6), 499–506. doi:10.1016/j.annemergmed.2005.06.012 PMID:16308063

Patel, R.S., Bachu, R., Adikey, A., Malik, M., & Shah, M. (2018). Factors related to physician burnout and its consequences: a review. *Behav Sci, 8*(11), 98.

Prades, J., Remue, E., van Hoof, E., & Borras, J. (2015). Is it worth reorganizing cancer services on the basis of multidisciplinary teams (MDTs)? A systematic review of the objectives and organization of MDTs and their impact on patient outcomes. *Health Policy (Amsterdam)*, *119*(4), 464–474. doi:10.1016/j.healthpol.2014.09.006 PMID:25271171

Reeves, S. (2016). Why we need interprofessional education to improve the delivery of safe and effective care. *Interface (Botucatu)*, *20*(56), 185–197. doi:10.1590/1807-57622014.0092

Reeves, S., Lewin, S., Espin, S., & Zwarenstein, M. (2010). *A Conceptual Framework for Interprofessional Teamwork*. John Wiley and Sons. Interprofessional Teamwork for Health and Social Care. doi:10.1002/9781444325027.ch4

Reeves, S., Perrier, L., Goldman, J., Freeth, D., & Zarenstein, M. (2013). Interprofessional education: Effects on professional practice and healthcare outcomes (update). *Cochrane Database of Systematic Reviews*, (3), CD00213. doi:10.1002/14651858.CD002213.pub3 PMID:23543515

Rich, M. W., Beckham, V., Wittenberg, C., Leven, C. L., Freedland, K. E., & Carney, R. M. (1995). A multidisciplinary intervention to prevent the readmission of elderly patients with congestive heart failure. *The New England Journal of Medicine*, *333*(18), 1190–1195. doi:10.1056/NEJM199511023331806 PMID:7565975

Rintoul, Y., Wynaden, D., & McGowan, S. (2009). Managing aggression in the emergency department: Promoting an interdisciplinary approach. *International Emergency Nursing*, *17*(2), 122–127. doi:10.1016/j.ienj.2008.11.005 PMID:19341998

Rizzo, V. M., Burnes, D., & Chalfy, A. (2015). A systematic evaluation of a multidisciplinary social work-lawyer elder mistreatment intervention model. *Journal of Elder Abuse & Neglect*, *27*(1), 1–18. doi:10.1080/08946566.2013.792104 PMID:24965802

Roland, D. (2015). But I told you she was ill! The role of families in preventing avoidable harm in children. *BMJ Quality & Safety*, *24*(3), 186–187. doi:10.1136/bmjqs-2015-003950 PMID:25628427

Rosenstein, A. H., & O'Daniel, M. (2005). Disruptive behavior and clinical outcomes: Perceptions of nurses and physicians. *The American Journal of Nursing*, *105*(1), 54–64. doi:10.1097/00000446-200501000-00025 PMID:15659998

Rummans, T. A., Clark, M. M., Sloan, J. A., Frost, M. H., Bostwick, J. M., Atherton, P. J., Johnson, M. E., Gamble, G., Richardson, J., Brown, P., Martensen, J., Miller, J., Piderman, K., Huschka, M., Girardi, J., & Hanson, J. (2006). Impacting quality of life for patients with advanced cancer with a structured multidisciplinary intervention: A randomized controlled trial. *Journal of Clinical Oncology*, *24*(4), 635–642. doi:10.1200/JCO.2006.06.209 PMID:16446335

Sarcevic, A. (n.d.). *Understanding teamwork in trauma resuscitation through analysis of team errors* (Dissertation). Rutgers University. Available at: https://pdfs.semanticscholar.org/f29e/2fc608d82a7c9dfd0550670c7b56c05f4ac7.pdf

Singer, S. J., Falwell, A., Gaba, D. M., Meterko, M., Rosen, A., Hartmann, C. W., & Baker, L. (2009). Identifying organizational cultures that promote patient safety. *Health Care Management Review*, *34*(4), 300–311. doi:10.1097/HMR.0b013e3181afc10c PMID:19858915

Smith CB, Phillips T, Smith TJ. (2017). Using the New ASCO Clinical Practice Guideline for Palliative Care Concurrent With Oncology Care Using the TEAM Approach. *Am Soc Clin Oncol Educ B.*, (37), 714-723. doi:10.1200/EDBK_175474

Sommers, L. S., Marton, K. I., Barbaccia, J. C., & Randolph, J. (2000). Physician, nurse, and social worker collaboration in primary care for chronically ill seniors. *Archives of Internal Medicine*, *160*(12), 1825–1833. doi:10.1001/archinte.160.12.1825 PMID:10871977

Steineman, S., Berg, B., Skinner, A., Ditulio, A., Anzelon, K., Teráda, K., ... Speck, C. (2011). In situ, multidisciplinary, simulation-based teamwork training improves early trauma care. *Journal of Surgical Education*, *68*(6), 472–2. doi:10.1016/j.jsurg.2011.05.009 PMID:22000533

Stewart, R. M., Myers, J. G., Dent, D. L., Ermis, P., Gray, G. A., Villarreal, R., Blow, O., Woods, B., McFarland, M., Garavaglia, J., Root, H. D., & Pruitt, B. A. Jr. (2003). Seven hundred fifty-three consecutive deaths in a level I trauma center: The argument for injury prevention. *The Journal of Trauma Injury Infection and Critical Care*, *54*(1), 66–71. doi:10.1097/00005373-200301000-00009 PMID:12544901

Strasser, D. C., Falconer, J. A., Stevens, A. B., Uomoto, J. M., Herrin, J., Bowen, S. E., & Burridge, A. B. (2008). Team training and stroke rehabilitation outcomes: A cluster randomized trial. *Archives of Physical Medicine and Rehabilitation*, *89*(1), 10–15. doi:10.1016/j.apmr.2007.08.127 PMID:18164324

Taplin, S. H., Weaver, S., Salas, E., Chollette, V., Edwards, H. M., Bruinooge, S. S., & Kosty, M. P. (2015). Reviewing cancer care team effectiveness. *Journal of Oncology Practice / American Society of Clinical Oncology*, *11*(3), 239–246. doi:10.1200/JOP.2014.003350 PMID:25873056

Teaster, P. B., Nerenberg, L., & Stansbury, K. L. (2003). A national look at elder abuse multidisciplinary teams. *Journal of Elder Abuse & Neglect*, *15*(3-4), 91–107. doi:10.1300/J084v15n03_06

Temel, J. S. (2010). Early palliative care for patients with metastatic non-small-cell lung cancer. *The New England Journal of Medicine*.

Tourigny, A., Durand, P.J., Bonin, L., Hébert, R., & Rochette, L. (2004). Quasi-experimental Study of the Effectiveness of an Integrated Service Delivery Network for the Frail Elderly. *Canadian Journal on Aging/La Revue canadienne du vieillissement, 23*(3), 231-246.

Trivedi, D., Goodman, C., Gage, H., Baron, N., Scheibl, F., Iliffe, S., Manthorpe, J., Bunn, F., & Drennan, V. (2013). The effectiveness of interprofessional working for older people living in the commuity: A systematic review. *Health & Social Care in the Community*, *21*(2), 113–128. doi:10.1111/j.1365-2524.2012.01067.x PMID:22891915

Von Korff, M., Gruman, J., Schaefer, J., Curry, S. J., & Wagner, E. H. (1997). Collaborative management of chronic illness: Essential elements. *Annals of Internal Medicine*, *127*(12), 1097–1102. doi:10.7326/0003-4819-127-12-199712150-00008 PMID:9412313

Walders, N., Kercsmar, C., Schluchter, M., Redline, S., Kirchner, H. L., & Drotar, D. (2006). An interdisciplinary intervention for undertreated pediatric asthma. *Chest*, *129*(2), 292–299. doi:10.1378/chest.129.2.292 PMID:16478844

Walter, H. J., Vernacchio, L., Trudell, E. K., Bromberg, J., Goodman, E., Barton, J., Young, G. J., DeMaso, D. R., & Focht, G. (2019). Five-Year Outcomes of Behavioral Health Integration in Pediatric Primary Care. *Pediatrics*, *144*(1), e20183243. doi:10.1542/peds.2018-3243 PMID:31186366

Weller, J., Boyd, M., & Cumin, D. (2014). Teams, tribes, and patient safety: Overcoming barriers to effective teamwork in healthcare. *Postgraduate Medical Journal*, *90*(1061), 149–154. doi:10.1136/postgradmedj-2012-131168 PMID:24398594

Whitcomb, M. E. (2009). Commentary: Flexner redux 2010: Graduate medical education in the United States. *Academic Medicine*, *84*(11), 1476–1478. doi:10.1097/ACM.0b013e3181bb25db PMID:19858793

Wolf, L., Delao, A., & Perhats, C. (2014). Nothing Changes, Nobody Cares: Understanding the Experience of Emergency Nurses Physically or Verbally Assaulted While Providing Care. *Journal of Emergency Nursing*, *40*. . doi:10.1016/j.jen.2013.11.006:1-6

Wong, A., Wing, L., Weiss, B., & Gang, M. (2015). Coordinating a team response to behavioral emergencies in the emergency department: A simulation-enhanced interprofessional curriculum. *The Western Journal of Emergency Medicine*, *16*(6), 859–865. doi:10.5811/westjem.2015.8.26220 PMID:26594279

World Health Organization (WHO). (2010). *Framework for action on interprofessional education & collaborative practice*. WHO.

Wright, A. A., & Katz, I. T. (2018). Beyond Burnout—Redesigning Care to Restore Meaning and Sanity for Physicians. *The New England Journal of Medicine*, *378*(4), 309–311. doi:10.1056/NEJMp1716845 PMID:29365301

You, P., Malik, N., Scott, G., & Fung, K. (2017). Current state of interprofessional educaiton in Canadian medical schools: Findings from a national survey. *Journal of Interprofessional Care*, *31*(5), 670–672. doi:10.1080/13561820.2017.1315060 PMID:28481135

Chapter 2
Moving From Vertical to Horizontal:
How to Mitigate Unconscious Bias With the IPE Team

Denise Lynn Schilling
Western University of Health Sciences, USA

Kelley Sharp
Ohio State University, USA

Reid Waldman
University of Connecticut, USA

ABSTRACT

Unconscious bias impacts the ability to engage with interprofessional education activities. This bias comes in many forms and occurs for a variety of reasons. This chapter reviews the types of bias that frequently plague IPE and reviews common theories explaining this bias. Theories discussed in this chapter include social identity theory, realistic conflict theory, and Allport's contact theory. The purpose of this chapter is to assist readers with improving IPE engagement and help promote healthier communication among members of the healthcare team.

DOI: 10.4018/978-1-7998-3066-5.ch002

SECTION 1

Healthcare providers, like most professionals, want to believe that they are bias-free. However, prevailing neuroscience research demonstrates that no one is truly bias-free as many biases are formed throughout life and held at the subconscious level, mainly through societal conditioning, parental conditioning and life experiences. These formative experiences determine how information is consciously and unconsciously processed and categorized. This processing of information is where bias is introduced and where stereotypes are created. How have you categorized information? Have your life experiences created stereotypes or unconscious biases?

Activity 1: What are the first 3 attributes such as characteristics and/or job responsibilities that you think of when you hear the following:

- Pharmacist
- Podiatrist
- Physical Therapist

When you reflected on Pharmacist did you think patient educator and/or administrator of immunizations? Pharmacists educate and counsel patients regarding smoking cessation, blood pressure measurement and cholesterol management and provide immunizations. The 2014 National Pharmacist Workforce Survey report 60% of pharmacists provided medication therapy management and 53% perform immunizations. Does the word podiatrist evoke thoughts of doctor, surgeon and/or wound care specialist? Podiatrists perform surgery, prescribe medications and often lead wound management teams (Bell, 2009). In contradistinction, when you think of Physical Therapist, were your first thoughts massage, sports, and assistive devices such as canes and walkers? Physical therapists have a clinical doctorate, they are front line providers, they work in dental medicine, women's health and the ICU, in addition to "providing cost-effective alternative treatment to many patients who currently undergo surgery and take costly prescription drugs" (APTA). These 3 professions provide an opportunity to begin exploring common stereotyping and bias. These simple and common stereotypes assigned to professions are a form of bias and are detrimental to effective interprofessional education and ultimately interprofessional practice.

What Is Bias?

Bias is defined as "prejudice in favor of or against one thing, person, or group compared with another, usually in a way considered to be unfair" (Oxford), "an attitude that you have that makes you treat someone in a way that is unfair or different from the way you treat other people"(Macmillan Dictionary) or "an inclination of temperament or outlook *especially*: a personal and sometimes unreasoned judgment" (Merriam Webster). The commonality in these definitions that applies directly to the potential for negative impact on building a successful IPE team is "unfair/unreasoned" judgement of "group/another" in this case imposing preconceived attributes to another profession either by personal characteristics or professional role/responsibilities.

There are 2 types of bias: explicit bias and implicit bias. Explicit bias is conscious bias meaning the biased individual is aware of his/her attitudes and feelings and the individual's associated behaviors are with intent. Explicit bias is processed neurologically at a conscious level as declarative, semantic memory, and in words (Amodio 2011, Smith 2000). While the individual is aware of his or her explicit bias, it still has its root in formative experiences during development like implicit bias. Explicit bias is typically the easiest form of bias to elicit as it is outwardly manifested; however, it is often difficult to change. Addressing explicit bias is a priori during IPE. Failure to do so will subsequently undermine team dynamic and interprofessional empowerment.

Implicit bias is unconscious bias meaning the biased individual is unaware that he or she is biased. In fact, implicit bias frequently directly contradicts the biased individual's espoused beliefs and values. Implicit bias must be addressed as it "automatically seeps into a person's affect or behavior and is outside of the full awareness of that person" and can thus interfere with clinical assessment, decision-making, and communication (Blair 2001). Interference in accurate assessment, decision-making and communication negatively impact interprofessional relationships that are critical to the successful development and delivery of interprofessional education. Unaddressed implicit bias moving from IPE to IPP can result in behaviors and communication that can undermine collaboration in health goals and the delivery of effective cohesive patient-centered care.

In healthcare, the term 'bias' is typically used to refer to both implicit stereotypes and prejudices, as provided by example in activity 1. It is important to note that biases by definition are not inherently bad but are nonetheless commonly inaccurate. Dispelling interprofessional bias underpins the success of IPE. Similarly, addressing interprofessional bias can be used as a segway into enhancing awareness of other personal biases which may interfere with patient care. (Green, 2013; Lapkin, Levett-Jones, & Gilligan, 2011; D'Amour, Ferrada-Videla, Rodriguez, and Beaulieu (2005). Ultimately, understanding the roles and responsibilities of other healthcare professionals promotes interprofessional empowerment and positively influences healthcare delivery.

SECTION 2

Generalization vs. Stereotyping: Are They Different?

Generalization is a sorting strategy that is used make sense of the large amount of information gathered day to day. The ability to compartmentalize and label information such as professional roles in healthcare allows for ease in cross professional communication and patient referrals; however, when oversimplification occurs and one assumes information without knowledge or evidence of accuracy, generalization becomes stereotyping. Generalizations are often the starting point for learning whereas stereotypes, right or wrong, are an endpoint. Stereotypes in interprofessional education are commonly explained through Social Identity Theory, Realistic Conflict Theory or Contact Hypothesis Theory.

Social Identity Theory

Social Identity Theory refers to a person's sense of identity (i.e. who they are) based on their group membership(s). As healthcare providers we are trained to introduce ourselves not only by name but also by our profession. Professionals are encouraged, and in some cases mandated, by CEU requirements to attend profession-specific conferences and to be active within their corresponding professional organizations. These profession-specific activities are critical to communication, professional development, patient care and safety and they also promote a sense of social identity. Without a focused effort one can easily become siloed within one's own profession which leads to the risk of developing stereotypes about other professionals based on minimal experience interacting with other professions.

Activity 2: Imagine that a registered nurse working on an inpatient rehabilitation unit is assigned an elderly patient recovering from a fractured hip. The patient currently lives alone in a single-family home but will need to be discharged to an assisted living facility for more advanced care. This patient not only requires nursing care but is also being cared for by social work, physical therapy, occupational therapy, and the pharmacy team.

- How is patient care impacted when one profession attempts to perform the roles of another profession?
- How can this registered nurse utilize interprofessional resources to optimize safe and effective patient-centered care?

If the nurse is unaware of each of these professions' scope of practice and abilities, the nurse might attempt to ambulate the patient without first conversing with the physical therapist or may attempt a medication reconciliation when the pharmacy team has already performed this task. Truly effective interprofessional teamwork is established by not only seeking accurate knowledge of other health care professions but also by identifying how team member's various roles overlap and complement each other. As healthcare professionals we must be aware of our own social identities, acknowledge our personal biases towards other professions, and then work diligently to learn more about other healthcare professions and their specific social identities

Realistic Conflict Theory

Although a foundational knowledge of one's professional identify is important, the practice of Social Identity theory alone is not enough to avoid interprofessional bias and/or conflict. Within a healthcare team there may be overlap within the professional roles of each team member. This overlap may produce conflict within the team, especially when determining patient fees, provider re-imbursement and allocation of resources. Have these logistics ever been the source of conflict between yourself and another professional? For example, how do the professional roles of Occupational Therapy, Physical Therapy, Recreational Therapy, Chiropractic, and Osteopathic Manual Manipulation differ? How does one choose which referral will best suit a patient's needs? Will reimbursement be equivalent for each referral to these various professions? Should one professional group be provided greater resources for patient care? The Realistic Conflict Theory states that when "two or more groups are competing over limited resources (either from real or perceived) prejudicial feelings and negative stereotypes can develop towards the other group. However, enhanced interprofessional education can reduce the conflict that results from this perceived competition because IPE exposure reinforces the tenant that all professions are working collaboratively towards a "common" goal, providing patient-centered care.

Contact Hypothesis Theory

Introduced in 1954, Allport's Contact Hypothesis Theory aligns with interprofessional education and continues to be relevant in clinical practice today. Originally developed to address social prejudice, Allport suggested that positive effects occur in contact situations characterized by four key conditions: equal status, intergroup co-operation, common goals, and support by social and institutional authorities. (Henry, PJ & Hardin CD, 2006). These four key conditions serve as pillars to successful, modern IPE implementation and sustainability in both practice and education.

SECTION 3

Implications of bias IPEC core competencies

- Values/Ethics for Interprofessional Practice
- Roles/Responsibilities
- Interprofessional Communication
- Teams and Teamwork

Take a moment to reflect on any past negative experiences to IPE or unsuccessful IPE attempts. What were the underlying issues? Bias and strong professional identity formation are often thought of obstacles to establishing effective IPE, but as we explore the implications of each of these factors, we encourage reframing as challenges to overcome not barriers. Barrier as defined by Merriam-Webster is: "something that prevents or blocks movement from one place to another.: a law, rule, problem, etc., that makes something difficult or impossible.: something that makes it difficult for people to understand each other." Thus, a perceived barrier typically suggests an insurmountable problem. On the other hand, challenge as defined by Merriam Webster is: "a stimulating task or problem". Thus, a perceived challenge suggests an opportunity to think outside the box, problem solve and create resolution. This simple reframing of situational perception from "barrier" to "challenge" reduces the inherent negative connotations of IPE and allows for productive and positive movement forward.

It is important to dissect the expected outcomes of IPE and individually examine the impact of bias on each of the 4 IPEC core competencies. The Interprofessional Education Collaborative, IPEC, was established in 2009 when six national education associations of schools of the health professions formed a collaborative group to 1) promote and encourage the advancement of interprofessional learning experiences, and 2) help prepare future health professionals for enhanced team-based care of patients and improved population health outcomes. The members of IPEC include representatives from allopathic and osteopathic medicine, dentistry, nursing, pharmacy, and public health education. In 2011, the IPEC published competencies for interprofessional collaborative practice to guide curricula development across health professions schools. In 2016, IPEC restructured the guidelines to establish 4 core competencies with the intent to guide and promote interprofessional collaboration between health care professionals and provide measurable behaviors for assessment. The core competencies for IPE are: Competency 1 - values/ethics, Competency 2 - roles and responsibilities, Competency 3 - interprofessional communication and, Competency 4 - teams and teamwork. (Core Competencies for Interprofessional Collaborative Practice:2016 Update)

Competency 1

Competency 1 - Values/Ethics for interprofessional practice, focuses on the ability to effectively work with individuals from other professions to maintain a climate of mutual respect. According to the realistic conflict theory, the numerous treatment options and the variety of healthcare providers that engage in the care of a medically complex patient produces a patient-care situation ripe for conflict among professions due to resource allocation limitations. To further illustrate the complexity of such a situation, each healthcare provider brings a specific passion for their profession and a perceived, and often rigid, view of what their profession will provide to patient care. The entrenched social identify of each profession provides further opportunity to challenge IPE and disrupt patient care. In order to address the potential challenges created by bias in the form of social identity and reality conflict, it is key to practice self-awareness (know yourself and your bias) and to work collaboratively with other professionals to identify shared values and to define the desired patient outcomes. The ability to openly view treatment from multiple professional perspectives to find shared goals and values will turn perceived challenges into shared successes.

Competency 2

In order to master this Competency 2- Roles and Responsibilities, one must examine one's own role and use knowledge of the roles of other professions to appropriately assess and address the health care needs of patients on both a micro and macro scale. Take a moment and reflect on your chosen health profession. Have your practice requirements changed since you entered the profession over time either in terminal degree obtained or actual patient care scope of practice? To maintain professional licensure are you required to engage in continuing education to maintain currency in practice? With the ever changing/expanding roles within each of our chosen professions how can anyone be expected to be an expert on the many other professions outside one's scope of practice? This continual evolution in professional roles requires on-going communication and a commitment to continued learning from interprofessional colleagues. Without the willingness to seek information from others and share expertise, it is easy for professional bias and subsequent competition between professions to occur. Remember, it is not possible to fully understand all professional roles, the various educational requirements of each profession, the many different scopes of practice and the legal frameworks by which each profession is allowed to practice; therefore, a simple declaration of "I don't know" is a safe, honest and productive starting point to increase knowledge and build a successful IPE climate.

Competency 3

Competency 3 - Interprofessional Communication, refers to the ability of a healthcare professional to communicate with patients, families, communities, and other professionals in a receptive and responsible manner. Effective interprofessional communication cultivates and supports a team approach to disease prevention, maintenance of patient health, selection treatment options. The art of interprofessional communication begins with active listening. When we listen with bias or listen to respond rather than hear the potential for successful collaboration, interprofessional education and patient-centered care is harmed. The implications of poor communication on IPE can cause irreparable damage to mutual respect. It is important to note that interprofessional communication extends beyond verbal communication to encompass non-verbal communication methods as well. Body language, eye contact, and hand gestures are critical components of interprofessional communication, and this non-verbal communication can easily be mis-interpreted; therefore, when engaging in interprofessional education or clinical practice, it is imperative to be cognizant of both verbal and non-verbal communication. Healthcare professionals work diligently to engage in patient communication that is clear, accurate, and culturally competent. This same level of intentional communication must be brought to interprofessional interactions ensuring that each professional "listens to hear" and engages in "courageous dialogues" in order to build productive interprofessional relationships and execute effective patient care. Successful IPE communication is honest, transparent, and focused on leaning about each other by identifying commonalities/opportunities for shared resources, utilizing differences to complement each other, and creating shared values/goals.

Competency 4

Competency 4 - Teams and Teamwork, refers to the ability to apply relationship-building values to enhance team performance team in order to plan, deliver, and evaluate patient- centered care, population health programs and policies that are safe, efficient, and equitable. Although isolated as a fourth and independent competency, effective teamwork is without a doubt the culmination of competencies 1, 2 and 3 and is the ultimate goal of interprofessional education and practice. There is no place for individually held social identities or realistic conflict issues within the healthcare team. When professional bias is not addressed the opportunities for team development and teamwork are lost and both the providers and their patients lose.

SECTION 4

Setting the Stage for IPE Success

How does one diminish/eliminate the inherent bias associated with social identity and realistic conflict in IPE?

Here are 8 simple strategies to mitigate unconscious bias:

1. Recognize and accept that everyone has biases. To have bias is to be human. Do not place a value-laden judgement on having bias, but instead honestly reflect, accept, and then address interprofessional bias.
2. Look beyond the surface – Held generalizations about other professions are similar to the structure of an iceberg, only the tip is visible above the water – look deeper. Learning about other professions is a journey and interprofessional development is a commitment.
3. Do not hesitate to say, "I don't know." You do not need to be the expert in everything. You are the expert of your profession – learn from others about theirs.
4. Communication is key! Engage in "courageous dialogues." A sense of discomfort and awkwardness is a sign of growth: embrace the challenge.
5. Healthcare is not a competition – the patient needs every member of the healthcare team. Each profession brings something to the patient – the time for each profession varies on the patient's needs. Your job is secure, and the patient is the priority.
6. Listen to your internal tapes identifying pre-conceived interprofessional bias- are these tapes accurate? Why are they playing? If inaccurate – begin to delete and re-program.
7. Focus on successes – opportunities can be gained when resources are shared. Celebrate each accomplishment as a team!
8. Remember – medicine is a team sport with the patient acting as your coach. Listen intently to the coach's message.

REFERENCES

Amodio, D., & Ratner, K. (2011). A memory systems model of implicit social cognition. *Current Directions in Psychological Science, 20*(3), 143–148. doi:10.1177/0963721411408562

Bell, D. Jr. (2009, July). The Role of Podiatry in Wound Management. *The Journal of the American College of Certified Wound Specialists, 1*(3), 78–79. doi:10.1016/j.jcws.2009.05.003 PMID:24527119

Bias. (2019). In *Macmillan dictionary*. Retrieved September 10,2019, from https://www.macmillandictionary.com/dictionary/british/biasMacmillan

Bias. (2019). In *Merriam-Webster.com*. Retrieved September 10, 2019, from https://www.merriam-webster.com/dictionary/biasmerriam-webster

Blair, I. V., Ma, J. E., & Lenton, A. P. (2001). Imagining stereotypes away: The moderation of implicit stereotypes through mental imagery. *Journal of Personality and Social Psychology, 81*(5), 828–841. doi:10.1037/0022-3514.81.5.828 PMID:11708560

(2005). Bluml, B Definition of Medication Therapy Management. *Development of Professionwide Consensus J Am Pharm Assoc., 45*, 566–572. doi:10.1331/1544345055001274

D'Amour, D., Ferrada-Videla, M., San Martin Rodriguez, L., & Beaulieu, M. (2005). The conceptual basis for interprofessional collaboration: Core concepts and theoretical frameworks. *Journal of Interprofessional Care, 19*(sup1), 116-131.

Eckel, F.M. (2014). Pharmacy Workforce Center's 2014 National Pharmacist Workforce Survey. *Pharmacy Times*.

FitzGerald, C., & Hurst, S. (2017). Implicit bias in healthcare professionals: A systematic review. *BMC Medical Ethics, 18*(1), 19. doi:10.118612910-017-0179-8 PMID:28249596

Green, B., & Johnson, C. (2015). Interprofessional collaboration in research, education, and clinical practice: Working together for a better future. *The Journal of Chiropractic Education, 29*(1), 1–10. doi:10.7899/JCE-14-36 PMID:25594446

Gunaldo, T. P., Brisolara, K. F., Davis, A. H., & Moore, R. (2017). Aligning interprofessional education collaborative sub-competencies to a progression of learning. *Journal of Interprofessional Care, 31*(3), 394–396. doi:10.1080/13561820.2017.1285273 PMID:28272902

Harper, J. C. (2019). IPEC's core competency 2 roles and responsibilities: What more do we need to implement these? *Journal of Nursing Education and Practice, 9*(7).

Henry & Hardin. (2006, Oct. 1). The Contact Hypothesis Revisited: Status Bias in the Reduction of Implicit Prejudice in the United States and Lebanon. *Psychological Science*.

Hogg, M. A. (2018). Social identity theory. In P. J. Burke (Ed.), *Contemporary social psychological theories* (pp. 112–138). Stanford University Press.

Interprofessional Education Collaborative. (2016). *Core competencies for interprofessional collaborative practice: Report of Expert Panel 2016 update.* Washington, DC: Interprofessional Education Collaborative. Retrieved 11-4-2019 from: https://ipecollaborative.org/uploads/IPEC-Core-Competencies.pdf

Lapkin, S., Levett-Jones, T., & Gilligan, C. (2011). The effectiveness of interprofessional education in university-based health professional programs: A systematic review. *Joanna Briggs Institute Library of Systematic Reviews*, *9*(46), 1917–1970. doi:10.11124/jbisrir-2011-103 PMID:27820537

McLeod, S. A. (2019, Oct 24). Social identity theory. *Simply Psychology*. https://www.simplypsychology.org/social-identity-theory.html

Oxford English Dictionary. (n.d.). *art, n. 1*. Oxford University Press.

Smith, E. R., & DeCoster, J. (2000). Dual-process models in social and cognitive psychology: Conceptual integration and links to underlying memory systems. *Personality and Social Psychology Review*, *4*(2), 108–131. doi:10.1207/S15327957PSPR0402_01

Stets, J.E., & Burke, P.J. (2000). Identity Theory and Social Identity Theory. *Social Psychology Quarterly, 63*(3), 224-237. http://links.jstor.org/sici?sici=0190-2725%28200009%2963%3A3%3C224%3AITASIT%3E2.0.CO%3B2-V

The Role of the Physical Therapist in National Health Care Reform. (n.d.). *APTA's Health Care*. https://www.apta.org/uploadedFiles/APTAorg/Advocacy/Federal/Health_Care_Reform/APTA_Position/RoleofPTinHealthCareReform.pdf

Chapter 3
Practical Insights Into the Group Process:
What Works and What Doesn't

Brenda J. Rogers
University of Missouri-Kansas City School of Medicine, USA

Brian Burghardt
University of Missouri-Kansas City School of Medicine, USA

ABSTRACT

The group process can be a highly effective and efficient method to address a problem, especially among persons with different professional backgrounds. Interprofessional collaboration can provide insight and solutions that extend beyond a single professional's knowledge. But collaboration has potential problems too, including determining how to effectively and respectfully work with people with different knowledge, experiences, and authority. This chapter reviews the benefits of group process as well as identifies the detriments of doing so and provides guidance on how to develop a successful group collaboration project.

INTRODUCTION

There are benefits and challenges to group process, which can both enhance and thwart efficient patient care. Groups can be dynamic, innovative, collaborative and determined to meet an objective; they can also be obstructive, dysfunctional, apathetic, disengaged and focused on individual needs. Creating an environment of effective and efficient groups is the primary goal, but achieving that goal requires

DOI: 10.4018/978-1-7998-3066-5.ch003

identifying the objective, nurturing the group members and developing a supportive and effective infrastructure. Within the healthcare field, group collaboration can range from focusing on an individual patient's needs to meeting the needs of a community. In 2010, the World Health Organization published the *Framework for Action on Interprofessional Education and Collaborative Practice*, a landmark document that recommended interprofessional collaboration as a solution to the global health workforce deficiency. (1) This document provides a foundation of action steps that can be applied to enhance existing community health needs in different locations around the world. From this document came the identification and recommendation for educating students in healthcare fields about the opportunities within interprofessional education. From that recommendation came the need to understand how groups work, leading to the study of group process. In medical education, there is an emphasis on interprofessional teams.

In 2011, the Association for American Colleges published recommendations from a panel of six national associations of schools of the health professions that identified interprofessional learning and experiences as a core competency expected of medical students. (2) This collaborative document, involving educators from allopathic medicine, dentistry, nursing, osteopathic medicine, pharmacy and public health, identified the value and need for interprofessional education in order to "prepare all health professionals to intentionally and effectively work together to build a safe and better, person-centered and community/population-oriented health care system." (2) A compelling reason for the emphasis on group work is the change in the healthcare environment.

Only a few decades ago the practice of medicine was very different. The physician was the leader of the healthcare team and dictated the evaluation and treatment of the patient. Ancillary healthcare services were instructed to follow the orders prescribed by the physician leader. Healthcare practice in the current era is markedly different, with healthcare providers of different training programs working side by side to meet the needs of the expanding patient population. The patient's healthcare team leader may be a physician, but may also be a nurse practitioner, physician's assistant, physical therapist, clinical nurse or another medically trained person. In our era, patient care also requires collaboration between medical specialties and ancillary care programs such as case management and social work. Some medical conditions that were terminal even just a decade ago, such as a genetic metabolic disorder, are not terminal anymore and require ongoing attention to care as these patients age and develop age-related medical conditions. An example is the patient who survives a major medical event, such as heart surgery, but still requires dental care. The cardiologist and dentist must work together to coordinate the patient's medications and approach to a dental procedure that will be safe for the patient. The transition to working as a collaborative team member in providing patient care has been challenging for some who are accustomed to the historical method of treatment, thus the importance of educating healthcare learners about working in groups in preparation for the future.

BENEFITS

When approaching a problem, there are many benefits to group process, particularly interprofessional group process endeavors, as compared to individual decision-making. Group process methodology is an approach to problem-solving that includes individuals from different professions or specialties coming together with an objective to solve the problem. During the group problem-solving endeavor, it is anticipated that resources are identified that contribute valuable information that would not be known to an individual attempting to solve the same problem. Benefits to a group process endeavor are the inclusion of diverse experience and educational roles in assessing a problem, knowledge gained from working with other professions, the inclusion of viewpoints from an array of backgrounds, utilization of a multidisciplinary approach to problem-solving and the opportunity to extrapolate knowledge gained in the process to situations beyond the local level.

Inclusion of diversity among the group members is valuable to the process and outcome. When developing an interprofessional group, including those from multiple specialties and backgrounds is important to broaden the knowledge and experience base of the group. Increased access to knowledge, experience, creativity, innovation, efficiency and better outcomes occurs when the group has representatives from a variety of backgrounds. In the book, *The Wisdom of Crowds*, author James Surowiecki provides ample examples that the intelligence, innovation and efficiencies of groups frequently outperform an individual despite the make-up of the individuals of the group. (3) He provides multiple examples that the summary of individual decisions grouped together outperforms even the most knowledgeable expert individual. The book offers explanations as to how this occurs, which includes utilizing diverse knowledge and educational skills among the individuals that compose a group. He emphasizes that the diversity of the group, including those from different socioeconomic and educational backgrounds as well as different political and religious belief systems are the reasons that a crowd, or group, outperforms an individual. His examples range from problems that solve a highly technical engineering problem, guessing the weight of the local fair ox, and predicting a political race outcome. In all these situations and more, the group's "collective intelligence" was superior to that of an individual by being more accurate, efficient and productive. In one example, a group, which included engineers, technicians and administrative support identified the solution to the electrical failure crisis of the Apollo 13 mission. By working together and with a clearly defined objective, the group formulated an innovative solution that resulted in the successful return of the Apollo 13 astronauts to Earth. In a second example, the average of 800 fair attendees who provided an individual guess of the weight of an ox was more accurate than any single entry. The individuals who participated included anyone who wished to submit an entry, regardless of knowledge about animals or estimating weight. And in a third example, information was shared about a group of volunteer voters managed by a company in Iowa has been extremely reliable in predicting political race outcomes; more predictable than any single individual or poll. The volunteer voters are comprised of people of different demographic backgrounds and who live throughout the United States. They are volunteers and are not selected; thus, the composition of the group is truly random. These examples, as well as many others in additional resources, provide objectivity, data and science to clearly establish that groups outperform individuals in making accurate, meaningful, capable and effective decisions.

Knowledge gained from working with those from other professions and the inclusion of viewpoints from an array of backgrounds are benefits to both the individual participating in a group process endeavor as well as to the recipient of the group's objective. Specifically, in the healthcare field, utilizing group process to address a problem is particularly beneficial when people from different professions combine. Interprofessional group process includes individuals from any profession that might impact a patient or healthcare system problem, resulting in a team that has capability and benefit beyond its individual members. Whereas studies have documented the power and ability of groups to problem-solve more effectively and accurately than individuals, the individuals who participate in such endeavors also conclude that group problem-solving can be beneficial. There is evidence that individual participants in medical education group process endeavors benefit from the experience. Knowledge gained by exposure to experiences and resources utilized by other medical disciplines can enhance and broaden the knowledge and abilities of each individual participant, as well as strengthen future working relationships and problem-solving by including knowledge obtained about the responsibilities of other professions. Qin, et all, reviewed 63 studies regarding cooperative versus competitive problem-solving efforts in a literature review and determined that in all studies the cooperative member teams outperformed individuals competing, and this applied to linguistic, non-linguistic, well-defined and ill-defined tasks. (4) In 2014, Johnson, et al, noted specific outcomes from cooperative learning that included improved psychological adjustment and social competence of the individual, the development of positive relationships and an effort to achieve. (5) Comments from undergraduate students who participated in group problem-solving endeavors reported that the skills learned during class assigned tasks were highly valued and recognized as skills valuable to post-graduation employability. (6) This is particularly important among healthcare students whose future practice requires skills to effectively work on an interprofessional team. Medical education requires a unique model of group learning that requires learners with different backgrounds and knowledge to collaborate, thus identifying the members of an interprofessional team is important.

Utilization of a multidisciplinary approach benefits the outcome of the group's problem-solving. Interprofessional teams, a type of group, are composed of representatives from differing clinical services who have a common objective. In healthcare education, that objective is typically the care of a patient or community. Traditionally, a patient's healthcare team was composed of individuals who played a specific role in the patient's treatment. Consider a patient hospitalized for pneumonia. The physician developed the treatment plan, the pharmacist provided medications to be used, the nurse administered the medications and the respiratory therapist provided pulmonary treatments. Although everyone may have a piece of information about the patient, the hierarchical decision making resulted in physicians adjusting the treatment plan in a manner that may or may not have included information from others. In current medical practice, individuals involved in the patient's care are allowed some autonomy to adjust the care, and decisions are based on information from the caregiver with the expertise. For the hospitalized patient with pneumonia, the physician will develop a treatment plan based on the initial assessment. The pharmacist may adjust the dose of medication, contacting the physician for approval to do so, based on additional patient information specific to that patient, such as laboratory values. The nurse may administer the intravenous antibiotic over a certain amount of time, varying that time depending upon the patient's condition; but the time frame falls within a pre-determined range that is approved by the team. The respiratory therapist may adjust the frequency of breathing treatments or the oxygen flow rate based on the patient's condition, with the autonomy to do so based on his/her expertise in respiratory therapy. The physician fulfils the team leader role as the person who oversees each component of care but allows other interprofessional members to act as per their expertise. Communication among the team members is very important in this patient's care, as all members must be knowledgeable about the patient's condition and care plan changes in order to meet the goal of patient improvement and hospital discharge. Family members and the patient him/herself may also actively participate in the care by assisting with care and/or information about the outcomes of treatment. When asked, patients and family members report a positive impact from interprofessional team involvement during hospital rounds, noting satisfaction of treatment and the overall hospital experience. (7) A second example of the benefit of collaborative care among interprofessional teams occurs in the dental office, where the dental hygienist and dentist share the treatment of a patient by each fulfilling a specific role. When healthcare students learn in an environment of interprofessional teams, are encouraged and expected to coordinate and collaborate on treatment plans, and are taught to communicate effectively, the patient benefits.

Group process offers the opportunity to extrapolate and extend processes and outcomes to a population broader than locally. Implementing a multidisciplinary healthcare group to address a problem can address the initial problem but may also establish a procedure and mindset that lends itself to problem solving beyond that individual patient problem. A solution to one problem might be utilized to address a larger system problem, or perhaps extend to benefit multiple institutions or communities. By instructing learners to engage and accept the benefit of group collaboration, subsequent larger systems-based problems can be addressed. Eye care in Canada is a good example of this. In Canada, there is a deficiency of ophthalmologists. Acknowledging this deficiency, optometrists and ophthalmologists have overcome issues of mistrust and misunderstanding to develop a mutually respectful relationship that has benefitted patients by improving access to care. The education of optometry students has adjusted to include the treatment of primary care eye disease. That has resulted in the ability of ophthalmologists to care for more complicated eye conditions without adversely affecting patient access to care despite a limited number of providers. (8) Green, et al, noted this when proposing that chiropractors could be of benefit to collaborate with care provided by a physician. "The team provides opportunities to learn and go beyond traditional ways of thinking and access to people we would not normally reach in order to serve a larger body of people." (9)

REQUIREMENTS

For group process to be successful in achieving a specific objective, the group needs certain elements. These four elements are (A) a clearly defined objective, (B) participation of all individuals, (C) decision-making capability and (D) organizational roles. (4) A clearly defined objective tends to result in an effective group working relationship; however, it is possible that the objective will change once the group discussion begins. Agreement of the objective(s) is important to keep members engaged as well as to be respectful of everyone's time. Determining the objective(s) at the first meeting sets the agenda for subsequent meetings and encourages the group to develop a plan of addressing the problem. Open-minded and respectful communication is necessary for effective group work; it encourages participation from each group member. Discouraging members from participating by intimidation, disregard or dismissal adversely affects the group's purpose and effectiveness. Participation by all members is key and should be encouraged and expected. In review of literature about group process, some promote the designation of a team leader prior to the development of the group and others suggest identification of the leader once the group has been formed. There are benefits to both. Identifying a leader prior to forming the group allows for the leader to determine team members that will assist in identifying and achieving the objective. The possible negative consequence to this is that valuable members might be overlooked due to an individual leader's narrowed focus. Requesting volunteers to form a group or having a non-team member assign people to a group can result in a multidisciplinary productive group. This type of group can select a leader when it first meets and is preferable for student learning as it encourages learning by being immersed into the group. Adequate training and support for the leader is important for the group's success. This may require a formal educational program or an available mentor external to the group to provide guidance among student leaders who might lack leadership experience. Providing this resource can assure the group is organized and utilizes meeting time efficiently. The leader has the responsibility for assuring respectful and effective communication among the team members.

Participation of all individuals in the group is the second element of a successful group and is imperative to an effective group process endeavor. This can occur in several ways, but ultimately the leader has the responsibility of encouraging individual participation. One method of encouraging individual participation is to require input from everyone by setting the expectation at the onset of the meeting sessions. We will later address the challenges of group process endeavors and lack of individual input due to fear, intimidation or disinterest. Recognition that these feelings can adversely affect a group dynamic requires that expectations and encouragement for individual participation are clearly expressed at the onset of the group's work. Developing a plan for how individual group members participate is an additional method to encourage everyone's participation. Group process is not successful in achieving the goal of multidisciplinary input if individuals do not engage. And the harm in lack of multidisciplinary dialogue is an outcome decision based on "group think." Group think, a term common in psychology literature, represents a decision based on the desire to conform and avoid conflict in deciding among group members and can lead to irrational or ineffective decisions. Teams who groupthink ignore individual creativity and discourage alternative solutions or thoughts that disagree with the mentality of most of the group. In these groups, the priority becomes avoiding conflict and agreeability rather than realistic plans to achieve the objective. (10)

Decision-making capability is a third element of effective group process. This includes two perspectives: how the group makes decisions as well as the implementation of the final decisions. At the onset of the group development, it is wise to determine how final decisions will be made. That could be by complete agreement, majority opinion or the leader may make a final determination based on the group discussion. The important factor is ensuring that each team member can share his/her thoughts and opinion for consideration. Developing an environment of support, respect, encouragement to participate and willingness to listen during group meetings results in team members who are empowered to offer opinions. Once decisions have been determined, the group must be able to enact its recommendations, or to entrust that proposed recommendations will be implemented by others who request the information. If it is unclear how the group's decisions will be utilized, there is the potential for the group to be less engaged and less interested in the outcome. Group members appreciate when their time and contributions are acknowledged using a recommendation and are subsequently more interested in the outcome and likely to participate in future group process endeavors.

Organizational roles are the fourth element essential to group process success. Optimally a group is comprised of members from multiple disciplines and backgrounds to provide diversity to the group. Within healthcare education, including members from different aspects of the healthcare system is recommended. Roles are imperative to ensure that the group is successful in accomplishing the objective(s) identified. There are primarily three categories of roles: task, maintenance and self-oriented. (11) Members who are attentive to the group's task focus on the work process needed; they are those who gather information to share, contribute ideas and/or resource information, share knowledge about prior experiences that are applicable to the group objective(s) and record progress as well as future tasks. Maintenance members are those who are dedicated to the group objective but also focus on involvement of the members to encourage effective working relationships among individuals within the group. By seeking harmony, compromise and respectful interactions among members, the maintenance members encourage individual participation in the group endeavors. Lastly, the self-oriented members are those who are less interested in the group's individual members and instead prioritize their needs and objectives. These members have value in sharing opinions and information that might be helpful in meeting the group objective(s), but they also have the potential to be disruptive and obstructive to working relationships. Recognizing that group process team members typically identify into one of these three roles allows the team leader to preemptively set expectations and continuously remind the group of those expectations.

ADDITIONAL REQUIREMENTS

There are other methods that might be considered when creating a group. Choi and Pak (12) suggest an alternate strategy that includes additional components to the four elements mentioned previously that are implemented in order to develop an effective team. They recommend a strategy entitled TEAMWORK to enhance effective multidisciplinary teamwork. The TEAMWORK acronym provides an easy-to-remember foundation upon which to develop a group. It includes the four foundational elements of a successful group as noted previously as well as additional components. TEAMWORK is an acronym for Team, Enthusiasm, Accessibility, Motivation, Workplace, Objectives, Role and Kinship. Team refers to the members that comprise the group. Enthusiasm refers to the commitment and involvement of team members. Accessibility is the method in which the group has access to each other, which could be in person, electronically by writing or including electronic video capability. Motivation refers to the incentives and rewards provided by involvement in the group process endeavor. Workplace refers to the institutional support required for the group to exist and be productive; this might be an instructor and course for a student project experience or administrative leaders of an organization. Objective is the purpose of the group process endeavor. Role refers to the responsibilities of the member participants both as individuals and collectively as the group. And kinship refers to the way in which the members communicate and interact with each other. Choi and Pak explain that each of these components is necessary to consider and address when developing a group project, as each is necessary for a group endeavor to be productive. (12)

The purpose of the group process endeavor is relevant to its composition and requirements for existence. In the workplace, the decision to create a group to identify solutions to a problem is commonly made with the intention of improvement. In healthcare education, however, the intention may emphasize the knowledge gained by involvement in a group endeavor more than the outcome. It is important for the group's leader and members to understand the purpose and responsibilities of the team. The team members might be selected or appointed, and this difference matters. Selected members are requested to participate and do so with the understanding of what is requested. Appointed members, such as might occur in a classroom setting, lends itself to members who may not be invested in the process or outcome. Using the TEAMWORK model gives the leader information to consider and reference when leading the team. A leader should understand the purpose of the team, the reason for member involvement, determine methods in which the group communicates, identify external support resources, motivate members to participate and clearly identify the objectives.

Consider the example of a group process endeavor in a healthcare system. A terminally ill patient of a specific religion recognized that he was likely to die in the very near future. He requested that prior to his death, that his bed be adjusted to face a different direction. Facing that direction, to the East, was important to his religious beliefs as part of the dying process. His request seems rather simple, however is complicated. His hospital room in the intensive care unit was arranged with electronic devices and equipment in a fixed position; turning the bed 180 degrees would necessitate moving that equipment. One of his healthcare providers, determined to meet the patient's request, assembled a multidisciplinary team to problem solve, with the objective being to move the patient's head so that he faced east while continuing to provide excellent medical care. The healthcare provider, a nurse who functioned as the team leader, created a team of nurses, a religious leader, a facilities/equipment representative, the patient and a family member, a social worker and a physician to embark on a group process endeavor. Each member had specific knowledge and experience that is relevant to this problem. And each member is motivated to assist a dying patient. Many solutions to the problem were suggested, and then members provided information on how each solution might or might not be implemented. Each member provided suggestions that involved compromise in order to meet the objective. Ultimately a solution was identified that met the objective that included compromises on medical care and the patient's needs but were acceptable to all. In this situation, the healthcare team decreased the frequency of checking vital signs and discontinued continuous electronic cardiorespiratory monitoring, and the patient agreed to temporary repositioning when use of fixed equipment could not be substituted. Subsequent to this group process endeavor, a process for meeting similar needs for other patients was implemented. Using one specific situation to apply widely to other situations is an example of the benefit of group process.

The value, benefit and importance of group process has been addressed. The requirements, items to consider when creating a group and the process of doing so have also been addressed. But there are barriers, challenges and limitations to group process also. In certain instances, utilizing a group to solve a problem is not appropriate. Individual task completion is critical to students attaining knowledge, problem-solving, learning time management and task completion, all of which are imperative to a career in healthcare. Individuals in health care must achieve life-long learning expectations and are individually responsible for attaining knowledge and experience necessary to function effectively. Examples include learning for knowledge board certification examinations and providing up-to-date health care by learning the most current information. There are other circumstances in which group process is a barrier to achieving an objective, such as making urgent or emergent patient care decisions. And there are instances in which group collaboration is appropriate to tackle a problem but that the process itself will encounter barriers and be ineffective.

BARRIERS

Group process is time and resource intensive. Both are required for a group process to be effective. Time utilized to participate in the group results in the inability to utilize that same time on another task or responsibility, therefore individuals participating in a group endeavor need to understand the sacrifice. Many resources are necessary for a group process project, including items such as physical space, informational paperwork, persons with relevant information and technical equipment. Identification of resources and assistance in obtaining them should occur either prior to or at the first group process session. Barriers to group process can occur at institutional, group and individual levels. Institutional challenges can include lack of resources, lack of administrative support, misunderstanding about the purpose and expectations of the group and differences in defining the outcome objective. Group challenges include lack of knowledge and expertise, lack of leadership, and dysfunction of the team. Individual barriers include lack of motivation, lack of perceived value, unequal power among team members, territorial issues and lack of respect towards other professions. (13)

Institutional lack of resources can be a barrier to an effective group task. Resources may include financial support, time to participate with the group that includes relieving members from competing responsibilities, physical space to meet, necessary electronic or computer resources, identification of knowledgeable and competent team members and recognition by the organization's administration of the value of the group's work. (13) Administrative support is important to support the group process by providing these resources, as administrators may have access to resources that the group members may not. It is also important for the administration to recognize and utilize the outcome of the group process to address the problem identified as a reason for the process. Otherwise the group effort can be deemed unworthy of the time, effort and work required of individual members. Misunderstanding the purpose of the group project is another barrier. Optimally, an organization's leaders have shared reasons for assimilating the group and plans for implementing the outcome with the group process team members at the onset of the project. Members should fully understand the purpose, expectations and post-utilization of the group's work at the onset of the endeavor. How the objective of the group is determined can occur in many ways and is another barrier to success. An organizational leader might determine a specific problem and assimilate a group to address that problem, which becomes the objective. Or an administrator might identify a system-based problem and create a group to evaluate a complex, multisystem problem. In that case, the group members determine how to evaluate the complex problem by determining multiple objectives for the group. In a school setting, identifying the purpose of the group can occur when a professor outlines the rationale and expectations of the project at the onset. A medical school course endeavor might have an objective of learning about the experience of group teamwork rather than utilization of the outcome, and this should be clarified for the group members. A multidisciplinary school endeavor has additional challenges, which include coordinating multiple school schedules and providing time to accomplish the project. If medical, nursing and pharmacy school students are all engaged in a group task, it is important that time and appropriate expectations for each academic unit are provided for the task to be valuable to each. Some schools create an extracurricular learning experience to minimize conflicts among differing school schedules. Learning by experiencing is valuable in preparing students for the post-educational workplace, thus including group process endeavors as part of the curriculum has value beyond achieving the final objective.

The group itself also has barriers to success. These include lack of knowledge and experience, lack of effective leadership, and dysfunctional team dynamics. (13) It is important that the members of the group are strategically selected in order to result in an effective endeavor. In an organization, members are selected based on knowledge and expertise that can be utilized to solve a specific problem. A group lacking persons with these skills may find itself frustrated, struggling and ineffective. In a healthcare school setting the group may be assigned based on roles to ensure involvement from multiple disciplines but may not be assigned based on knowledge or experience. It is likely part of the group process endeavor to identify the value of those skills and seek them as resources to assist. When the members of the group determine the needs and either obtain resources among the existing members or utilize an alternate resource, the group is more likely to be successful. Although the group's members each contribute to the function of the group, a leader with experience is important. The leader's skills are necessary to ensure that the group functions effectively. In an educational program, faculty members may need to provide the identified leader with training and guidance. Using well trained and enthusiastic faculty to serve as role models for student learns participating in interprofessional group tasks requires administrative support too. Experience and age do not necessarily result in improved leadership quality, thus training and guidance within an institution's group process may also be necessary. A successful leader recognizes the group's challenges, identifies resources, sets clear expectations, motivates each person to participate and fulfil his/her role and determines how to settle conflict. Each of these leader responsibilities is utilized in assuring that the group functions effectively. A dysfunctional group is a barrier to group process. Group dysfunction may be due to a myriad of reasons, but individual barriers may be contributors.

Individual barriers include lack of motivation, lack of perceived value, unequal power among team members, territorial issues and lack of respect towards other professions. (13) Lack of motivation and disinterest results in team members who are not engaged, do not fulfil their responsibilities and do not contribute to the success of the group. In fact, such individuals may interfere with the group's success by being disruptive or distracting. Misunderstanding the value of participating in the group endeavor is also a barrier to a productive team member. Understanding but disregarding the value is another possible barrier. A team member may feel intimidated by others, and this results in a team member who does not fully contribute to the group. This may occur due to individual personality characteristics or may occur due to the perceived value of the roles of the individual members. Barriers unique to interprofessional collaboration among health care workers include bias towards professions, lack of respect towards other professions and misunderstanding of knowledge among differing professions. These attitudes can result in territorial issues among individuals that comprise the group as well as a lack of respect towards other professions. (13) An interprofessional collaboration includes individuals from a "melting pot of professions, and each profession has its own unique history, culture, attitudes, values, customs, and beliefs." (9) It becomes important for the leader to set expectations of interpersonal working relationships, motivate all team members to participate, explain the benefits of each profession's expertise, and encouraging each member to share information. Territorial issues may occur when an individual from one profession believes his/her knowledge and/or experience should be recognized for greater value than that of another. It is imperative that the group leader clearly state that each profession has a valuable contribution to the group to avoid conflict and a poorly functioning team.

Finally, some urgent settings may not lend themselves to the use of group process. In the healthcare setting, an example of ineffective use of group process to meet an objective is the trauma patient. If a patient experiences a life-threatening occurrence, the emergency room personnel will activate the trauma team. Members of the team include physicians, nursing, respiratory therapy, laboratory, pharmacy, chaplains and social work. Each member has a pre-assigned role with specific responsibilities, and each member fulfils that role without the need for guidance from others. The leader's role is to observe and aid those who request it. The objective, treating the patient and saving his/her life, does not change. There is no need for group member discussion or encouragement of participation of each member; that is determined prior to the onset of the team activation. The team functions because the objective, roles and responsibilities have been pre-determined and practiced.

TACKLING BARRIERS

Interprofessional conflict among team members can derail the success of a project, so addressing this potential barrier is quite important. Combining group project members from different disciplines within heatlh care is valuable in addressing a specific problem from different perspectives and lends itself to unique problem-solving by utilizing knowledge and resources from different disciplines. Lack of knowledge or misunderstanding about the education, knowledge and skills of each discipline can result in confusion, lack of inclusion of a resource or dismissal of a potential solution. When beginning an interprofessional group task among different health care providers, beginning with learning about the educational background and roles of each of the group team members can diminish or eliminate this potential barrier. A faculty member or trained group leader can lead this portion, emphasizing the value of each discipline and setting the expectation that each team member contribute to the group's work. An individual may feel intimidated or devalued by those perceived to be in an educational program of a different status, which is consistent with the outdated belief of the hierarchy among health care disciplines. It is imperative that the group leader sets expectations about participation and input from everyone, sets guidelines regarding encouraging comments from all and disallows interruptions while another is speaking. Competing thoughts or plans should be encouraged and discussed, with the leader referencing the group's objective during the discussion to foster participation.

Group process relies upon the thinking methods of its individual members. There is a possibility for individual members to consciously avoid conflict by accepting comments from others rather than disagreeing or sharing questions. By avoiding comments that might be different than opinions from others, the individuals of the group may make decisions to avoid conflict rather than to discuss different opinions in order to identify the best decision. The process may result in a group conclusion that is not rational or practical. This is the group think entity described by Irving Janis, a research psychologist, who described the phenomenon in the 1970's after analyzing flawed military decisions. (10) In his evaluation of these decisions, Janis noted that group members were sometimes reluctant to contribute an opinion or share a differing sentiment due to intimidation, fear of repercussion or to avoid conflict. Therefore, the group's final decision was determined without valuable information from some members. The decision was subsequently incorrect, irrational and not helpful. To address this possibility and avoid arguing, Edward De Bono proposed a thought process that encourages an individual to consider multiple perspectives of a situation prior to making a decision. (14) His "Six Thinking Hats" theory proposes that an individual should use five stages of thinking about a problem. Those stages are assigned colors and correspond to thinking stages of neutrality/data analysis, emotions, caution, positivity, creativity and organization. (14) De Bono encourages that everyone should utilize all these perspectives when working as a group by preparing thoughts and information relevant to each stage, or hat. When the leader declares a color, each team member shares information related to that color hat. For example, the leader states that "white hat" thinking should begin the discussion. De Bono has defined the "white hat" to represent neutrality, objectivity, facts and figures. (14) During this portion of the group discussion, all members will share objective facts and figures. Once each team member has shared information, the leader will change to a different "hat," or thinking stage. After the six stages have been discussed, the leader will conclude the session with a summary and make a decision.

To decide, the discussion may require a different sequence of colored hat speaking information based on the topic. For example, exploring a topic may require a different sequence of discussion than problem solving, settling a dispute or decision-making. The leader determines the sequence based on the goal of the group. This method has the benefit of encouraging participation of all members, although some members may be more comfortable with one thinking stage than another and thus may contribute more during one portion. An alternate method to encourage participation of each team member is to assign roles.

To ensure participation by all members, assigning roles to each member can be implemented by the leader. Assigning roles is a method to formalize the role of a team member. Roles are characteristics expected of member and may not align with the member's opinion. The role is assigned for one specific meeting, with the plan to change roles in subsequent meetings. The roles are pre-assigned, allowing members to prepare ahead of the meeting, and it is expected that each member participates in the assigned role. This method ensures that alternate opinions and options are considered and can avoid groupthink decisions.

Roles and their responsibilities may include:

- Leader – a facilitator, the leader sets the agenda, monitors the meeting to ensure each group member participates and reminds the group of the objective(s). This role does not change.
- Supporter – one who supports the proposed idea by highlighting the benefits
- Doubter – one who opposes the proposed idea by identifying risks or problems
- Visionary – one who reminds the team of the potential application and impact beyond the current objective
- Pragmatist – one who assesses the fine details of the proposal, such as how to accomplish one step or how to accommodate a lacking resource
- Collaborator – one who reminds the group of the need to use a wealth of resources available and inquires members to obtain information about missing resources
- Mediator – one who monitors the interactions and comments of the group members, with the goal of all to be respectful and helpful

Using this method places individuals into a role that they may not find comfortable but guarantees that the proposal will be viewed from different perspectives. This meeting type is particularly beneficial when used among interprofessional student group process tasks. In addition to providing alternate perspectives, it also eliminates the possibility of intimidation due to territorial issues or status roles. Hierarchical attitudes or beliefs are less apparent as roles are assigned based on random assignment rather than knowledge or skills. Following the first meetings in which information from all roles are shared and discussed, the leader assigns new roles to continue the discussion at subsequent meetings. The goal of assigning roles is to make certain that all members can share information in a non-intimidating environment, and therefore provide information representative of the member's specialty. By being inclusive, role assignment results in achieving a goal that assures input from multiple disciplines.

Figure 1. Role Assignment Model

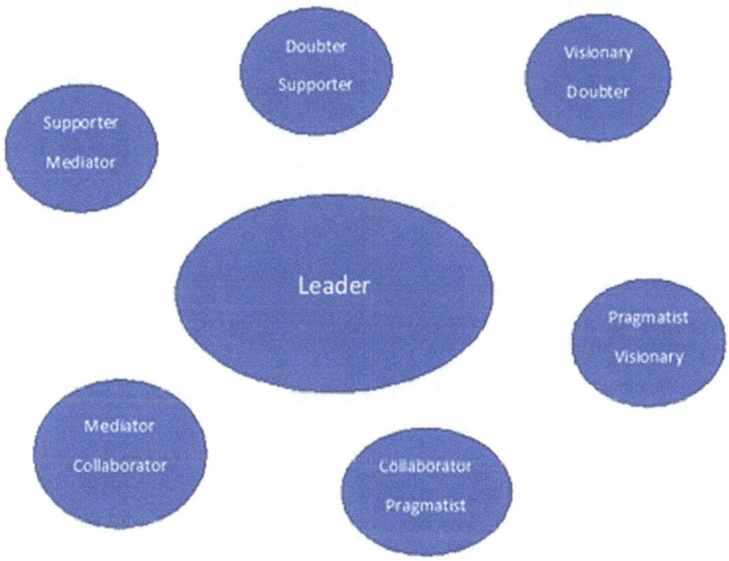

In this model, each shape represents a team member. The Leader position remains unchanged. Member roles change randomly, as represented by the member's first role identified at the top of the circle and subsequent role identified at the bottom.

CONCLUSION

In summary, group process is an educational, effective and productive method of achieving an objective when used in the appropriate setting. Participation in a group process experience can be beneficial or challenging for members; therefore, it is important to carefully consider the purpose. Identifying the benefits and barriers to a group process should occur prior to developing the group in preparation for a successful venture. Benefits of group process include the inclusion of differing perspectives, implementation of knowledge that extends beyond an individual and the potential to apply a problem's solution to a broad population. Determining the requirements needed to compose an effective team requires thoughtful preparation and can utilize elements that include individuals, motivation, external support, objectives and roles, among others. Barriers to successful group process projects include lack of resources, ineffective or dysfunctional teams and unequal power of participants as well as others. When used in an educational setting, group process participants learn how to work in a multidisciplinary setting in addition to achieving an objective. That knowledge, in an educational setting, prepares learners for the healthcare workplace and is extremely valuable beyond the group's objectives.

Table 1. Summary of Group Process Benefits and Challenges

Benefits	Challenges
Diversity in decision-making	Time and resource intensive
Inclusion of a variety of viewpoints	Lack of support and/or resources
Opportunity to extrapolate beyond local situation	Lack of knowledge and/or experience
Multidisciplinary approach to problem-solving	Dysfunctional team dynamics
Gain knowledge regarding other disciplines or professions	Unequal power among participants
	Potential for conflict avoidance impacting participant decision-making

REFERENCES

Budning, A., & El-Defrawy, S. (2016). Interprofessional collaboration in eye health care. *Canadian Journal of Ophthalmology*, *51*(3), 130–132. doi:10.1016/j.jcjo.2016.04.007 PMID:27316255

Choi, B., & Pak, A. (2007). Multidisciplinarity, interdisciplinarity, and transdisciplinarity in health research, services, education and policy: 2. Promotors, barriers, and strategies of enhancement. *Clinical and Investigative Medicine. Medecine Clinique et Experimentale*, *30*(6), E224–E232. doi:10.25011/cim.v30i6.2950 PMID:18053389

De Bono, E. (2016). *Six Thinking Hats*. Penguin UK.

Green, B. N., & Johnson, C. D. (2015). Interprofessional collaboration in research, education, and clinical practice: Working together for a better future. *The Journal of Chiropractic Education*, *29*(1), 1–10. doi:10.7899/JCE-14-36 PMID:25594446

Jackson, D., Sibson, R., & Riebe, L. (2014). Undergraduate perceptions of the development of team-working skills. *Education + Training*, *56*(1), 7–20. doi:10.1108/ET-01-2013-0002

Janis, I. L. (1972). *Victims of Groupthink: A Psychological Study of Foreign-Policy Decisions and Fiascoes*. Houghton Mifflin.

Johnson, D. W., Johnson, R. T., & Smith, K. A. (2014). Cooperative Learning: Improving University Instruction By Basing Practice On Validated Theory. *Journal on Excellence in University Teaching*, *25*(4), 1–26.

Lalis, T., Anson, J., & Greenfield, D. (2014). Barriers and enablers that influence sustainable interprofessional education: A literature review. *Journal of Interprofessional Care*, *8*(4), 305–310. doi:10.3109/13561820.2014.895977 PMID:24625198

Qin, Z., Johnson, D. W., & Johnson, R. T. (1995). Cooperative Versus Competitive Efforts and Problem Solving. *Review of Educational Research*, *65*(2), 129–143. doi:10.3102/00346543065002129

Rea, K. E., Rao, P., Hill, E., Saylor, K. M., & Cousino, M. K. (2018). Families' Experiences With Pediatric Family-Centered Rounds: A Systematic. *La Revue de Pediatrie*, *141*(3), 2–13. doi:10.1542/peds.2017-1883 PMID:29437931

Schmitt, M., Blue, A., Aschenbrener, C., & Viggiano, T. (2011). Core Competencies for Interprofessional Collaborative Practice: Reforming Health Care by Transforming Health Professionals' Education. *Academic Medicine*, *86*(11), 1351. doi:10.1097/ACM.0b013e3182308e39 PMID:22030650

South Dakota School of Mines and Technology Student Activities and Leadership Center. (n.d.). *Understanding Group Process*. Retrieved from https://www.sdsmt.edu/uploadedFiles/Content/Campus_Life/Student_Activities/Organizations/Understanding%20Group%20Process.pdf

Surowiecki, J. (2005). *The wisdom of crowds: Why the many are smarter than the few*. Abacus.

World Health Organization. (2010). *Framework for Action on Interprofessional Education and Collaborative Practice*. Retrieved from https://www.who.int/hrh/resources/framework_action/en/

Chapter 4
The Positive Impact of Intentional Curricular Design on Interprofessional Learning

Nurry Pirani
University of Missouri-Kansas City School of Medicine, USA

Steven D. Waldman
University of Missouri-Kansas City School of Medicine, USA

Kara Zweerink
University of Missouri-Kansas City School of Medicine, USA

Valerie Chuy
University of Missouri-Kansas City School of Medicine, USA

Saqib Hassan
University of Missouri-Kansas City School of Medicine, USA

Debra Wekesa
University of Missouri-Kansas City School of Medicine, USA

Marcella Riley
University of Missouri-Kansas City School of Medicine, USA

ABSTRACT

Interprofessional education has been gaining traction in the educational and professional climate today. As a shift has been made to incorporate the collaboration of health professionals into education, benefits in overall quality of education and patient care have been observed. Students who are involved in IPE are able to

DOI: 10.4018/978-1-7998-3066-5.ch004

learn about other careers, learn the limitations of their own career, cement existing knowledge, develop relationships with members of various fields, improve teamwork skills, and enhance their job satisfaction. Patients have also benefited from the new IPE implementation. As a result of increased collaboration, there has been a reduction in patient errors and overall improved quality of care among programs who participate in IPE.

INTRODUCTION

Interprofessional education, defined as "educational experiences shared by members or students of different health professions," has been gaining traction in the educational and professional climate today. As a shift has been made to incorporate the collaboration of health professionals into education, benefits in overall quality of education and patient care have been observed. Students who are involved in IPE are able to learn about other careers, learn the limitations of their own career, cement existing knowledge, develop relationships with members of various fields, improve teamwork skills, and enhance their job satisfaction. Patients have also benefited from the new IPE implementation. As a result of increased collaboration, there has been a reduction in patient errors and overall improved quality of care among programs who participate in IPE. Additionally, as members of healthcare teams feel more empowered, better recommendations are provided for patient care. The improved relational benefits provided by IPE allow for reduced communication gaps in patient care, less delayed diagnosis, and fewer poor outcomes. The comprehensive needs of a patient are also better addressed using a team approach and the overall healthcare environment tends to be more patient centered when IPE is emphasized.

However, while the positive impact of IPE is apparent, there are many barriers that hinder the implementation of IPE programs. Logistically, equal representation of healthcare professionals in programs, addition of new content into an already crowded curriculum, and the lack of experience of educators in teaching IPE have all posed concerns. Psychosocial barriers have also arisen, as the healthcare hierarchy and "self-sufficient" mentality that has permeated health education is not easily broken. Furthermore, finding funding for programs is an obstacle for IPE implementation. Still, these barriers can be overcome. Through faculty training conferences, skills sessions, and integration of IPE into current individual skills programs, many of the logistical concerns can be addressed. Psychosocial barriers can be attended to by ensuring students interact with one another and are forced to collaborate in simulation settings. Financial barriers can also be addressed through the development of long-term, more stable programs and providing paid faculty to specifically teach IPE programs. Additionally, through implementing a six-step plan involving problem identification, needs assessments, goals and objectives, educational strategies, implementation, and evaluation and feedback, curriculum can be strengthened and improve IPE program success. Incorporating the core IPE competencies of values and ethics, interprofessional communication, roles and responsibilities, and teams and teamwork will also help guide curricular development and ensure the full benefits of IPE are reaped in the future.

Throughout history, medical professionals have strived to provide patients with the best care possible. The overall goals of the medical profession are stated as "the relief of pain and suffering, the promotion of health and the prevention of disease, the forestalling of death and the promoting of a peaceful death, and the cure of disease when possible and the care of those who can not be cured."(Callahan, 1998) In order to achieve these goals, health care providers are trained through rigorous curriculum and countless hours of clinical experience.

However, an increase in isolated career-based knowledge is not the only way to improve patient care. The field of healthcare consists of many different professions, all of which must work in harmony to care for patients. Therefore, increasing the efficiency of the collaboration between members of different healthcare fields can help to vastly improve quality of care. This teamwork, like other skills in the medical field, must be learned. It is vital for schools to have intentionally designed and appropriately taught interprofessional curriculum. As the field of interprofessional education grows and improves, medical professionals will be better able to perform their duties as providers and give patients the best care possible.

INTERPROFESSIONAL EDUCATION (IPE)

Interprofessional education can be defined as "educational experiences shared by members or students of different health professions."(WHO Study Group on Multiprofessional Education of Health Personnel (Ed.),1988) Instead of providers viewing their fields in isolation, the focus has shifted to ensuring that medical professionals utilize and value the skills of one another and work as a team. This shift in viewpoint truly began to take hold in the 1960s, as institutions in the United States and UK began small scale "initiatives" in community and local care settings to ensure teamwork was used to meet patient needs.(Barr H (2009) However, the IPE movement truly began to gain force when the World Health Organization (WHO) began to push for interprofessional collaboration in the 1970s and 1980s. In their article titled "Continuing Education for Physicians", a WHO expert committee called for an interprofessional education program that would "not replace programs for individual health professions, but should offer a new opportunity for members of health care teams to learn together how to solve problems in which all have a common interest."(World Health Organization, G. (Switzerland),1973) This report pushed medical professionals beyond simply using their own expertise and called them to elevate their practice by also utilizing the expertise of others to achieve the goal of patient care. A second article released by WHO further defined and explored multiprofessional education. This report discussed the role of IPE in ensuring that a patient is seen as both a person and a part of society. Additionally, WHO began to call for instruction of IPE at an institutional level. (WHO Study Group on Multiprofessional Education of Health Personnel (Ed.),1988)

Though IPE began to gain more recognition during the 1980s, there was a lot of disagreement on the exact goals and implementation of interprofessional programs. Many institutions viewed IPE as a means to improve workforce relations, while others sought improved patient care and teamwork through the program. Additionally, there was disagreement about the timing and quantity of interprofessional education. Some argued that it should be integrated into medical curriculum in order to provide healthcare professionals with comprehensive and early exposure to IPE. Others thought that simply having occasional presentations on IPE in the workplace would be sufficient.(Fransworth, T. J., Seikel, J. A., Hudock, D., & Holst, J. 2015)

This discrepancy in views on IPE led to a need to clearly define the goals and practices of interprofessional education. This was done in part by the development of the Centre for the Advancement of Interprofessional Education (CAIPE) in 1987. This organization officially defined IPE as "occasions when two or more professions learn with, from and about each other to improve collaboration and the quality of care."(About Us, 2019) They also began to develop educational systems to improve the quality of IPE. More clarity was provided when WHO released a report in 2008 that called for health professionals to shift from the current coordination model of IPE to a collaborative model.(*World Health Organization, 2008).*

This provided further evidence that IPE should not only be focused solely on helping healthcare workers co-exist, but should teach them to strive to work alongside and problem solve with one another. WHO also helped to define the educational parameters of IPE by calling for the coordination of interprofessional health education systems on an institutional, cultural, and environmental level. (The WHO Framework for Action, 2010) This charged institutions such as schools and hospitals to provide a curriculum that addresses widespread IPE issues while adjusting for regional concerns.

As the idea of IPE continued to gain notoriety and traction, many institutions began to integrate interprofessional education into their curriculum. Today, there are more than 30 medical schools nationwide that include IPE as part of their curriculum. As schools seek to make their graduates more competent team members and health professionals, programs continue to be developed to ensure the highest quality of education possible.

EDUCATIONAL BENEFITS OF IPE

As the development of IPE in the curricular setting continues to expand, the benefits of IPE are becoming more apparent. One of the key benefits from interprofessional education comes from the core of the discipline itself-the opportunity for students to learn how the roles of other healthcare providers work. Healthcare is a very diverse field, with team members ranging from physicians to pharmacists to nurses to social workers. With so much diversity among care teams, it is easy to miss out on the perspectives and knowledge of other team members as providers perform their specific roles. Interprofessional education allows students to expand on the knowledge they gain from their specific curriculum and learn the roles of their teammates in patient care. This will allow students to be better providers in the future and improve their ability to utilize their fellow healthcare workers as resources in patient care.

Interprofessional education also allows for students to gain a fuller understanding of the limitations of their own roles in the healthcare system.(Illingworth, P., & Chelvanayagam, S, 2007) As students are granted the opportunity to work and interact with one another, they are better able to recognize the values and the strengths of other professions. In seeing this, students realize that they will not always have the best tools and skills to deal with every situation. Seeing these limitations within their roles allows students to see the need for other medical professionals. An example of this principle lies in the physician and nurse relationship; both fields provide patient care in different ways. Physicians must integrate a vast array of both subjective and objective information into a patient care plan. However, this plan cannot be made without input from what the nurses may have seen or experienced during the day and overnight. The physician cannot maintain the patient load that is required of them and spend the same amount of time with each and every patient as nurses do. So, simply put, nurses will inevitably have a better grasp on the overall subjective experience of the patient. Additionally, the time constraints placed on a physician does not allow them the ability to perform basic care activities such as provide medicationing for patients or drawing blood every few hours, nor do the duties of a nurse allow them the time to come up with a comprehensive care plan for every patient or interpret all physical exam findings relevant to a disease or disease course. As students work together in IPE settings, they are exposed to the realities of their own patient care abilities, and they learn to respect and utilize the unique roles of others.

Though it is easy to confine interprofessional education to a classroom model, learning to interact and collaborate with peers is a skill that must be extended beyond the typical lecture hall. According to the *American Journal of Pharmaceutical Education*, "the goal of IPE is for students to learn how to function in an interprofessional team and carry this knowledge, skill, and value into their future practice, ultimately providing interprofessional patient care as part of a collaborative team and focused on improving patient outcomes."(Buring, S. M., Bhushan, A., Broeseker, A., Conway, S., Duncan-Hewitt, W., Hansen, L., & Westberg, S, 2009) With this goal in mind, interprofessional education is not a topic that should be taught solely in a classroom setting. Interprofessional education should be introduced repeatedly throughout an individual's training in order to be truly successful. It is never too late for interprofessional education to occur. This continued learning provides students with the ability to cement the knowledge and skills they are developing in practical, real world situations. By providing continued learning with context, previous education can be better utilized, and students can reach a higher level of functioning in their respective practices.

Integrating interprofessional education into future practice provides educational benefits beyond the retention of knowledge. These educational experiences allow for the "development of personal relationships"(Carney, P. A., Thayer, E. K., Palmer, R., Galper, A. B., Zierler, B., & Eiff, M. P., 2019) among members of various professions. This development allows for an ease of communication to occur between all participants in IPE. The comfortable environment created by this improved communication level takes some of the burden off individual providers by allowing them to feel they are able to ask for assistance from their peers. "(Carney, P. A., Thayer, E. K., Palmer, R., Galper, A. B., Zierler, B., & Eiff, M. P., 2019) In a patient care setting, asking for help or asking questions is a key feature to providing adequate care.

Interprofessional education also helps improve job satisfaction. "(Carney, P. A., Thayer, E. K., Palmer, R., Galper, A. B., Zierler, B., & Eiff, M. P., 2019) By allowing individuals to feel that they are not working in isolation but as part of a team, IPE paves the way for a feeling of comradery in the workplace. As different members of the healthcare team are able to meet up and exchange viewpoints and discuss patient care, members feel more valued and therefore experience a higher degree of satisfaction in their work. "(Carney, P. A., Thayer, E. K., Palmer, R., Galper, A. B., Zierler, B., & Eiff, M. P., 2019) This discussion also allows for multiple viewpoints to be considered and increases the quality of patient care.

Overall, the development of the skills necessary for teamwork permeates the educational benefits of IPE. As seen through IPE curriculum, "sharing information about the roles of team members, determining professional responsibilities and boundaries, and learning about how different professions can work together to optimize their strengths in providing patient care all contribute to the development of professionals working together towards a common goal (eg, optimizing patient care)." (Buring, S. M., Bhushan, A., Broeseker, A., Conway, S., Duncan-Hewitt, W., Hansen, L., & Westberg, S, 2009) This full understanding of everyone's role within the healthcare team allows for patient care to be performed effectively and efficiently. In turn, a lack of understanding leads to shortcomings in a provider's role in patient care. IPE helps prevent role confusion and animosity that would later lead to the failure of students to function effectively in the workforce.

PATIENT CARE BENEFITS OF IPE

The benefits of the IPE programs are not limited to the learners themselves. The patients treated by care teams also benefit from interprofessional education. According to the Agency for Healthcare Research and Quality, the ability to provide safe healthcare requires that healthcare workers with varying roles and clinical responsibilities act together in the best interest of the patient." KJ, J., & HC, C. (n.d.), 2020). In 2000, the IOM published a report that revealed medical errors are the leading cause of adult death in the United States(L.T. Kohn, J.M. Corrigan, M.S. Donaldson, 2000). This fueled a push to move from a physician centric model of care to a more team-based approach to care. The Institute of Medicine (IOM) recognizes IPE as an important mechanism to improve the overall quality of care.(Institute of Medicine Committee on the Health Professions Education Summit, 2003) A key recommendation highlighted in the IOM's 2003 report entitled "Health Professions Education: A Bridge to Quality" was that "all health professionals should be educated to deliver patient-centered care as members of an interdisciplinary team.(Institute of Medicine Committee on the Health Professions Education Summit, 2003) This would help to address the quality of care problems highlighted in the 2000 IOM report. Interprofessional collaboration begins with interprofessional education. When healthcare students are trained to work effectively as members of a team of varying disciplines, they are well positioned to collaborate in a similar way in the workplace. According to the World Health Organization, "interprofessional health- care teams understand how to optimize the skills of their members, share case management and provide better health-services to patients and the community. The resulting strengthened health system leads to improved health outcomes." The team-based approach to care fostered by IPE promotes several behaviors which, when executed, have the potential to positively impact patient care as outlined below.(World Health Organization, 2010, Benefits of IPE/C. (n.d.). 2020)

1. Empowering team members to participate in care

Before the prominence of Interprofessional education, the physician made the majority of decisions regarding patient care. With increasing emphasis on collaboration, other care providers from varying disciplines play an integral role in patient care and are encouraged to make recommendations for patients within the scope of their practice.

2. Reducing communication gaps

When healthcare professionals work independently there are opportunities for missed communication, delayed clinical diagnosis and adverse outcomes. IPE promotes collaboration and an environment where communication is a central theme. With better channels of communication, healthcare professionals are encouraged to share suggestions for patient management and treatment plans. In such a team approach, continuity of care is maintained across disciplines.

3. Promoting comprehensive patient care

Each healthcare discipline contributes a special set of skills and knowledge to a patient care team. When members of different disciplines collaborate, the team is able to form a more comprehensive view of the patient and hence needs assessments as well as management options are more comprehensive.

4. Promoting patient-centered care

When each discipline works separately and takes turns assessing patients and developing care plans, it is more likely that important diagnoses can be missed and care delayed. It is easier to provide patients with the best possible care when there is interprofessional collaboration. In this collaborative environment, the goal of patient care is continually discussed and there is an improvement in patient safety.

As mentioned previously, there is sufficient evidence to show that care provided by an Interprofessional team improves overall team efficiency, effectiveness, patient satisfaction, and health outcomes.(Reeves, S., Pelone, F., Harrison, R., Goldman, J., & Zwarenstein, M, 2017, Coleman K, Reid R, 2013) Research has also shown that collaborative practice can improve access to and coordination of health-services, promote appropriate use of specialist clinical resources, and ensure patient care and safety.(Naylor, C., Griffiths, R., & Fernandez, R., 2004) Research has also shown that collaborative practice can decrease patient complications, length of hospital stays and medical errors.(Naylor, C., Griffiths, R., & Fernandez, R., 2004, Mcalister, F., Stewart, S., Ferrua, S., & Mcmurray, J, 2004)

While evidence supports that working in a collaborative environment has a positive impact on patient care, more work could be done to evaluate specifically how IPE impacts health outcome in the inpatient and outpatient setting. There is not currently a method in place to assess or track the benefits of IPE to patient care when compared to other models of patient care. According to Illingworth and Chelvanayagam, "there appears to be little agreement as to what is expected of service users and carers when it comes to their involvement in course design, delivery and evaluation."(Illingworth, P., & Chelvanayagam, S, 2007) They encourage the use of users' expertise to provide a "more comprehensive knowledge of how existing services really work, and the positive or negative impact users have in practice." (Illingworth, P., & Chelvanayagam, S, 2007)

CURRENT SHORTCOMINGS INTERPROFESSIONALLY

While the benefits of IPE and collaboration are numerous, the institution of this curriculum is not always simple. Barriers to interprofessional education—logistically, psychosocially, and structurally—have become increasingly apparent with more attempts to implement theoretical models into medical school curriculum.

One shortcoming of current IPE programs is logistical: how do you coordinate different academic schedules and calendars, add new or expanded content to an already crowded curriculum, and standardize the faculty? In a 2017 study done by the National Institutes of Health, 16 United States medical schools were surveyed to look for how they can improve integration of "social and behavioral science education," including interprofessional education, into health professional training. (West C, Graham L, Palmer RT, 2016) All the schools were tested based on essential IPE education components including "values and ethics, roles and responsibilities, communication, and teamwork for a total of 42 items." (West C, Graham L, Palmer RT, 2016) It was found that the top two challenges of the IPE education were structural and financial support. In terms of structural support, problems arose when institutes had to build workshops into existing curricular time and find faculty that would be available during that same time, especially with groups that had clerkship obligations year-round. Additionally, in organizing a large-scale IPE event, the logistics of moving all the students through a simulation event proved to become difficult in comparison to group discussion.

Another issue that programs encounter is ensuring equal and appropriate representation and participation across professionals. This can be seen in a 2013 review of Saint Louis University's (SLU) IPE program. This program intentionally integrates courses that teach "teamwork inpatient/client-centered care" into student curriculum. The challenges and benefits of each course was accessed across disciplines. Eliot K, Carlson J, Breitbach A, Gockel-Blessing E, Kienstra K, 2013. One of the main challenges was trying to include diverse programs in the healthcare professions. In the case of SLU, 8 different healthcare professional programs all had variability in how many students were in each professional program each semester, differing from 10 to 100 students. With such large population diversity between classes, it is almost impossible to ensure equal representation of different healthcare professions in IPE events.

Limited faculty experiences teaching interprofessional concepts and content provides another obstacle to the development of successful IPE programs. While faculty and educators may understand the importance of IPE, the ability to teach interprofessional practice and facilitate groups still stands as a barrier to effective learning.(Schapmire TJ, Head BA, Nash WA, 2018) Schools drastically vary in the faculty development for IPE. Some have non-existent approaches to IPE faculty development, while other institutions have regulated measures put in place to train faculty.(West C, Graham L, Palmer RT, 2016) There is, overall, a lack of guidance in how to train staff who don't have experience guiding IPE events. Additionally, there is often not a set group of instructors who consistently run IPE events. Many institutions rely on limited and inconsistent faculty and developmental instruction, which can lead to an unreliable regulation of group activities and discussion. While some institutions have discussions about IPE in workshops such as Academy of Educators and occasional Educational Grand Rounds (EGRs), these educator development opportunities are often limited. Many of these workshops simply "meet with faculty briefly (approximately 1 hour) to discuss how to run these [IPE] sessions. (West C, Graham L, Palmer RT, 2016)" For these institutions in the "letting go," or planning stage, further work is needed to identify an IPE-specific faculty that consistently works to develop and participate in IPE-related workshops.(Palatta A, Cook BJ, Anderson EL, Valachovic RW, 2015) Due to IPE's focus on team-based group discussion and simulation, faculty development and training is necessary to facilitate learning and active participation.

Another barrier to interprofessional education involves psychosocial and cultural Issues that can limit the potential of interprofessional education to improve student collaboration in the future. This can be seen in the tendency of individuals navigate through the traditional health care hierarchy via silo mentality. Silo mentality is a mentality in which individuals in one profession are isolated from other professions due to a reluctance to share information with another division. A silo mentality acts as a significant barrier to collaboration among healthcare professions.(Wang R, Shi N, Bai J, Zheng Y, Zhao Y, 2015) If interprofessional education is not introduced early enough or addressed effectively, this shift from silo mentality to collaboration is often faced with resistance. In a study conducted by the *International Journal of Nursing Studies*, students from eight healthcare groups were surveyed about interprofessional attitudes. Results supported the need to introduce healthcare students to interprofessional education at the start of their education.(Coster S, Norman I, Murrells T, et al, 2008) This was based on the students' overall readiness for IPE and their strong professional identities at the start of their education. On the other hand, the study also suggested that students who started out with negative attitudes about interprofessional learning tended to still have these negative attitudes post-IPE. Poorly facilitated programs can further reinforce these negative attitudes and interaction between students from different disciplines. (Coster S, Norman I, Murrells T, et al, 2008) Relational issues limiting IPE effectiveness are also perpetuated by lack of interaction between different healthcare groups secondary to the current layout of the educational system. The traditional educational system discourages multidisciplinary teamwork. For example, in medical school, physicians are typically isolated into classes with only their medical school peers. In these classes, they receive two years of basic science education followed by two years of clinical science experience. This leads to a hierarchical mentality where the "physician is…regarded as the leader of the healthcare team" and where health care students make assumptions about themselves, patients, and other players in the healthcare system.(Olsen L, Saunders RS, McGinnis JM, 2011) Uniprofessional teaching, largely unchanged since the 19th century, combined with "reinforcement during training," makes it difficult for United States medical students to separate themselves from a culture of self-sufficiency and superiority. (Olsen L, Saunders RS, McGinnis JM, 2011)

Following structural challenges, the other major challenge of interprofessional education is financial support. Regarding funding for interprofessional education, several institutions reported issues with receiving funding needed to expand IPE-centered exercises to all students and obtaining funding to develop a virtual platform to make IPE more accessible. For many programs, it becomes difficult to sustain financial support. Interprofessional programs are frequently initiated with grant funding and/or other support that tends to be time limiting-meaning this funding will typically last around two to three years. When being interviewed by The Interprofessional Education Consortium, eleven of the thirteen IPE programs fell into this category.(Stuart Foundation, 2002) Though uncommon, university departments can also support interprofessional education by assigning paid faculty designated to teach courses specifically for the program. Two of the programs interviewed by the Interprofessional Education Consortium reported this. However, this is rare, as most IPE programs are not established within the core curriculum of the professional schools. Outside of this, two of the IPE programs reported that they were forced to start IPE without funding and it was through "unpaid efforts of faculty and others" that they were able to support events. (Stuart Foundation, 2002) In order for programs to maintain funding after the first few years, programs tend to have one of two options: donated support or grants/funding activities. (Stuart Foundation, 2002) Donated support, in order to be sustainable, has to be done for extended periods of time; grants can be temporary or a more long-term option, depending on the grant's duration. Long term programs that have permanently incorporated themselves into the educational curriculum of the multiple professional schools tend to be more stable financially.(Stuart Foundation, 2002)

OVERCOMING BARRIERS

Though many practical barriers exist to the successful development of IPE curriculum, these barriers are not insurmountable. It is important to shift the focus to what policies and practices can be implemented to improve the system. Many of the problems discussed center around structural and financial barriers in various IPE programs, and there are many ways that universities can be supported to overcome these barriers.

Structural problems largely center around the lack of faculty training as well as the psychosocial and cultural issues which are frequently found across various IPE programs around the country. Faculty training is particularly important as the heart of an interprofessional education program is its curriculum. Unlike traditional disciplines (education, social work, psychology), IPE is a relatively new field whose knowledge base has not yet been widely agreed upon or published. Thus, defining curriculum content and designing methods for its delivery are particularly complex challenges. (Stuart Foundation, 2002) In addition to the relatively recent nature of the field, it is important to keep in mind that, currently, many health professionals have had little or no exposure to IPE activities during their own training, and many clinical sites in which faculty oversee training lack robust or explicit examples of interprofessional team-based care.(Hall, L & Zierler, 2015) According to a guide published in the *Journal of Interprofessional Care,* IPE leaders from various institutions used an initial 3.5-day faculty development conference to ensure common grounding in key IPE knowledge. This shared experience proved to be an important foundation upon which participants could develop and deploy a strategy for preparing faculty to participate in their curriculum, often using techniques modeled during the initial training. Immediately following the training, faculty members experienced deep and enduring learning, allowing many of them to replicate the curriculum at their home institution in the following months. (Stuart Foundation, 2002,) Such conferences and training sessions are simple and affordable ways to help ensure staff receive a consistent and adequate training needed to practically teach IPE.

Addressing the faculty role in implementing IPE programs into curriculum is only part of the issue—responsibility falls upon the students and professionals who are partaking in the courses as well. In order to understand their role, the notion of "silo mentality" must be re-visited.(Clark K, 2018, Barnsteiner, J. H., Disch, J. M., Hall, L., Mayer, D., & Moore, S. M. 2007) As previously mentioned, silo mentality is a mentality in which individuals in one profession are isolated from other professions due to a reluctance to share information with another division. A study in the American Journal of Pharmaceutical Education highlights the fact that many healthcare professions students had entered their respective professional courses with a stable set of traditional (largely negative) stereotypes of other professionals, which shaped their early interprofessional interactions.(Thurston, M. M., Chesson, M. M., Harris, E. C., & Ryan, G. J. 2017)

The essence of interprofessional education (IPE) requires interaction and active engagement among different health disciplines. It simply is not enough to teach students and practitioners about collaboration; rather, we need to create learning environments and experiences that place them in the context of realistic clinical situations to understand and appreciate differences and contributions of other disciplines. In doing so, the notion that there is a division between different aspects of the health care professions can be addressed and bridged. Much of the problem revolves around unclear definitions of specific roles, which, when combined with the idea of the "hospital hierarchy," creates and environment in which cooperation and effective communication is increasingly difficult. Specific ways to address this include the use of interprofessional leadership. (Clark K, 2018) Leadership of IPE efforts should be collaborative, reflecting shared decision-making and respect for the unique contributions of each profession.(Hall, L & Zierler, 2015) A study conducted among nursing students demonstrated the importance of "realistic" training in learning together and the benefits realized by breaking down stereotypes and by appreciating both individual roles and those of others.(Wang R, Shi N, Bai J, Zheng Y, Zhao Y) This can perhaps erase much of the internal bias or false premonitions that students may have towards interprofessional roles. A balance must be achieved, however, between the role of well-trained faculty and the students participating in the event. The faculty should be equipped to facilitate the events and direct the students, but the students themselves should play very active and important leadership roles during the event.

While collaborative sessions and education are undoubtedly important for the cohesion of different professionals in the workplace, simply allowing various professions to collaborate in an IPE event which occurs a couple of times a year may not be enough to effectively integrate these practices into the workplace. To combat the potential harm of infrequent IPE opportunities, targeted programs which are catered towards the specific roles of professionals can be integrated into each field's respective curriculum. Future healthcare workers can learn the skills needed for their future professions in a collaborative instead of isolated environment. Formal education that includes integrated, interprofessional learning about teamwork, collaboration, problem-solving, and decision-making beyond the confines of one's own discipline leads to an improved ability to navigate the complexity of the current healthcare environment.

(Barnsteiner, J. H., Disch, J. M., Hall, L., Mayer, D., & Moore, S, 2007) By integrating IPE into pre-existing curriculum, not only can healthcare outcomes be improved, but the conundrum of incorporating this education into various busy and full schedules can perhaps be solved. While many classes are directed towards learning one's own role in a hospital setting, exploring the differences and similarities among professional groups as a part of the interprofessional learning process helps learners to build a solid foundation of understanding upon which future health care partnerships can be built. These concepts do not necessarily have to be studied with the same rigor and stress as other concepts, but some degree of learning about others' roles may be an effective complement to interactive IPE programs. Interprofessional education targeted at students and delivered by educators skilled in the philosophy and strategies of IPE can help to transform health care into another highly regarded, safety-critical industry.(Barnsteiner, J. H., Disch, J. M., Hall, L., Mayer, D., & Moore, S, 2007)

It is important to keep in mind, however, that the timing of the education is important as well. Introducing this curriculum at an early stage can actually be detrimental to students. Studies conducted by unstall-Pedoe et al. found that the more mature and experienced learners were more favorably disposed towards IPE than the younger and less experienced learners.(Thurston, M. M., Chesson, M. M., Harris, E. C., & Ryan, G. J, 2017) This can be attributed to the fact that at that stage of their education, young students have had very little experience interacting with other professions in the hospital environment. Some clinical experiences, such as the docent program at the University of Missouri-Kansas City, which begins during students' first year of education and provides students with excellent interaction with doctors and patients, do not always need to provide experience collaborating with different professions in the hospital. This delay allows students to better understand and find comfort in their own roles before learning to incorporate the roles of others. Additionally, implementing IPE later in the educational experience allows to learn these important skills near a time when they can immediately apply it to their daily lives. Students will be better able to retain information as it will be quickly followed by practical use.

CURRICULAR SUGGESTIONS

While addressing specific barriers to instituting an IPE program in general is incredibly important to educational success, this alone is not enough to develop a successful program; it is also important to have well designed curriculum. This can be accomplished by taking a general six step approach to medical curricular design. (Thomas, P. A., Kern, D. E., Hughes, M. T., & Chen, B. Y, 2016)

Step one is to identify problems and perform a general needs assessment. During this phase of curricular development, it is important to look at what is lacking in the healthcare system currently. The goal is to identify and analyze how the current approach to patient care differs from the ideal approach. In relation to IPE, the need for healthcare professionals to work cohesively as a team to achieve optimal patient care is a strong overarching problem. Idealistically, providers would be able to communicate with and utilize the knowledge of other professionals effectively and with respect.

Once the general problems are identified, step two in curricular development is to perform a targeted needs assessment. It is important to see how the needs of specific target groups differ from that of the overarching healthcare system. Here is where problems, barriers, and needs of students and specific institutions are taken into account. For example, the time burden of adding extracurricular demand on students or financial burdens of IPE on an institution should be considered.

Step three is to develop goals and objectives. After needs have been identified, it is important to come up with goals and objectives in the new curriculum to meet these needs. As a general rule, it is easiest to start with a broad approach and move to more specific goals. For example, the broad goal of the IPE curriculum may be to improve interprofessional relationships, while a more specific goal in that category might be to ensure that the medical and nursing students develop an understanding and respect for one another's roles. It is also important that the goals set up are measurable. There needs to be a way to evaluate these goals in the future to ensure the purpose of the curriculum is being met.

After goals are set, step four is to develop educational strategies. The content and methods of the curriculum must be meticulously designed so that the educational material developed meets to goals of the curriculum. Lessons plans must be made, and specific lectures, simulations, and activities developed to provide students and educators alike with a well structured, uniform curriculum.

Step five is to implement the developed curriculum. After the curriculum is designed, the next step is to put it to the test. As educational intervention occurs, it is important to have the resources and support needed to implement to program. Additionally, any barriers to success should be identified and managed.

The final step of curricular development is to evaluate and give feedback on the implemented curriculum. No new system is instituted without flaw, and evaluating the new curriculum and providing feedback to instructors and students alike will ensure that programs progress and improve in the future.

IPE COMPETENCIES

When following these general steps in curricular development, it is important to keep the core competencies of IPE in mind. These competencies are values and ethics, interprofessional communication, roles and responsibilities, and teams and teamwork.(Morano, C. L. (2017)

The values and ethics competency centers around respect and shared values. Professionals should aim to respect the cultures and the dignity of both their coworkers and patients. In addition, individuals should value the roles of their peers on the healthcare team and develop a culture of respect and trust in the workplace. In turn, honesty and integrity should be at the core of the relationships in IPE scenarios.

Interprofessional education involves communicating with "patients, families, communities, and professionals in health and other fields in a responsive and responsible manner that supports a team approach to the promotion and maintenance of health and the prevention and treatment of disease". Healthcare workers must be able to communicate and interact in a way that will provide the best care possible for their patients. Through active listening and the sharing of ideas respectfully, each member of the team can provide valuable input and learn from others to better patient care.

The competency of roles and responsibilities involves each member of a healthcare team recognizing and engaging in their specific roles, while allowing others to do the same. As health professionals embrace their unique roles in a cohesive manner, all of the diverse needs of a patient can be met in the most effective way possible. Accepting both the responsibilities and limitations of each specific role also teaches members to rely on and respect one another.

Teams and teamwork focus on applying "relationship-building values and the principles of team dynamics to perform effectively in different team roles to plan and deliver patient-/population-centered care that is safe, timely, efficient, effective, and equitable." (Morano, C. L. (2017) This competency emphasizes coming together as a group to problem solve. By integrating the collective knowledge of many different types of professionals, unique ideas and creative solutions can be brought up in medical practice, leading to improved patient care. Additionally, working cohesively as a unit and preventing toxic, overly-competitive environments helps promote efficiency and prevent errors in overall practice.

These competencies, when considered in the goals phase of curricular development, can be used as a guide to IPE program creation.

CONCLUSION

Overall, it has become increasingly clear that IPE has incredible value in the field of healthcare. Through collaborative learning and the sharing of knowledge, the ability to use the resources offered by a healthcare team is promoted. This helps to enrich the educational opportunities of students and ensure that workforce relations and in turn patient care operate at the optimal level.

However, the development of effective IPE curriculum does not occur without barriers. When designing curriculum, it is important to ensure that potential problems such as logistical issues regarding integration of IPE into curriculum, psychosocial and cultural issues, and structural issues are addressed appropriately. Additionally, curriculum must be designed in a strategic manner that ensures that the core competencies of IPE are met while addressing healthcare needs, developing intentional curriculum, and providing room for feedback. Developing curriculum in this intentional manner will help to ensure the success and growth of IPE programs allow program graduates to be more effective future practitioners.

REFERENCES

AboutUs. (2019, October 22). Retrieved from https://www.caipe.org/about-us

Barnsteiner, J. H., Disch, J. M., Hall, L., Mayer, D., & Moore, S. M. (2007). Promoting interprofessional education. *Nursing Outlook*, *55*(3), 144–150. doi:10.1016/j.outlook.2007.03.003 PMID:17524802

Barr, H. (2009). Interprofessional education as an emerging concept. In *Interprofessional education: Making it happen*. Palgrave Macmillan. doi:10.1007/978-1-137-08028-8_1

Benefits of IPE/C. (n.d.). Retrieved from https://education2practice.org/benefits-of-ipec/

Buring, S. M., Bhushan, A., Broeseker, A., Conway, S., Duncan-Hewitt, W., Hansen, L., & Westberg, S. (2009). Interprofessional education: Definitions, student competencies, and guidelines for implementation. *American Journal of Pharmaceutical Education*, *73*(4), 59. doi:10.5688/aj730459 PMID:19657492

Callahan, D. (1998). Managed Care and the Goals of Medicine. *Journal of the American Geriatrics Society*, *46*(3), 385–388. doi:10.1111/j.1532-5415.1998.tb01060.x PMID:9514393

Carney, P. A., Thayer, E. K., Palmer, R., Galper, A. B., Zierler, B., & Eiff, M. P. (2019). The benefits of interprofessional learning and teamwork in primary care ambulatory training settings. *Journal of Interprofessional Education & Practice*, *15*, 119–126. doi:10.1016/j.xjep.2019.03.011

Clark, K. M. (2018). Interprofessional education: Making our way out of the silos. *Respiratory Care*, *63*(5), 637–639. doi:10.4187/respcare.06234 PMID:29703797

Coleman, K., & Reid, R. (2013). Continuous and team-based healing relationships: improving patient care through teams. In K. E. Phillips & V. Weir (Eds.), *Safety Net Medical Home Initiative Implementation Guide Series* (2nd ed.). Qualis Health and The MacColl Center for Health Care Innovation at the Group Health Research Institute.

Coster, S., Norman, I., Murrells, T., Kitchen, S., Meerabeau, E., Sooboodoo, E., & d'Avray, L. (2008). Interprofessional attitudes amongst undergraduate students in the health professions: A longitudinal questionnaire survey. *International Journal of Nursing Studies*, *45*(11), 1667–1681. doi:10.1016/j.ijnurstu.2008.02.008 PMID:18423644

Eliot, K., Carlson, J., Breitbach, A., Gockel-Blessing, E., & Kienstra, K. (2013, Fall). From buy-in to integration: Melding an interprofessional initiative into academic programs in the health professions. *Journal of Allied Health*, *42*(3), e67–e73. PMID:24013253

Fransworth, T. J., Seikel, J. A., Hudock, D., & Holst, J. (2015). History and Development of Interprofessional Education. *Journal of Phonetics and Audiology*, *1*(101). Advance online publication. doi:10.4172/2471-9455.1000101

Hall, L. W., & Zierler, B. K. (2015). Interprofessional Education and Practice Guide No. 1: Developing faculty to effectively facilitate interprofessional education. *Journal of Interprofessional Care*, *29*(1), 1, 3–7. doi:10.3109/13561820.2014.937483 PMID:25019466

Illingworth, P., & Chelvanayagam, S. (2007). Benefits of interprofessional education in health care. *British Journal of Nursing (Mark Allen Publishing)*, *16*(2), 121–124. doi:10.12968/bjon.2007.16.2.22773 PMID:17353824

Institute of Medicine Committee on the Health Professions Education Summit. (2003). Health Professions Education: A Bridge to Quality. National Academy Press.

KJ, J., & HC, C. (n.d.). *Teamwork Training*. Retrieved from https://www.psnet.ahrq.gov/primer/teamwork-training

Kohn, L. T., Corrigan, J. M., & Donaldson, M. S. (Eds.). (2000). To Err is Human: Building a Safer Health System. National Academy Press.

Mcalister, F., Stewart, S., Ferrua, S., & Mcmurray, J. (2004). Multidisciplinary strategies for the management of heart failure patients at high risk for admissionA systematic review of randomized trials. *Journal of the American College of Cardiology*, *44*(4), 810–819. doi:10.1016/S0735-1097(04)01123-4 PMID:15312864

Medicine. (2011). *Team-Based Care and the Learning Culture*. National Academies Press.

Morano, C. L. (2017). *Perspectives on interprofessional education and practice*. NASW Press.

Naylor, C., Griffiths, R., & Fernandez, R. (2004). Does a multidisciplinary total parenteral nutrition team improve patient outcomes? A systematic review. *Journal of Parenteral and Enteral Nutrition*, *28*(4), 251–258. doi:10.1177/0148607104028004251 PMID:15291407

Palatta, A., Cook, B. J., Anderson, E. L., & Valachovic, R. W. (2015). 20 Years Beyond the Crossroads: The Path to Interprofessional Education at U.S. Dental Schools. *Journal of Dental Education*, *79*(8), 982–996. PMID:26466391

Reeves, S., Pelone, F., Harrison, R., Goldman, J., & Zwarenstein, M. (2017). Interprofessional collaboration to improve professional practice and healthcare outcomes. *Cochrane Database of Systematic Reviews*. Advance online publication. doi:10.1002/14651858.CD000072.pub3 PMID:28639262

Schapmire, T. J., Head, B. A., Nash, W. A., Yankeelov, P. A., Furman, C. D., Wright, R. B., Gopalraj, R., Gordon, B., Black, K. P., Jones, C., Hall-Faul, M., & Faul, A. C. (2018). Overcoming barriers to interprofessional education in gerontology: The Interprofessional Curriculum for the Care of Older Adults. *Advances in Medical Education and Practice*, *9*, 109–118. doi:10.2147/AMEP.S149863 PMID:29497345

Stuart Foundation. (2002). Creating, Implementing, and Sustaining Interprofessional Education (Vol. 3). San Francisco, CA: Author.

The WHO Framework for Action. (2010). The WHO Framework for Action. *Journal of Interprofessional Care*, *24*(5), 475–478. doi:10.3109/13561820.2010.504134 PMID:20718593

Thomas, P. A., Kern, D. E., Hughes, M. T., & Chen, B. Y. (2016). *Curriculum development for medical education: a six-step approach*. Johns Hopkins University Press.

Thurston, M. M., Chesson, M. M., Harris, E. C., & Ryan, G. J. (2017). Professional stereotypes of interprofessional education naive pharmacy and nursing students. *American Journal of Pharmaceutical Education, 81*(5). Advance online publication. doi:10.5688/ajpe81584 PMID:28720912

Wang, R., Shi, N., Bai, J., Zheng, Y., & Zhao, Y. (2015). Implementation and evaluation of an interprofessional simulation-based education program for undergraduate nursing students in operating room nursing education: A randomized controlled trial. *BMC Medical Education, 15*(1), 115. doi:10.118612909-015-0400-8 PMID:26155839

West, C., Graham, L., Palmer, R. T., Miller, M. F., Thayer, E. K., Stuber, M. L., Awdishu, L., Umoren, R. A., Wamsley, M. A., Nelson, E. A., Joo, P. A., Tysinger, J. W., George, P., & Carney, P. A. (2016). Implementation of interprofessional education (IPE) in 16 U.S. medical schools: Common practices, barriers and facilitators. *J Interprofessional Educ Pract Online, 4*, 41–49. doi:10.1016/j.xjep.2016.05.002 PMID:28184380

WHO Study Group on Multiprofessional Education of Health Personnel. (Ed.). (1988). *Learning together to work together for health: Report of a WHO Study Group on Multiprofessional Education of Health Personnel: the team approach*. World Health Organization.

World Health Organization. (1973). *Continuing Education for Physicians. Report of a WHO (World Health Organization) Expert Committee*. Technical Report Series No. 534.

World Health Organization. (2010). *Framework for action on interprofessional education and collaborative practice*. WHO.

Chapter 5
Building Interprofessional Competencies Into Medical Education and Assessment

Susan Elaine Mackintosh
Western University of Health Sciences, USA

Emmanuel Katsaros
Western University of Health Sciences, USA

ABSTRACT

The goal of allopathic and osteopathic medical education is to develop the medical student into a competent and caring physician. As the evolving healthcare system continues to evolve and intersect with an increased breadth and depth of medical knowledge and an aging and more complex patient population, the emerging physician must now rely more on a team-based approach to patient-centered healthcare. Integrating interprofessional competencies into the span of the medical education and assessment process via the core competencies and the Entrustable Professional Activities has the potential to help instill not only the knowledge and skills required to practice as a member of an interprofessional healthcare team, but can also help to normalize the culture and thus the expectation of practicing collaboratively with all members of the health team toward the goal of improved patient outcome.

DOI: 10.4018/978-1-7998-3066-5.ch005

INTRODUCTION

The ultimate goal of allopathic and osteopathic medical education is to transform the matriculating student from a novice healthcare practitioner student into a highly competent and effective physician. The emerging physician is expected to be prepared to thrive in the healthcare environment and become an exemplary physician who practices safe and effective medicine. This task has become more difficult as the novice physician will encounter not only an increasingly complex healthcare environment, but an environment that now intersects with an aging and more complicated patient population and a marked increase in the breadth and depth of medical knowledge. In this "brave new world" of healthcare, medical education must now incorporate the concept of "no man is an island" as a foundation of training throughout the span of the medical education process. Teaching future physicians to not just function as a member of a healthcare team, but to incorporate the foundations and concepts of teamwork, which includes the patient, in every aspect of care is no longer a luxury reserved for rare cases or certain scenarios like a rapid response team. It must now become critical as a core principle of practice and by extension, medical education. Therefore, it is important that the concepts of interprofessional education, eventually culminating in interprofessional collaborative practice, must be imbedded as a core thread throughout the medical education process possibly in addition to the opportunity to engage in a centralized interprofessional education exposure with different healthcare professions students. The ensuing discussion assumes that healthcare practitioner students are provided an opportunity to engage in a curriculum that studies interprofessional roles and relationships but will additionally explore opportunities to enhance and reinforce interprofessional education core competencies throughout the medical education process.

This chapter will explore critical phases of the process: 1) the vehicle of transforming an entering medical student into a novel physician, which is the journey through the curriculum of the medical education institution, and is traditionally comprised of a pre-clinical (didactic) and a clinical phase, and 2) the juxtaposition of a medical student to entry into graduate medical education (GME). In each phase, the exploration will focus through the lens of teamwork/interprofessional education leading to interprofessional collaborative practice with a focus on patient-centered/relationship centered care. It should be noted that the clinical phase of medical education may somewhat be viewed as a bridge as the students are still expected to be ingrained with the competencies, but will also be expected to start demonstrating satisfactory progress toward achievement of the entrustable professional activities (EPA) ultimately leading toward achievement of the prescribed milestones as a final measurement of their preparedness to enter GME. While the focus of this chapter is on undergraduate medical education, it should be noted that the continuum of medical education does continue throughout the GME process and programs are encouraged to provide opportunities for both students and resident physicians to expand their knowledge and skills for interprofessional collaborative practice.

For the sake of this discussion, the medical education process will primarily focus on core competencies with transition to providing more opportunities to demonstrate entrustment during the clinical phase of the medical education training, and the intersect toward demonstrating readiness for GME will concentrate more on the EPAs demonstrating satisfactory progress of the milestones. It is recognized that there is an element of artificiality in this distinction as throughout the continuum of the medical education process to include GME, there are elements of competencies and milestones that are interwoven throughout the entire span of the process.

Core Competencies for Interprofessional Collaborative Practice

In 2011, the Interprofesional Education Collaborative (IPEC) sponsored an expert panel that created the Core Competencies for Interprofessional Collaborative Practice,(Interprofessional Education Collaborative Expert Panel (2011)). This document was updated in 2016, (Interprofessional Education Collaborative (2016)), but each version identifies four core competencies (domains) that must be included for interprofessional collaborative practice and by extension, must be taught to healthcare practitioner students during their medical education process. The four main competencies include 1) Values/Ethics for Interprofessional Practice, 2) Roles and Responsibilities, 3) Interprofessional Communication, and 4) Teams and Teamwork. Within each main domain, several sub-competencies were integrated as critical skills or knowledge sets that are necessary to achieve the overarching main competency. For sake of clarity, this discussion will focus on the 2016 version. The overarching goal of this discussion will focus on natural and potential areas of overlap and alignment between the IPEC Competencies and the core competencies for both allopathic and osteopathic medical education and the EPAs. Table 1 demonstrates each domain with a few examples of sub-competencies expected from each domain. The table is not inclusive of each domain's sub-competencies. By providing examples, it is anticipated that the institution will explore this document in further detail to examine these expectations.

PHASE I (Pre-Clinical and Clinical Education-Undergraduate Medical Education)

The initial process, transforming the beginning medical student into an emerging new physician, primarily occurs through the progression of the curriculum. The foundation of the curriculum focuses on core competencies. As the student advances

Table 1. IPEC Competency Domains

IPEC Domain	Values/Ethics for Interprofessional Practice	Roles and Responsibilities	Interprofessional Communication	Teams and Teamwork
Sub-competency examples	VE 3: Embrace the cultural diversity and individual differences that characterize patient, populations and the health team.	RR 1: Communicate one's roles and responsibilities clearly to patients, families, community members, and other professionals.	CC 1: Choose effective communication tools and technique, including information systems and communication technologies, to facilitate discussions and interactions that enhance team function.	TT 1: Describe the process of team development and the roles and practice of effective teams.
	VE 4: Respect the unique cultures, values, roles/responsibilities, and expertise of other health professions and the impact these factors can have on health outcomes.	RR 2: Recognize one's limitations in skills, knowledge, and abilities.	CC 2: Communicate information with patients, families, community members, and health team members in a form that is understandable, avoiding discipline-specific terminology when possible.	TT 3: Engage health and other professionals in shared patient-centered and populations-focused problem-solving.
	VE 6: Develop a trusting relationship with patients, families, and other team members.	RR 4: Explain the roles and responsibilities of other providers and how the team works together to provide care, promote health, and prevent disease.	CC 4: Listen actively, and encourage ideas and opinions of other team members.	TT 5: Apply leadership practices that support collaborative practice and team effectiveness.
	VE 9: Act with honesty and integrity in relationships with patients, families, communities, and other team members.	RR 6: Communicate with team members to clarify each member's responsibility in executing components of a treatment plan or public health intervention.	CC 8: Communicate the importance of teamwork in patient-centered care and population health programs and policies.	TT 9: Use process improvement to increase effectiveness of interprofessional teamwork and team-based services, programs and policies.

(Interprofessional Education Collaborative (2016))

through the curriculum, they should be provided increasing opportunities to demonstrate command of the Entrustable Professional Activities (EPA), especially in the clinical phase of their training. This discussion will explore the components of the competencies and EPAs through the lens of interprofessional patient-centered care and will examine opportunities to embed and assess the Core Competencies for Interprofessional Collaborative Practice as part of the foundation of the medical education/assessment process. The assumption is that as a student obtains mastery of the competencies and ultimately demonstrates satisfactory achievement of the EPAs, they should be ready to enter GME and by extension of the nature of this discussion, ready to engage in interprofessional collaborative practice.

Core Competencies for Allopathic and Osteopathic Medical Education and Their Alignment with IPEC Competencies

Allopathic and Osteopathic Medical Education

Throughout the span of medical education, students are expected to demonstrate proficiency in several major competencies. While the competencies below are from the American Association of Medical Colleges (AAMC) document, Core Entrustable Professional Activities for Entering Residency, (Obeso V, Brown D, Aiyer M, Barron B, Bull J, Carter T, Emery M, Gillespie C, Hormann M, Hyderi A, Lupi C, Schwartz ML, Uthman M, Vasilevskis EE, Yingling S, Phillipi C, (2017)), there is definite overlap between allopathic and osteopathic education. Institutions of both osteopathic and allopathic medical education may consider these as mutual goals. Key differentiation between osteopathic and allopathic medical education competencies will be noted in each section. The competencies include:

1. Patient Care (PC)
2. Knowledge for Practice (KP)
3. Practice-Based Learning and Improvement (PBLI)
4. Interpersonal and Communication Skills (ICS)
5. Professionalism (P)
6. Systems-Based Practice (SBP)
7. Interprofessional Collaboration (IPC)
8. Personal and Professional Development (PPD)

As with the IPEC Competencies, each of these main competencies for medical education is comprised of several sub-competencies that must be achieved to demonstrate proficiency for the primary competency. While there is a specific competency for Interprofessional Collaboration, which is dedicated toward the principle of instilling interprofessional knowledge, skills, and attitudes, each of the other competencies provides an opportunity to reinforce the principles of interprofessional education culminating in interprofessional collaborative practice. The primary goal of this section will be to explore some of those natural intersects with the intent of fostering a creative spirit for institutions of medical education to examine and implement other opportunities to embed and adopt a curriculum that augments interprofessional education and a culture that will eventually lead to interprofessional collaborative practice.

Patient Care

Within the domain of Patient Care, there are 11 sub-competencies as described in the AAMC document that must be achieved to demonstrate competency of the whole. While arguments could be made that each one could nurture a culture of interprofessional education/collaborative practice, several provide an absolute opportunity to integrate interprofessional concepts. Some examples of such opportunities include 1) developing and carrying out patient management plans; 2) providing appropriate referral of patients, including ensuring continuity of care throughout transitions between providers or settings: and following up on patient progress and outcomes; 3) providing healthcare service to patients, families, and communities aimed at preventing health problems or maintaining health; and 4) performing supervisory responsibilities commensurate with one's roles, abilities, and qualifications. (Obeso V, et al (2017))

The core competency of Patient Care for osteopathic medical education has similar goals that must be demonstrated for proficiency of this competency. There are six sub-competencies that each have several goals toward achievement of the area of focus. As examples, sub-competency 4 specifically describes forming a patient-centered, interprofessional, evidence-based management plan, and sub-competency 6 describes objectives toward achieving the overall goal of documentation, case presentation, and team communication. Specifically, one of the objectives noted in sub-competency 6 is to communicate verbally and in writing with other members of the interprofessional collaborative team, including those from other health professions, in order to provide effective and comprehensive patient-centered care. (Osteopathic Core Competencies for Medical Students, 2012)

While an argument can be made that virtually all four of the IPEC domains can be integrated into this particular competency for both allopathic and osteopathic medical education, a specific example exists in the domain of the Roles/Responsibilities (RR). A prime example of an overlap with this domain is RR 1, which states the healthcare team member should communicate one's roles and responsibilities clearly

Table 2. Examples of Allopathic and Osteopathic Patient Care Competencies and Sub-competencies

Examples of Allopathic Sub-competencies	Examples of Osteopathic Sub-competencies	Example(s) of Specific Objective in Osteopathic Sub-competency
1.6: Develop and carry out patient management plans	4. Form a patient-centered, interprofessional, evidence-based management plan	Formulate a plan that provides relief of the patient's physical, psychosocial, and psychological distress
1.8: Providing appropriate referral of patients, including ensuring continuity of care throughout transitions between providers or setting and following up on patient progress and outcomes	6. Documentation, case presentation, and team communication	Communicate verbally and in writing with other members of the interprofessional collaborative team, including those from other health professions, in order to provide effective and comprehensive patient-centered care
1.9: Providing healthcare service to patients, families, and communities aimed at preventing health problems or maintaining health		
1.11: Performing supervisory responsibilities commensurate with one's roles, abilities, and qualifications		

to patients, families, community members, and other professionals. (Interprofessional Education Collaborative (2016))

Each institution must creatively explore their own opportunities for overlapping the Patient Care competency with the IPEC competencies; however, an example of an activity could be as simple as integrating notes from other healthcare professionals with encouragement for students and residents to reach out and explore opportunities to communicate with the various members of the healthcare team on how to collaboratively work together toward patient management. This competency is also a perfect opportunity to reinforce that the patient is not only a member of the healthcare team, but is the center of the team, thus the term patient-centered care.

Knowledge for Practice

Knowledge for Practice has 6 sub-competencies that fall under an overarching goal to demonstrate knowledge of established and evolving biomedical, clinical, epidemiological, and social-behavioral sciences, as well as the application of this knowledge to patient care. This particular competency provides a wealth of opportunities for the curriculum to encompass interprofessional practices and awareness. As an example, sub-competency number 2.5 is to apply principles of social-behavioral sciences to provision of patient care, including assessment of the impact of psychosocial-cultural influences on health, disease, care-seeking, care compliance, and barrier to and attitudes toward care. While there are many potential applications for this sub-competency, prime examples could include exposure to such professions as mental health, social services, and a global approach to public health. (Obeso V, et al (2017))

Osteopathic medical education has several similar expectations under the competency of Medical Knowledge. This competency is comprised of three main sub-competencies. The sub-competency of physician interventions describes many opportunities for the student to gain understanding of not only interprofessional competencies across the healthcare team, but also intraprofessionally to help the student comprehend the team approach to engaging with the various specialties in medicine. A specific example is recognizing the limits of personal medical knowledge. There are also goals in this sub-competency that have strong public health alignment such as to outline preventive strategies across stages of the life cycle and describe and list risk factors for preventable diseases. (Osteopathic Core Competencies for Medical Students, 2012)

Table 3. Examples of Allopathic and Osteopathic Knowledge for Practice/Medical Knowledge Competencies and Sub-competencies

Examples of Allopathic Sub-competencies	Examples of Osteopathic Sub-competencies	Example(s) of Specific Objective in Osteopathic Sub-competency
2.5: Apply principles of social-behavioral sciences to provision of patient care, including assessment of the impact of psychosocial-cultural influences on health, disease, care-seeking, care compliance, and barrier to and attitudes toward care	2.Apply current best practices in osteopathic medicine	Retain knowledge of medical science appropriate for osteopathic patient care
2.6: Contribute to the creation, dissemination, application, and transition of new healthcare knowledge and practices	3. Physician interventions	• Use scientific concepts to evaluate, diagnose, and manage clinical patient presentations and population health • Recognizing the limits of personal medical knowledge

While many of the IPEC domains could also overlap with this competency, a specific example is under the Teams and Teamwork Sub-Competency (TT). TT3 state the practitioner should engage health and other professionals in share patient-centered and population-focused problem solving. (Interprofessional Education Collaborative (2016)) As with the competency of Patient Care, it is imperative that the institution creatively explores possibilities for such overlap with the IPEC competencies, but a specific example could be to introduce the concept of One Health, (Centers for Disease Control and Prevention, One Health) which is the intersect of human health, animal health and environmental health factors.

Practice-Based Learning and Improvement

The ten sub-competencies under Practice-Based Learning and Improvement (PBLI) coalesce to address the over-all goal of demonstrating the ability to investigate and evaluate their care of patients, to appraise and assimilate scientific evidence, and to continuously improve patient care based on constant self-evaluation and lifelong learning. As with the other competencies, there are multiple opportunities for the institution to explore ways to integrate interprofessional competencies toward achieving this goal. One example is Sub-competency 3.4, which discusses the importance of systematically analyzing practice using quality-improvement methods and implementing changes with the goal of practice improvement. Sub-competency 3.9, which is to obtain and utilize information about individual patients, populations of patients or communities from which patients are drawn to improve care, also has very strong potential to reinforce principles of interprofessionalism. (Obeso V, et al (2017))

While this particular competency has a slightly different focus in the osteopathic medical education core competencies to include an emphasis on research, there is still a strong potential to integrate principles of interprofessional education and interprofessional collaborative practice. Of the five sub-competencies, number 5 is to describe and apply systematic methods to improve population health. (Osteopathic Core Competencies for Medical Students, 2012)

As with the previous competencies, there are several opportunities for integrating the IPEC competencies. Specifically, in both the allopathic and osteopathic medical education system, this particular arena addresses the concept of the importance of public health and population health. The IPEC domain of Roles and Responsibilities alone provides many opportunities to reinforce the interprofessional team in this particular aspect. A prime example is RR 10, which is to describe how professionals in health and other fields can collaborate and integrate clinical care and public health interventions to optimize population health. (Interprofessional Education Collaborative (2016)) Principles of public health/population health are instilled in virtually every medical student. By extrapolation, this particular concept could easily reinforce the importance of other healthcare and non-healthcare professions that contribute to the overall public health goals. A specific example of an opportunity

Table 4. Examples of Allopathic and Osteopathic PBLI Competencies and Sub-competencies

Examples of Allopathic Sub-competencies	Examples of Osteopathic Sub-competencies	Example(s) of Specific Objective in Osteopathic Sub-competency
3.4: Systematically analyze practice using quality-improvement methods and implement changes with the goal of practice improvement	5. Describe and apply systematic methods to improve population health	• Describe public health surveillance and vital statistics • Identify opportunities for advocacy, health promotion, and disease prevention in communities served, and respond appropriately
3.9: Obtain and utilize information about individual patients, populations of patients or communities from which patients are drawn to improve care		

is to explore The 10 Essential Public Health Service as described by the Centers for Disease Control and Prevention (Centers for Disease Control and Prevention, Public Health Professionals Gateway). The medical education institution could find many opportunities to introduce roles and responsibilities of various agencies, departments, and professions toward achieving the goals of public health.

Interpersonal and Communication Skills

There are multiple sub-competencies under this general competency that provide an excellent back drop to not only achieve interprofessional practice skills, but that can enhance the achievement of the overall goal to demonstrate interpersonal and communication skills that result in the effective exchange of information and collaboration with patients, their families, and health professionals. In fact, this particular competency has significant overlap with interprofessional competencies as defined by IPEC. Of the seven sub-competencies listed in this specific competency, several of them directly address communication with other members of the healthcare team and patients and their families. Examples include sub-competency 4.2, which is to communicate effectively with colleagues with one's profession or specialty, other health professionals, and health-related agencies; and sub-competency 4.4, which indicates the medical student should strive to acquire skills where they can eventually act in a consultative role to other health professionals. (Obeso V, et al (2017))

For osteopathic medical education, this same competency has several sub-competencies describing goals to work collaboratively and effectively not only with the patient, but with other members of the health care team. Sub-competency number four specifically addresses the importance of working effectively with other health professionals as a member or leader of a health care team. (Osteopathic Core Competencies for Medical Students, 2012)

Table 5. Examples of Allopathic and Osteopathic Interpersonal and Communication Skills Competencies and Sub-competencies

Examples of Allopathic Sub-competencies	Examples of Osteopathic Sub-competencies	Example(s) of Specific Objective in Osteopathic Sub-competency
4.2: Communicate effectively with colleagues with one's profession or specialty, other health professionals, and health-related agencies	4. Work effectively with other health professionals as a member or leader of a health care team	Collaborate with other health care professionals in the care of the patient demonstrating effective personal skills and interpersonal dynamics
Act in a consultative role to other health professionals		

These competencies could overlap with virtually any of the four IPEC domains. A prime example is one of the sub-competencies in the Teams and Teamwork Domain. Sub-competency TT3 is to engage health and other professionals in shared patient-centered and population focused problem-solving. (Interprofessional Education Collaborative (2016))

While there are numerous opportunities where institutions could integrate and reinforce the IPEC competencies during the course of medical education, perhaps an excellent example would be utilization of simulation. Team-based Objective Structured Clinical Examination (TOSCE) scenarios provide a wealth of opportunities to interject opportunities for teaching and assessing students on both intraprofessional and interprofessional communication skills. The article by Dickter et al, *Development of the Ambulatory Team Observed Structured Clinical Evaluation (ATOSCE),* (Dickter D, Stielstra S, Mackintosh S, Garner S, Finocchio VA, Aston SJ) describes the process of creating a scenario that requires significant communication amongst the health care team to navigate the patient through the ambulatory health care setting. While this scenario was developed by an interprofessional team, exercises such as this could easily be created for utilization in a medical school curriculum, but with the intent of reinforcing interpersonal and communication skills across the entire health care team.

Professionalism

The overall goal of the professionalism competency is to demonstrate a commitment to carrying out professional responsibilities and an adherence to ethical principles. The six sub-competencies have a natural overlap and alignment with the IPEC domain on values and ethics with many potential areas for intersecting the two competency sets. While all six of the sub-competencies could easily parallel this specific IPEC domain, a prime example is sub-competency 5.1., which is to demonstrate compassion, integrity, and respect for others. (Obeso V, et al (2017)). This particular sub-competency alone could tie in the relationship between the competencies for medical education along with the competencies for interprofessional education and practice as a backbone of interprofessionalism is respect for not only patients, but other members of the health care team.

For osteopathic medical education, the competency of professionalism has significant overtones that intersect with the IPEC domains and with the AAMC competencies. Each of the nine sub-competencies addressed in the document provide several goals that easily promote interprofessional awareness and action. One of the sub-competencies specifically addresses the importance of accountability to patients, society, and the profession, including the duty to act in response to the knowledge of professional behavior of other. (Osteopathic Core Competencies for Medical Students, 2012)

Table 6. Examples of Allopathic and Osteopathic Professionalism Competencies and Sub-competencies

Examples of Allopathic Sub-competencies	Examples of Osteopathic Sub-competencies	Example(s) of Specific Objective in Osteopathic Sub-competency
5.1: Demonstrate compassion, integrity, and respect for others	4. ACCOUNTABILITY - Demonstrate accountability to patients, society, and the profession, including the duty to act in response to the knowledge of professional behavior of others.	• Effectively communicate to colleagues when transferring responsibility for medical care. • Properly report and disclose medical errors and "near misses" that can lead to improvements in the quality of care provided
5.4 Demonstrate sensitivity and responsiveness to patient needs that supersedes self-interest		

A prime example of overlap with the IPEC domains for both allopathic and osteopathic competencies is the entire section on Values and Ethics for Interprofessional Practice. This entire area discusses the importance of creating a culture of mutual respect and shared values, but also addresses the importance of competence, trust and ethical conduct with patients and other members of the health care team. (Interprofessional Education Collaborative (2016))

While the subject of medical error is an unpleasant area of focus, it could be utilized as an important teaching tool to address interprofessional competencies. Providing an opportunity for students to do a root cause analysis of errors that breached ethical boundaries, or where strict levels of competence were not maintained could be utilized to help the learner analyze how such errors can contribute to poor outcomes and subsequently provide opportunities to learn how to mitigate such mistakes in future scenarios. Examples of situations such as a mock deposition or a morbidity and mortality case could focus on an opportunity to reverse engineer errors that may have occurred as a result of issues such as a lack of competence, lack of communication, breach of ethical boundaries, and violation of trust.

Systems-Based Practice

The overall goals of the Systems-Based Practice (SBP) competency is to demonstrate an awareness of and responsiveness to the larger context and system of health care, as well as the ability to call effectively on other resources in the system to provide optimal healthcare. Each of the six sub-competencies can strongly be aligned to the goals of all four of the IPEC domains and provides the medical education institution the perfect opportunity to reinforce the principles of interprofessional education and practice within the context of the primary medical education curriculum. For example, sub-competency 6.1 describes the importance of working effectively in various health care delivery settings and systems relevant to one's clinical specialty. Sub-competency 6.2 likewise discusses the coordination of patient care within the health care system relevant to one's clinical specialty. (Obeso V, et al (2017))

The osteopathic core competencies details five main sub-competencies that also provide many opportunities to explore and strengthen interprofessional collaborative practice. As an example, sub-competency five states that it is important for the student to demonstrate knowledge of and the ability to implement safe, effective, timely, patient-centered, equitable systems of care in a team-oriented environment to advance populations' and individual patients' health. (Osteopathic Core Competencies for Medical Students, 2012)

Several of the IPEC domains can intertwine with both the allopathic and the osteopathic core competencies. As a prime example, under the domain of Interprofessional Communication, the first sub-competency, CC1, states that the student should choose effective communication tools and techniques, including information systems and communication technologies, to facilitate discussion and

Table 7. Examples of Allopathic and Osteopathic SBP Competencies and Sub-competencies

Examples of Allopathic Sub-competencies	Examples of Osteopathic Sub-competencies	Example(s) of Specific Objective in Osteopathic Sub-competency
6.1: Work effectively in various healthcare delivery settings and systems relevant to one's clinical specialty	5. Demonstrate knowledge of and the ability to implement safe, effective, timely, patient-centered, equitable systems of care in a team-oriented environment to advance populations' and individual patients' health	• Recognize, properly report, and utilize methods known to be effective in the reduction of medical errors • Demonstrate respect for and the ability to work with other health care providers to advance the health of individual patients and populations
6.2: Coordinate patient care within the health care system relevant to one's clinical specialty		

interactions that enhance team function. (Interprofessional Education Collaborative (2016))

These particular competencies are a perfect vehicle to address issues such as patient safety and quality of care. Introducing evidence-based tools such as TeamStepps (Agency for Healthcare Research and Quality, TeamSTEPPS®) could easily combine the achievement of the medical school curriculum along with the knowledge and skillset required to provide team-based effective care in an interprofessional setting.

Interprofessional Collaboration

This competency is completely geared toward educating the student about the importance of interprofessional practice. The overall goal of the competency is to demonstrate the ability to engage in an interprofessional team in a manner that optimizes safe, effective patient and population-centered care. Each of the four specific sub-competencies is in alignment with the four main IPEC domains. (Obeso V, et al (2017))

While Interprofessional Collaboration is not one of the original seven core competencies for osteopathic medical education, it should be noted that it is addressed in the Osteopathic Core Competencies for Medical Students document and does have absolute overlap with all the IPEC domains. Additionally, it is interwoven throughout all the competencies. (Osteopathic Core Competencies for Medical Students, 2012)

As this particular competency is entirely geared toward the achievement of interprofessional collaborative practice, it will not be addressed in this modality. It is hoped the goals of this particular competency can be achieved either through the institutions formal interprofessional education program and/or through integration with the other competencies as discussed throughout this chapter.

Personal and Professional Development

The overarching goal of this competency is to demonstrate the qualities required to sustain lifelong personal and professional growth. Each of the eight sub-competencies drives toward a future physician who not only values the importance of lifelong learning, but also embraces a well-balanced life and personal and professional relationships. The competency also drives home the importance of teamwork. In essence, the goal of a team-centered approach to healthcare could be reinforced in educational activities geared toward the implementation of this competency with a focus on maximally utilizing the team to assure all members of the healthcare team achieve balance in their personal and their professional lives and responsibilities. (Obeso V, et al (2017))

Although this is not a specific competency listed for osteopathic medical education, it should be noted that it is also interwoven throughout the other competencies. As an example, under the competency of professionalism, there is a specific sub-competency for continuous learning. Of the several goals within that particular sub-competency, on specifically highlights the importance of recognizing limits of personal knowledge and skill by consulting colleagues when necessary. (Osteopathic Core Competencies for Medical Students, 2012)

As with other competencies for medical and osteopathic medical education, virtually all of the four IPEC domains can intersect with the importance of personal and professional development. On example is under the domain of Roles and Responsibilities (RR). RR3, which is to engage diverse professional who complement

Table 8. Examples of Allopathic and Osteopathic Personal and Professional Development Competencies and Sub-competencies

Examples of Allopathic Sub-competencies	Examples of Osteopathic Sub-competencies	Example(s) of Specific Objective in Osteopathic Sub-competency
8.5: Demonstrate trustworthiness that makes colleagues feel secure when one is responsible for the care of patients	No specific Competency for Personal and Professional Development: Correlation can be found as an example in Competency of Professionalism: 5. Continuous Learning	• Recognize limits of personal knowledge and skill by consulting colleagues when necessary
8.6: Provide leadership skills that enhance team functioning, the learning environment, and/or the health care delivery system		

one's own professional expertise as well as associated resources, to develop strategies to meet specific health and healthcare needs of patients and populations. (Interprofessional Education Collaborative (2016))

Many opportunities exist for continuing professional development from an interprofessional vantage point. Examples could include activities such as interprofessional case presentations or journal clubs where students can continue to evolve in their own professional knowledge and skills but will also be afforded the opportunity to learn with, from and about their healthcare colleagues.

Osteopathic Medical Education

While the above eight competencies represent educational goals of both allopathic and osteopathic medical education, it is important to address the additional competencies for osteopathic medical education. The 2012 rendition of the Osteopathic Core Competencies for Medical Students describes the original seven core competencies for osteopathic medical education, which are Osteopathic Principles and Practices, Medical Knowledge, Patient Care, Interpersonal and Communication Skills, Professionalism, Practice-Based Learning and Improvement, and Systems-Based Practice. (Osteopathic Core Competencies for Medical Students, 2012). All but Osteopathic Principles and Practice closely align with the AAMC competencies. Additionally, the Osteopathic Core Competencies for Medical Students describes the Healthy People Curriculum Task Force's Clinical Prevention and Population Health Curriculum Framework, which includes the concept of Interprofessional Education. As the focus of this chapter is on the competencies that are similar between allopathic and osteopathic medical education, the only specific difference that will be discussed in this chapter is the competency of Osteopathic Principles and Practice and how that particular area could also provide an arena for reinforcement of Interprofessional collaboration. However, it is encouraged that both schools and colleges of osteopathic and allopathic education examine opportunities for overlap in the Healthy People Curriculum Task Force's Clinical Prevention and Population Health Curriculum Framework. The remaining competencies in the document include Counseling for Health Promotion/Disease Prevention, Cultural Competencies, Evaluation of Health Sciences Literature, Environmental and Occupational Medicine (OEM), Public Health Systems, Global Health, and the above mentioned Interprofessional Collaboration. (Osteopathic Core Competencies for Medical Students, 2012). Many of these concepts are found embedded in the aforementioned competencies and could provide very rich and diverse opportunities for institutions of medical education to explore opportunities for reinforcing interprofessional competencies.

Osteopathic Principles and Practices

The competency of Osteopathic Principles and Practices (OPP) is comprised of 8 main domains each with additional sub-competencies as part of that domain. Some of the examples of the larger domains include "Approach the patient with recognition of the entire clinical context, including mind-body and psychosocial interrelationships; Use the relationship between structure and function to promote health; and Collaborate with OMM specialists and other health care providers to maximize patient treatment and outcomes, as well as to advance osteopathic manipulations research and knowledge. (Osteopathic Core Competencies for Medical Students, 2012). Each of these, along with the other 5 domains, could provide the osteopathic medical education institution opportunities to promote and support teaching the osteopathic medical student how to engage other members of the healthcare team as part of the overall plan.

Table 9. Examples of Osteopathic OPP Competencies and Sub-competencies

Sub-competency	Objective(s) in Sub-competency
1. Approach the patient with recognition of the entire clinical context, including mind-body and psychosocial interrelationships	• Recognize and treat each patient as a whole person, integrating body, mind, and spirit
2. Use the relationship between structure and function to promote health	• Utilize knowledge of the clinical sciences to formulate a treatment plan, emphasizing the correction of clinical manifestations resulting from somatic dysfunction.
7. Collaborate with OMM specialists and other health care providers to maximize patient treatment and outcomes, as well as to advance osteopathic manipulation research and knowledge	• Recognize the role of and demonstrate a commitment to the utilization of other health care professionals in the diagnosis and treatment of the patient

The other competencies for osteopathic medical education; to include Medical Knowledge, Patient Care, Interpersonal and Communication Skills, Professionalism, Practice-Based Learning, and Systems-Based Practice, (Osteopathic Core Competencies for Medical Students, 2012), are presented in different formats from those detailed through the AAMC documentation. However, all competencies have similar overlaps with not only the AAMC competencies, but also with the IPEC domains.

Summary of Competencies

The goal of this section is not to define a new curriculum geared strictly toward interprofessional education, but to foster a spirit of creativity for institutions of allopathic and osteopathic medical education to explore opportunities to reiterate the concepts and idealism of interprofessional collaborative practice while in the midst of their medical education curriculum. It is not geared to replace any type of institutional interprofessional curriculum, but to instead augment that curriculum by fostering a culture within the medical education home program where interprofessional practice and collaboration is viewed as the norm as opposed to an add on curriculum. The ideas presented thus far in this chapter are only designed to provide fuel for thought for various institutions to create and look for opportunities to promote interprofessionalism as part of their identity as they educate future allopathic and osteopathic physician. As the competencies are the backbone of the process in creating our future physicians and osteopathic physicians, they provide an excellent opportunity to not only provide the educational activities, but to also explore ways for formative evaluation processes. It is incumbent upon the institutions of allopathic and osteopathic education to explore additional opportunities to reinforce the principles of interprofessional education and interprofessional collaborative practice utilizing methods, tools and opportunities that is conducive to their respective curriculums and cultures. The ideas and examples provided (Table 10) are meant only to foster creativity and as a platform for institutions of allopathic and osteopathic medical education to generate their own creative ideas on how to integrate interprofessional concepts in their curriculum.

It is also recognized that competencies in medical and osteopathic medical education will continue to evolve as will the interprofessional education/collaborative practice competencies, so it will be necessary that this intentional practice continues to evolve. In time, the offerings in this book may not be up to date with respect to specific competency numbers and headings, but it is encouraged that the institution continue to explore opportunities as the competencies continue to evolve.

Clinical Education: The Bridge to Entrustable Professional Activities

As described in the introductory section of this narrative, during the Clinical Education phase of training, traditionally the third and fourth year or medical education, the student is still expected to attain knowledge and skills toward mastery of the core competencies; however, they are also expected to start attaining skills, knowledge, and behaviors that will prepare them for demonstration of acceptable attainment of the EPAs. Many have questioned the utility of EPAs in undergraduate medical education. For instance, some argue that entrustment for unsupervised tasks involving

Table 10. Alignment of Competencies and Resources

Allopathic Competency	Osteopathic Competency	Example of IPEC Competency	Example of resource or activity
Patient Care	Patient Care	Roles and Responsibilities	Exposure to documentation from other healthcare professions
Knowledge for Practice	Medical Knowledge	Teams and Teamwork	One Health
Practice-Based Learning and Improvement	Practice-Based Learning and Improvement	Roles and Responsibilities	The 10 Essential Public Health Service
Interpersonal and Communication Skills	Interpersonal and Communication Skills	Teams and Teamwork	Simulation-Team-based OSCE
Professionalism	Professionalism	Values and Ethics	Root-cause Analysis of Medical Error
Systems-Based Practice	Systems-Based Practice	Interprofessional Communication	TeamStepps
Personal and Professional Development	Embedded in other competencies	Roles and Responsibilities	Interprofessional Case Presentations
N/A	Osteopathic Principles and Practice	Roles and Responsibilities	Education on benefit of osteopathic manipulative medicine
Interprofessional Education	Embedded in other competencies	All domains	Institutional IPE program

patients are not appropriate for unlicensed learners (Chen HC, van der Broek, W.E. S, ten Cate,O; 2015). Chen et al. (2015) report, however, that international support for a competency based medical education exists, in part, because educators are concerned that core competency domains do not fully capture valid outcomes for patient care. Indeed, the authors state that competencies do not account for the necessary integration of the competency domains or assess the proper application of the domains to the care of patients. EPA's can address the concerns of competencies because EPAs focus on the work that needs to be done for patients and require an integration of competency domains for the task to be accomplished successfully.

Competencies to Entrustable Professional Activities (EPAs)

The culminating goal of any medical education program, whether it be osteopathic or allopathic, is to assure that the graduate is prepared in terms of knowledge, behavior, attitudes and skills to enter the next phase of their training, which is graduate medical education. In undergraduate medical education, the EPAs can be designed as summative assessments, where the learner integrates competencies during the completion of a patient related task. Successful completion of these tasks allows the learner to move through stages of medical education until graduation, and thereby assuring the learner and the GME program that the new graduate has achieved the necessary skillsets to make this transition and is prepared to become a competent resident physician.

Before addressing how the EPAs can also be utilized to assure the advanced medical student or new physician is ready to enter and engage in graduate medical education, it is important to understand the alignment of the competencies with the EPAs. Competencies are measurable abilities of a healthcare provider. These abilities can be knowledge, skills or attitudes. EPAs are units of professional practice, such as performing physical exams or documenting clinical encounters, that are assessed for a learner's level of entrustment to perform the professional activity safely and independently. (Obesco, V). Competencies and EPAs are interrelated. EPAs require proficiencies in the competencies, but competencies are best assessed as a learner is performing an EPA. Although many competencies can be assessed during the preclinical years, the EPAs ideally require their evaluation during an actual professional encounter on a clinical rotation. Since competencies are best assessed through the lens of EPAs, achieving proficiency in each competency is best evaluated in the clinical portion of a medical education.

As described in the previous section, in addition to acquiring a command of the major competencies, students are expected to demonstrate proficiency in thirteen EPAs. The EPAs below are from the AAMC document but are identical to the osteopathic EPAs. The important difference between the two documents are that AACCOM incorporated considerations of osteopathic principles and philosophy, and techniques into the EPAs generated by the AAMC. Otherwise the bulk of the documents are identical. The EPAs include:

EPA 1: Gather a history and perform a physical examination
EPA 2: Prioritize a differential diagnosis following a clinical encounter
EPA 3: Recommend and interpret common diagnostic and screening tests
EPA 4: Enter and discuss orders and prescriptions
EPA 5: Document a clinical encounter in the patient record
EPA 6: Provide an oral presentation of a clinical encounter
EPA 7: Form clinical questions and retrieve evidence to advance patient care
EPA 8: Give or receive a patient handover to transition care responsibility
EPA 9: Collaborate as a member of an interprofessional team
EPA 10: Recognize a patient requiring urgent or emergent care and initiate evaluation and management
EPA 11: Obtain informed consent for tests and/or procedures
EPA 12: Perform general procedures of a physician

EPA 13: Identify system failures and contribute to a culture of safety and improvement

Both of the allopathic and osteopathic initial documents outlaying the EPAs, describe "functions" for each EPA. These functions are subunits of the task described in each EPA. While EPA 9, "collaborate as a member of an interprofessional team," appears to best relate to interprofessional education, most of the EPAs, as illustrated by some of their functions, relate to interprofessionalism and its teaching.

The following are examples of the functions of the EPAs that relate to inteprofessionalsm, which may be used by educators to design a curriculum that embeds interprofessionalsm into curriculum and into the mindset of students as they progress through their medical education and eventual practice. Because the AAMC and American Association of Colleges of Osteopathic Medicine (AACOM) EPAs and its functions are identical with the exception of the incorporated osteopathic considerations, all references to the EPAs and its functions are taken from both documents. (Basehore et al. 2016(; Flynn T, et al. 2015).

EPA 1: Gather a history and perform a physical examination

Obtaining a history and information of patients are not only derived from patients themselves, but from family and other health care professionals caring for a patient. Information in a patient history may be obtained from pharmacists, nurses or physical therapists. AAMC and AACOM describes one function of EPA 1 as "identify and use alternate sources of information to obtain history when needed, including but not limited to family members, primary care physicians, living facility, and pharmacy staff."

EPA 2: Prioritize a differential diagnosis following a clinical encounter

Two functions of EPA 2 are directly related to IPE: "Engage with supervisors and team members for endorsement and verification of the working diagnosis in developing a management plan" and "explain and document the clinical reasoning that led to the working diagnosis in a manner that is transparent to all members of the health care team" are functions that illustrate the importance of interprofessional collaboration. Poor communication with other health care providers, the patient, and the family, results in poor teamwork that can affect patient care. For instance, quality teamwork in the ICU has been associated with shorter hospital days and decreased mortality (Baggs JG, Schmitt MH, Mushlin AI, et al. 1999).

EPA 4: Enter and discuss orders and prescriptions

Physician orders that are to be carried out by other health care team members require that the orders are clear and align with the common regards to safety and efficacy understood by all health care providers carrying out the orders. This EPA is certainly collaborative by requiring physicians not only to communicate with other professionals, but to address concerns and suggestions by these professionals so that there is a mutual understanding of management decisions. One function offers a nuance to ordering by asking the learner to "demonstrate working knowledge of the protocol by which orders will be processed in the environment in which they are placing the orders." Communication with unit secretaries on a medicine floor, nurses and other professionals is critical to understanding the protocols of any given health care facility or department.

EPA 5: Document a clinical encounter in the patient record

The function: "Accurately document the reasoning supporting the decision making in the clinical encounter for any reader (e.g., consultants, other health care professionals,

patients and families, auditors)" underscores the importance of IPE. The document must be an accurate and honest description of the patient's condition and the physician's opinion of a patient's condition to, in part, earn respect and trust from team members. In order to carry out this function, a learner must know the roles and function of each member of the health care team. When understanding a member's role, a physician can include key information relevant for the team member to allow for safe and efficient care.

EPA 6: Provide an oral presentation of a clinical encounter

In EPA 6, learners are asked to "adjust the oral presentation to meet the needs of the receiver of the information," and "assure closed-loop communication between the presenter and receiver of the information to ensure that both parties have a shared understanding of the patient's condition and needs.To accomplish this, the learner must recognize each team member's unique contribution to a patient's care and adapt the presentation to allow that member to work most effectively. The learner must actively listen to illicit and take recommendations and recognize both verbal and nonverbal cues that may be important to clarify history, exam findings, assessments or plans. Also, during a learner's presentations, respect must be demonstrated to other members of the team to strength working relationships.

EPA 7: Form clinical questions and retrieve evidence to advance patient care

As the learner discovers evidence-based material that may affect a patient's care, EPA 7 asks the learner to "communicate one's findings to the health care team (including the patient/family)." . The IPEC competency of Interprofessional Communication include the sub-competency CC3, "expresses one's knowledge and opinions to team members". This EPA relates to communication and demonstrates respect for members and reinforces the idea of team and teamwork.

EPA 8: Give or receive a patient handover to transition care responsibility.

Although not explicitly stated in the AACOM or AAMC EPA documents, EPA 8 can be relevant to multiple care team members of a patient transferring care to another setting, such as home care or a rehabilitation facility. A physician must be able to succinctly communicate a patient's history during a hospitalization, express concerns, make recommendations or give orders to any number of health care providers, such as nurses, nurse practitioners, physical therapists, physical therapists, and case managers etc. The physician should also ask and create an atmosphere that allows members to make suggestions and ask questions.

EPA 9: Collaborate as a member of an interprofessional team

EPA 9 encompasses all of the IPEC competencies, but while most of the EPAs incorporates many aspects of collaboration, EPA 9 stresses the importance and highlights the characteristics of collaborative skills when working with other professionals. EPA 9 can be assessed in terms of the IPEC competencies and is the case with most of the EPAs.

EPA 10: Recognize a patient requiring urgent or emergent care and initiate evaluation and management

Urgent or emergent situations may occur during the care of a patient, and it will require a physician to, as written in EPA 10, "engage team members required for immediate response, continued decision making, and necessary follow-up to optimize patient outcomes." The physician must communicate with team members about the history and status of the patient and participate in any codes. When participating in a code they must be knowledgeable about the role of all the team members involved in the code.

EPA 13: Identify system failures and contribute to a culture of safety and improvement

The culture of safety and improvement is the responsibility of all health care workers. A physician or any learner has a responsibility to "speak up" about any systems problems that lead to errors or poor patient care. Contributing to the teamwork necessary to improve a system is also a provider's responsibility, and therefore, knowing the roles of all team members, contributing to a health team environment, and communicating properly are all imperative elements for this EPA.

Designing a Curriculum: Assessing Competencies Though EPAs to Achieve Milestones

These EPAs can be used as part of a summative evaluation to assess learners' competencies. The competencies are part of milestone assessments to determine students' overall progression during their medical education. EPAs can be adapted in a preclinical setting, such as an OSCE, or team-based workshop to evaluate various competencies. An example of the relationship between competencies, EPAs and milestones are illustrated in (Figure 1). Crosswalks are useful during the preclinical phase, phase 1, to determine the optimal courses, workshops or labs to best evaluate a particular competency. If a student successfully achieves a certain number of milestones based on competencies, then the learner may progress through the curriculum and eventually is able to move to the clinical phase, phase 2, of medical education.

The overall performances on EPAs and all of their associated competencies require that they be performed in a variety of environments to accurately assess entrustment. For Phase 2, one may design another crosswalk to determine which rotations are best suited for evaluation of particular EPAs (Table 11). The task of the EPA may vary slightly depending on the workplace context and other factors. (Linsenmeyer, M; Wimsatt L, Speicher, M; Powers, et al. 2018). Once again, milestones are checked as the learner continues through clinical rotations, eventually achieving entrustment to perform all of the EPAs and surpassing the threshold of competencies necessary to graduate to residency, where the same process will continue.

The interdependency of health care professionals requires an educator to select competencies that relate to interprofessionalism and to assess learners' ability to collaborate with those outside of their profession. These competencies, for instance, may be selected from AACOM, AAMC and IPEC. Peer reviewed tools have been used to assess competencies in medical education while the learner performs a learning activity in phase 1 or engages in a professional encounter in phase 2. Some examples of these assessment tools are illustrated below.

The Communication and Teamwork Skills (CATS) tool has been used to assess communication among interprofessional teams. CATS is completed by trained evaluators that directly observe the learner interact with a team. It assesses communication, coordination, cooperation, and situational awareness. The tool has been used in clinical teams in the operating room and during hospital rounds and has also been used during the preclinical phase in simulated environments. (Havyer,R.D.; Nelson, D.R.: Wingo, M.T.; Comfre, N.I.; Halvorsen, A.J.; McDonalds, F.S.; Reed,D.A, 2016) This tool is helpful in assessing IPEC Interprofessional Communication Competency, and the AAMC and ACCOM Interpersonal and Communication Skills competency during a leaners' involvement with EPAs 6, 9, 10 and 13.

Understanding one's role and the role of others on a team is a significant part of roles and responsibilities IPEC competencies and is significant part of AACOM and AAMC competencies of Interpersonal Communication, Patient Care, and Systems-Based Practice (Havyer et al . The readiness for Interprofessional Learning Scale (RIPLS) is often referenced as the tool to measure these competencies. It measures students' readiness for interprofessional learning and teamwork and consists of three main subscales on teamwork and collaboration, professional identity, and roles and responsibilities. This tool has been used in the classroom among medical students and fellows.

The teamwork Mini Clinical Evaluation Exercise (T-MEX) allows for evaluation of team relationships, self-awareness, and responsibility in a team, and it is also

Figure 1. IPEC competency evaluated through corresponding EPAs and Milestones derived from IPEC sub-competencies.

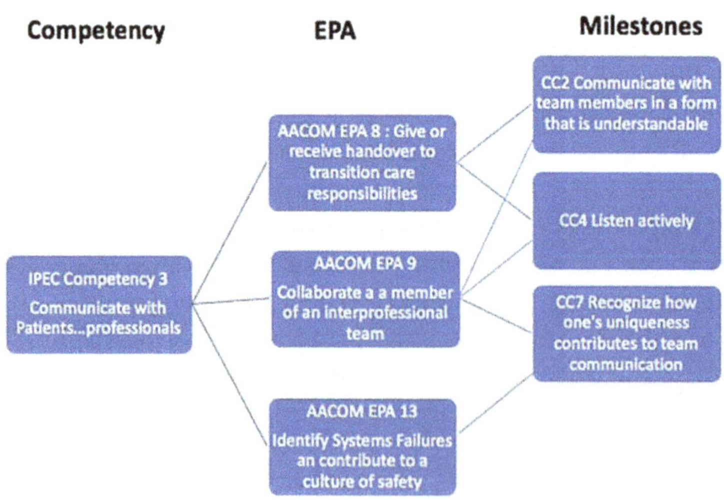

ideal for patient care, interprofessional communication, and systems-based practice competencies. The tool does not require training to use but has not been used in multiple settings. The use of this tool had been documented in the literature to assess students in the real world setting during clinical encounters (Olupeliyawa, A; Balasooriya, C; Hughes, C.; O'Sullivan, O, 2014).

EPA 9: Collaborate as a member of an interprofessional team

Table 11. Crosswalk of AAMC and AACOM EPA 9 Interprofessional Team Competency and the rotations chosen to best assess the EPA's corresponding sub-competencies

Core Sub-competency	Description	Emergency Medicine	Critical Care	Sub-Internship
IPC3	Communicate one's role to others	X	X	X
IPC4	Roles/ Responsibilities of providers	X	X	X
IPC5	Effective Communication tools	X	X	
IPC6	Give Feedback		X	X
IPC7	Shared Patient-Centered Problem Solving	X	X	X

CONCLUSION

There is no question that the primary charge of institutions of medical education is to develop exemplary future physicians. It is not incumbent upon the institutions to assure their students/graduates are experts in all healthcare professions. However, with the increasing complexity of the shifting paradigms of the healthcare systems, it is imperative that students are provided with ample opportunities to learn to work together with their healthcare professions colleagues toward the goal of team-based patient-centered care. Including elements of interprofessionalism in the medical school curriculum will not only provide additional learning opportunities but will also help break through the status quo to reinforce and normalize a culture of interprofessional collaborative practice.

Many aspects of interprofessional education and collaborative practice are still evolving and there is much room and opportunity to continue to explore and implement practices. Even within the profession, there are still some examples where there is room to continue to study and validate both educational and assessment tools. For example, relatively few valid and reliable assessment tools have been published to assess EPAs in undergraduate medical education and that is strictly within the realm of medical education (Basehore, P M; Mortensen, LH; Katsaros, EP et. Al. 2017). This fact becomes even more pronounced when parameters are adjusted to now also include teaching and assessing interprofessional concepts within the medical education curriculum.

While the quadruple aim has not specifically been addressed in this document, the vehicles of interprofessional education and collaborative practice are ideally suited to help achieve the goals of the quadruple aim It is hoped that as the healthcare professions students and ultimately the evolving healthcare practitioners continue to collaborate, these goals will come closer to fruition. The goals of improving patient outcome and experience, improving the population health, reducing per capita costs of healthcare and improving the well-being of the entire healthcare team are achievable. While we still have "Miles to Go Before We Sleep", the vision that as we narrow the gaps and increase integration of interprofessionalism into medical education and assessment, are within our grasp.

REFERENCES

Agency for Healthcare Research and Quality. (n.d.). *TeamSTEPPS®*. https://www.ahrq.gov/teamstepps/index.html

Baggs, J. G., Schmitt, M. H., Mushlin, A. I., Mitchell, P. H., Eldredge, D. H., Oakes, D., & Hutson, A. D. (1999). Association between nurse-physician collaboration and patient outcomes in three intensive care units. *Critical Care Medicine*, *27*(9), 1991–1998. doi:10.1097/00003246-199909000-00045 PMID:10507630

Basehore, P., Soper, E., Getz, R., Graneto, J., Hover, M., Kalousek, K., Katsaros, E., Kaufmann, J., Langenau, E., Linsenmeyer, M., Mehdi, S., Sexton, P., & Told, T. (2016). *Osteopathic Considerations for Core Entrustable Professional Activities (EPAs) for Entering Residency*. American Association of Colleges of Osteopathic Medicine. http://www. aacom.org/docs/default-source/med-ed-presentations/core-epas.pdf ? sfvrsn=20

Basehore, P. M., Mortensen, L. H., Katsaros, E. P., Linsenmeyer, M., McClain, E. K., Sexton, P. S., & Wadsworth, N. (2017). Entrustable Professional Activities for Entering Residency: Establishing Common Osteopathic Performance Standards in the Transition From Medical School to Residency. *The Journal of the American Osteopathic Association, 117*(11), 712–718. doi:10.7556/jaoa.2017.137 PMID:29084324

Centers for Disease Control and Prevention. (n.d.). *Public Health Professionals Gateway*. https://www.cdc.gov/publichealthgateway/publichealthservices/essentialhealthservices.html

Chen, H. C., van der Broek, W. E. S., & ten Cate, O. (2015). The Case for Use of Entrustable Professional Activities in Undergraduate Medical Education. *Academic Medicine, 90*(4), 431-436. https://www.cdc.gov/onehealth/index.html

Dickter, D. N., Stielstra, S., Mackintosh, S., Garner, S., Finocchio, V. A., & Aston, S. J. (2013). Development of the Ambulatory Team Observed Structured Clinical Evaluation (ATOSCE). *Medical Science Educator, 23*(S3, 3S), 554–558. doi:10.1007/BF03341676

Flynn, T., Carraccio, C., & Cleary, L. (2014). *Core Entrustable Professional Activities for Entering Residency: Curriculum Developers*. Association of American Medical Colleges. https:// members.aamc.org/eweb/upload/Core%20 EPA%20 Curriculum%20Dev%20Guide.pdf

Havyer, R. D., Nelson, D. R., Wingo, M. T., Comfre, N. I., Halvorsen, A. J., McDonalds, F. S., & Reed, D. A. (2016). Addressing the Interprofessional Collaboration Competencies of the Association of American Medical Colleges: A Systematic Review of Assessment Instruments in Undergraduate Medical Education. *Academic Medicine, 91*(6), 865–888. doi:10.1097/ACM.0000000000001053 PMID:26703415

Interprofessional Education Collaborative. (2016). *Core competencies for interprofessional collaborative practice: 2016 update*. Interprofessional Education Collaborative.

Interprofessional Education Collaborative Expert Panel. (2011). *Core competencies for interprofessional collaborative practice: Report of an expert panel*. Interprofessional Education Collaborative.

Linsenmeyer, M., Wimsatt, L., Speicher, M., Powers, P., Miller, S., & Katsaros, E. (2018). Assessment Considerations for Core Entrustable Professional Activities for Entering Residency. *J Am Osteopath Assoc., 118*(4), 243-251. Doi:10.7556/jaoa.2018.049

Obeso, V., Brown, D., Aiyer, M., Barron, B., Bull, J., Carter, T., Emery, M., Gillespie, C., Hormann, M., Hyderi, A., Lupi, C., Schwartz, M. L., Uthman, M., Vasilevskis, E. E., Yingling, S., & Phillipi, C. (Eds.). (2017). For Core EPAs for Entering Residency Pilot Program. Toolkits for the 13 Core Entrustable Professional Activities for Entering Residency. Washington, DC: Association of American Medical Colleges. aamc.org/initiatives/coreepas/publicationsandpresentations

Olupeliyawa, A., Balasooriya, C., Hughes, C., & O'Sullivan, O. (2014). Educational impact of an assessment of medical students' collaboration in health care teams. *Medical Education*, *48*(2), 146–156. doi:10.1111/medu.12318 PMID:24528397

Osteopathic Core Competencies for Medical Students. (2012). *American Association of Colleges of Osteopathic Medicine*. https://www.aacom.org/docs/default-source/core-competencies/corecompetencyreport2012.pdf?sfvrsn=4

Chapter 6
How to Use Technology and Telehealth to Enhance the Interprofessional Community of Practice

Steven D. Waldman
University of Missouri-Kansas City School of Medicine, USA

Corey W. Waldman
University of Texas-San Antonio School of Medicine, USA

Reid A. Waldman
UConn Health, USA

Judith Ovalle Abuabara
University of Missouri-Kansas City School of Medicine, USA

ABSTRACT

The widespread availability and use of digital technology including the internet, cell phones, remote electrocardiogram, PACS (picture archiving and communication) systems, and video chat platforms such as Facetime and Zoom have fueled the growth of telehealth. In 2013, only about 350,000 Americans utilized telehealth technology as part of their care plan, and most of these patient interactions involved the use of telephone consults. By the end of 2018, that number had jumped to over 7,000,000. Coupled with the exponential increase in the use of telehealth technology has been a rapid decrease in the cost of telehealth technology and HIPAA compliant telehealth platforms. The ease of use and relative affordability of these technologic advances make telehealth technology an ideal tool to enhance the interprofessional community of practice.

DOI: 10.4018/978-1-7998-3066-5.ch006

INTRODUCTION

The widespread availability and use of digital technology including the internet, cell phones, remote electrocardiogram, PACS (picture archiving and communication) systems, and video chat platforms such as Facetime and Zoom have fueled the growth of telehealth. In 2013, only about 350,000 Americans utilized telehealth technology as part of their care plan and most of these patient interactions involved the use of telephone consults. By the end of 2018, that number had jumped to over 7,000,000. The recent Covid-19 pandemic has led to an explosive increase in the use of telehealth, with virtual visits expected to exceed one billion interactions by the end of 2020.(Coombs, 2020) Coupled with the exponential increase in the use of telehealth technology has been a rapid decrease in the cost of telehealth technology and HIPAA compliant telehealth platforms.

Table 1. Advantages of telehealth

· Increased access to care · Improved patient engagement · Improved patient satisfaction · Improved patient autonomy · Improved clinical outcomes · Decreased costs · Improved clinical workflows · Enhanced ability for collaborative practice

The ease of use and relative affordability of these technologic advances make telehealth technology an ideal tool to enhance the interprofessional community of practice. Advantages of telehealth are summarized in Table 1 and include the expansion of access to care for remote and disadvantaged patients, improved patient engagement, improved patient satisfaction, reduced costs, improved clinical workflows, enhanced ability for collaborative practice, and most importantly, improved clinical outcomes. Because privacy and anonymity may be important to some individuals seeking help for mental health problems, telehealth has the potential to help alleviate this issue by allowing patients to receive care in the privacy of their own home. As the interprofessional healthcare team has gained experience and confidence in the use of telehealth technology, specialized applications of telehealth programs such as remote hypertension improvement programs, behavioral telehealth, and "hospital at home" programs have the potential to further leverage the benefits of telehealth. (Weinstein, Krupinski, & Doarn, 2018) (Table 2)

Table 2. Telehealth applications for behavioral health

Domain	Potential Telehealth Solutions
Interprofessional Collaboration	Real-time patient/provider and provider/provider interactive communication
Assessment	Store and forward video of patient behaviors
Medication Management	Automated text reminders to take medicines
Individual Talk Therapy	Real-time patient/provider interactive communication
Group Therapy	Real-time patient/provider interactive group communication
Support Groups For Relapse Prevention	Real-time patient/provider interactive group communication
Education	Webinars using video chat technology

Telehealth Defined

The World Health Organization defines telehealth as "*the delivery of health care services, where distance is a critical factor, by all health care professionals using information and communication technologies for the exchange of valid information, for diagnosis, treatment and prevention of disease and injuries, research and evaluation, and for the continuing education of health care providers, all in the interest of advancing the health of individuals and their communities*".(WHO, 2016) While the term telemedicine is often used interchangeably with the term telehealth, some experts suggest that telehealth describes the use of technology to communicate with patients and other members of the interprofessional healthcare team, while telemedicine describes the use of telehealth technology to actually provide patient care, e.g. virtual clinical visits, virtual consultation, remote monitoring, etc. (Wickland, 2020)

Clinical Applications of Telehealth Technology

With each advance in digital technology, telehealth continues to evolve, becoming more sophisticated in both scope and breadth. Currently, there are four basic types of telehealth technology commonly used by the interprofessional healthcare team: (1) Real-time patient/provider and provider/provider interactive communication; (2) Store-and-forward telehealth; (3) Remote monitoring; and (4) Telephone/email/text patient/provider and provider/provider communication.(Table 3) Each type of telehealth has it unique attributes and limitations, but all have in common the ability to allow the interprofessional healthcare team to enhance the care of their patients. (Tsai, J, Cheng M, Tsai, H, Hung, H, & Chen, Y, 2019)(Chakrabarti, O, 2019)

Table 3. The four common telehealth modalities

(1) Real-time patient/provider and provider/provider interactive communication (2) Store-and-forward telehealth (3) Remote monitoring (4) Telephone/email/text patient/provider and provider/provider communication

REAL-TIME PATIENT/PROVIDER AND PROVIDER/PROVIDER INTERACTIVE COMMUNICATION

Real-time patient/provider and provider/provider interactive communication, which is also know simply as real-time telehealth allows patients and providers to utilize video chat or videoconferencing software to hear and see each other in real time. Real-time telehealth has many advantages over telephone/email/text communications in that it restores many of the visual clues absent in telephone/email/text communications. This is important in that much of our communication involves non-verbal cues, with eye contact and facial expression among the most important as they create social bonds and shared understanding. It is also postulated, that the use of multiple senses with real-time patient/provider and provider/provider telehealth has the potential to heighten concentration and allow participants to better understand and retain information. This advantage can be enhanced by the fact that real-time telehealth allows the participants the benefit of the use visual aids to facilitate understanding and improve patient and learner education.

It is important to note that consumer video chat and video conferencing platforms such as Skype and Facetime may not be appropriate for most telehealth applications as they may not protect patient privacy or meet all of the privacy protections required by the Health Insurance Portability and Accountability Act(HIPAA), although some of these restrictions have been temporarily relaxed during the current pandemic. (AHIMA, 2020) It should be remembered that a patient may waive his or her privacy protections under HIPAA and a healthcare professional may disclose otherwise protected healthcare information if the provider believe that it is in the best interest of the patient, making the use of consumer video chat and video conferencing platforms acceptable in these narrow circumstances.

Store-and-Forward Telehealth

Store and forward telehealth technology is a technique by which patients and members of the interprofessional health care team can share medical information such as laboratory reports, imaging studies, medical records, videos, scientific articles, and patient and learner educational materials. Patients can also take pictures of rash, laceration, etc. and forward the image to their healthcare provider for advice. Also known asynchronous telehealth, store and forward the use of telehealth technology has really exploded with the ubiquity of smart phones. It helps busy healthcare providers leverage their clinical workflow and improve collaboration and communication because it allows the patient, primary care provider, specialists, and other members of the interprofessional healthcare team to review the information received at a time that is convenient for them. Store and forward telehealth technology enhances patient access to the care team even if members of the team are in separate locations and different time zones. This technology has its best application in the specialties of radiology, dermatology, and ophthalmology, although it is being used with increasing frequency by primary care providers and other members of the interprofessional healthcare team.

Remote Patient Monitoring

Remote patient monitoring, which is also known as telemonitoring, is a telehealth technology that allows members of the interprofessional healthcare team to remotely monitor patient vital signs, electrocardiogram, pulse oximetry, and glucose levels. Remote patient monitoring has been shown to reduce re-hospitalizations in patients which certain chronic illnesses including diabetes, cardiac arrythmias, uncontrolled hypertension, chronic obstructive lung disease, stroke, pneumonia, and patients who have been recently discharged from intensive care units. .(Weinstein, Krupinski, & Doarn, 2018) Studies suggest that remote patient monitoring encourages patients to become a more active participant in their healthcare and a more constant stream of data flowing to healthcare providers allows clinical intervention at an earlier point in time. This data allows providers to not only accurately and objectively measure what's going on with a given patient which is a distinct advantage when caring for patients who are unwilling or unable to provide the provider accurate feedback. (Hoppe, K, Williams, M, Thomas, N, Zella, J, Drewry, A, Kim, K, Havighurst, T, & Johnson, H, 2019)

Telehealth and the Interprofessional Care Team

Collaboration has been defined as "a mutually beneficial process involving active participation from autonomous individuals whose relationships are governed by negotiated shared norms and visions". While collaboration is the glue that holds the interprofessional care team together, it is the combined specialized skill sets and insights of each team member that has the power to really improve the health care experience for the patient by making the entire interprofessional healthcare team and the patient partners in the process. When all participants share a vision that is driven by the values, preferences, and preferences of the patient, improved outcomes and patient satisfaction can be expected.(Lipscome, C & Zupec, J, 2020) It is important to note that the interprofessional healthcare team will be most successful if the team views themselves as a single entity working collaboratively as a single entity for the benefit of the patient rather than individual experts who may be separated by practices, professions, and locations who practice in parallel. Furthermore, team leadership needs to be dynamic and situationally driven. A patient who has recently undergone organ transplant may be best served by having the transplant surgeon as team leader early on, with a pharmacist assuming the leadership role when management of immunosuppressant medications is the focus of the patient's care.

Because telehealth facilitates communication between the patient and the interprofessional healthcare team and the patient as well as communication between team members, this enhanced communication and connectivity has the potential to yield care that is personal, flexible, and transparent to all participants. As mentioned above, telehealth introduces efficiency and flexibility into the provision of healthcare. Done properly, telehealth can improve outcomes and patient satisfaction and engagement while at the same time reducing costs (Tietze M, Woods, S, Brown, G, Brown S, 2020).

REFERENCES

AHIMA. (n.d.). *Telehealth and Relaxed HIPAA Enforcement During COVID-19.* Retrieved from https://journal.ahima.org/ahima-special-update-telehealth-and-relaxed-hipaa-enforcement-during-covid-19/

Chakrabarti, O. (2019). Telehealth: Emerging evidence on efficiency. *International Review of Economics & Finance*, *60*, 257–264. doi:10.1016/j.iref.2018.10.021

Coombs, B. (n.d.). *Telehealth visits are booming as doctors and patients embrace distancing amid the coronavirus crisis*. Retrieved from https://www.cnbc.com/2020/04/03/telehealth-visits-could-top-1-billion-in-2020-amid-the-coronavirus-crisis.html

Hoppe, K., Williams, M., Thomas, N., Zella, J., Drewry, A., Kim, K., Havighurst, T., & Johnson, H. (2019). Telehealth with remote blood pressure monitoring for postpartum hypertension: A prospective single-cohort feasibility study. *Pregnancy Hypertension*, *15*, 171–176. doi:10.1016/j.preghy.2018.12.007 PMID:30825917

Porter, C., & Zupek, J. (2020). Use of Telehealth Experiences To Facilitate Interprofessional Education. *American Journal of Health-System Pharmacy*, *17*. doi:10.1093/ajhp/zxaa033 PMID:32179887

Tietze, M., Woods, S., Brown, G., & Brown, S. (n.d.). *Telehealth: Delivering on Interprofessional, Analytic and Patient Safety/Quality With Community Based Partnerships*. Retrieved from https://community.ania.org/HigherLogic/System/

Tsai, J., Cheng, M., Tsai, H., Hung, H., & Chen, Y. (2019). Acceptance and resistance of telehealth: The perspective of dual-factor concepts in technology adoption. *International Journal of Information Management*, *49*, 34–44. doi:10.1016/j.ijinfomgt.2019.03.003

Weinstein, R., Krupinski, E., & Doarn, C. (2018). Clinical Examination Component of Telemedicine, Telehealth, mHealth, and Connected Health Medical Practices. *The Medical Clinics of North America*, *102*(3), 533–544. doi:10.1016/j.mcna.2018.01.002 PMID:29650074

Wockland, E. (n.d.). *Is There A Difference Between Telemedicine and Telehealth?* Retrieved from https://mhealthintelligence.com/features/is-there-a-difference-between-telemedicine-and-telehealth

World Health Organization. (n.d.). *Global Health Observatory data*. Retrieved from https://www.who.int/gho/goe/telehealth/en/

Chapter 7
Geriatric Interprofessional Education:
A Practical Guide for Health Professions Educators

Tina M. Meyer
https://orcid.org/0000-0002-8435-0563
College of Health Sciences, Western University of Health Sciences, USA

Janice Hoffman Simen
College of Pharmacy, Western University of Health Sciences, USA

ABSTRACT

Older persons commonly experience complex health needs that are best met by a multifaceted healthcare team. Most healthcare disciplines provide geriatric competencies specific to their professions which support the development of IPE curricula. The American Geriatric Society provided a list of formal geriatric competencies that are useful to curriculum designers and health professions educators. The chapter provides ideas for imbedding commonly occurring geriatric concepts and clinical assessment tools that are relevant to all disciplines for the creation of interprofessional learning activities.

DOI: 10.4018/978-1-7998-3066-5.ch007

"To care for those who once cared for us is one of the highest honors". Tia Walker (Tina Meyer, DHSc, MS, PA-C; Janice Hoffman, EdD, Pharm, APh, BCGP, FASCP)

AGING

All indications affirm that the population is aging. There are currently more than 46 million persons over the age of 65 living in the US. By 2050, the number is expected to grow to nearly 90 million. Rising obesity rates, economic disparities, increasing diversity and high rates of divorce among aging persons set the stage for increasingly complex challenges as future generations of healthcare providers strive to meet their needs. The old-age dependency ratio is projected to have far-reaching effects on the ability to adequately provide for aged persons. By 2020, the US Census Bureau National Population Projections (2017) expects there will be 3.5 working-age adults for every retirement-age person. Elders are increasing while resources are decreasing.

INTERPROFESSIONAL TEAM-BASED CARE IN GERIATRICS

In the early 1900's Nascher coined the term *geriatrics* to emphasize the need to distinguish senility as a special circumstance of aging. Following WW1 and II, several social forces drove the process of geriatrics forward. Chief among them was the increasing life expectancy due to improved economies and the availability of antibiotics and intravenous fluids. Large numbers of wounded and disabled soldiers required long term care to which the medicine, nursing, and social work professions responded by training their members to better care for patients. Great Britain led in the care of the elderly in the first half of the 20th century developing chronic hospitals separate from acute care facilities. Marjory Warren, a young physician ultimately organized patients into five categories based on their functional level and care needs. Warren's work made its way to the US and was taken up by T. Franklin Williams (Forciea, 2014). Team-based care was integral to the care divisions derived by Warren. Similarly, the hospice concept championed by Dame Cicely Saunders in the 1950's advanced many nuances and benefits of team-based care. Saunders believed that the best care of persons with terminal conditions was patient-centered and required attention to physical, mental, emotional and spiritual needs. This was best accomplished in a loving home environment. With the establishment of St.

Christopher's Hospice in the UK in 1967 true interprofessional care began to take shape (Fisher, 2018).

GERIATRIC IPE CURRICULA

Older persons commonly experience complex health needs that are best met by a multifaceted healthcare team. Most health care disciplines provide geriatric competencies specific to their professions which support the development of IPE curricula. The *American Geriatric Society* (2019) provided a list of formal geriatric competencies that are useful to curriculum designers and health professions educators. A patient-centered interprofessional approach is essential to achieving the highest level of care. Although no clear statement of best practices in geriatric IPE have been identified, a review of literature revealed that *Adult Learning Theory* and *Self-Determination Theory* were the most commonly applied teaching strategies in health professions IPE curricula. The hallmark of quality IPE ensures that students learn from and about one another. Real world collaboration is simulated when students learn from and experience one another (Keijsers, et al., 2016). Other learning theories frequently included in IPE curricula involve *Contact Theory, Social Identity Theory, Social Learning Theory* and *Situated Learning Theory*. Team-based, multi and inter-professional care remain the norm in hospice, long-term care and rehabilitation environments. Benefiting from the tertiary model of expertise in conditions commonly affecting older adults, hospice, physical medicine and rehabilitation units maximize patient-centered team functioning through shared care philosophy, collaborative leadership, and maintaining team dynamics, relationships and effective communication. These environments and the health conditions they commonly address provide many ideas for IPE learning activities (Turk & Nitu-Maquise, 2015).

THE GERIATRIC TEAM

In 2010 the *World Health Organization* defined interprofessional education as two or more professions combined to learn about and from one another to enable collaboration and improve health outcomes. The interprofessional geriatric team is ideally comprised of professionals with expertise in the physical, emotional, social, psychological, spiritual, medical, ethical, legal, financial, and other areas. Team members must be adept at collaboration to achieve the goals of care. No interprofessional team is complete without robust participation from the patient and family. Every encounter is an opportunity to increase health literacy, discover needs, fears, and wishes, and to better understand the many contexts affecting the health and wellbeing of patients and families. Providing for the highest possible levels of autonomy and quality of life in all areas of the aging experience is the priority. In addition to care planning and coordination, team members must maintain constant attention through the transitions of care including: a) caregiver support, b) navigation through healthcare systems, benefits programs and community resources, c) abuse surveillance and prevention, d) health promotion and safety, and e) end-of-life care options.

IMBEDDING GERIATRIC CONCEPTS INTO IPE LEARNING ACTIVITIES

Outside the confines of geriatric specialization, many commonly held concepts set the stage for valuable interprofessional learning activities that are relevant to all health professions. Preserving function and autonomy are core concepts that drive the care of older adults. Having achieved old age, the focus of care shifts from prevention and cure to quality and comfort. Learners from all health disciplines must come to operationalize these concepts from their unique perspectives. The combined effects of the aging process, disease, environmental and lifestyle factors are integral to the normal aging process. Geriatricians speak of the *Rule of Thirds* (Sloane, 1992) when determining the cause of decline in function. Approximately one third of overall decline is due to disease, one third to disuse, and the remaining third to normal aging. Nearly every professional who regularly cares for older adults has heard the mantra, *go, but go slow* when prescribing drug treatments. In general, aging is associated with atrophy, such that providers of elder care often become concerned when the liver or spleen is easily palpated. Similarly, lung changes on spirometry signal concern because it is widely accepted that intrinsic capacity of the lungs is adequate to overcome the changes associated with aging.

According to 2015 data from the *National Council for Aging*, one in four elders in the US experience a fall annually resulting in more than 2.8 million injuries at a cost of $50 billion. Commonly applied tools to assess fall risk include a) *Fall risk management*, b) *Timed Up and Go, c) Gait Speed*, d) *Resistance to Nudge* and others. Many standardized instruments exist to assess the functional, cognitive, psychological, social, and economic status of older adults. These tools are valuable in documenting improvements or declines that herald the need for changes in the care plan. Some assessments do not require medical background or training and may be applied by non-clinicians, care givers, and family members. Introducing assessment tools into the IPE curriculum provides learners from all disciplines with insights to resources that improve the care of elders and impower patients and families through education.

The effects of aging on the body. The rate of decline of function in most organs is approximately 1% annually after the age of 40. The result is that by age 70, the global loss of function is approximately 30% of the individuals peak in young adulthood (Walston, 2016). Hearing and vision are often exceptions to the general rule with decline commonly beginning by about age 25. Lean muscle mass begins to decline at approximately age 30. As a result, older adults may have as much as one-third more fat compared to their younger baseline. The change from lean to fat tissue has far reaching effects on medication management. Height loss of approximately one-half inch every 10 years begins about age 40 and accelerates after age 70 for a total loss of 1-3 inches. Men often gain weight up to age 55 and then begin to lose as they age. Women frequently gain weight to about age 65. Fat is lighter than lean muscle and likely accounts for majority of weight loss in the 6th and 7th decades (Shah & Villareal, (2017). Healthcare providers must remain alert to physiologic changes of aging in addition to changes associated with specific disease processes. An elder with congestive heart failure (CHF) and chronic kidney disease (CKD) stage 3 or 4, will likely not benefit from a thiazide diuretic because the kidneys are not functional at the proximal tubules. Therefore, loop diuretics are an alternative therapy when diuretics are needed to unload excessive fluid.

Normal aging includes decline in sensory function that may affect appetite and weight control. During hunger receptors are activated which stimulate the olfactory bulb and cortex. The smell of food stimulates appetite. Upon tasting desired foods, the appetite is further enhanced. When olfaction and taste are reduced the body may not signal the need or the desire to eat (Zoon, et al., 2016). Additional to these biological changes, many medications such the ACE-I class of drugs an alter the sense of taste and smell.

Low vision impacts the ability to read a prescription label resulting in possible medication compliance issues. Hearing loss may make it difficult to comply with care instructions. When instructions are not adhered to the savvy geriatric provider refrains from automatically assuming that the patient is willfully non-compliant.

Learning activities addressing common effects of aging. Health professions students should practice ways to accommodate for sensory changes during the geriatric IPE curricula:

- Ensure instructions are both verbal and written. If possible, involve a family member or caregiver in the process to assist the patient;
- When providing written instructions, us a larger font size (20 or above) and a san serif style;
- Assess the patient with weight loss carefully. Ask about taste and smell as well as monitor electrolytes, lipids and albumin levels. Consult with a dietician or nutritionist to assist with weight issues;

Table 1. Functional Systems and Functional Changes.

Functional Systems	Functional Changes
Sensory Losses	• Reduced sense of taste, smell, sight, hearing, touch
Oral Health Status	• Xerostomia - dry mouth caused by hyposalivation • Dentures and periodontal problems
Gastrointestinal	• Hypochlorhydria – low level of stomach acid • Constipation
Metabolic/Endocrine	• Decreased glucose tolerance • 15-20% decline in resting metabolic rate & thyroid function • Decrease in hormones-estrogen, testosterone, growth with decrease bone density, sexual function, muscle mass and strength
Renal	• Mass and weight of kidneys decline (atrophy) • Decreased glomerular filtration rate (GFR) • Electrolyte imbalances • Urinary incontinence
Cardiovascular	• Loss of elasticity in blood vessels and decreased relaxation phase of the heart cycle with increase of peripheral resistance and isolated systolic hypertension • diminished baroreceptors causing orthostatic hypotension and syncope • ♂: cholesterol peak ~60 y.o. • ♀: total cholesterol + LDL continue to rise until ~70 y.o.

· Monitor vital signs and complete a physical exam on every visit;
· Monitor labs routinely and more often if the patient is symptomatic of a change; for example:
  ◦ Warfarin therapy requires a monthly INR;
  ◦ When diuretics are taken electrolytes and renal function (chem 7) should be evaluated at least twice annually or more often as indicated;
  ◦ When Angiotensin-Converting Enzyme Inhibitors (ACEi) or Angiotensin Receptor Blockers (ARB) are prescribed electrolytes, especially changes in potassium, and renal function must be monitored regularly.

The *Comprehensive Geriatric Assessment* (CGA) is a multidisciplinary process that assesses five broad domains of health: Physical medical conditions, mental health conditions, functional abilities, social circumstances, and environment. Standardized scales may be applied by the team members within each of the domains and are useful in detecting changes over time. Multidimensional input from all team members produces an accurate problem list and provides for the information needed to prioritize needs and drive an integrated treatment plan. While learners may not yet possess the clinical expertise to fully master the complexities of the CGA, valuable learning activities may be derived from it as part of an IPE geriatric curriculum.

Functional assessments include basic activities of daily living, (BADL's) instrumental activities of daily living, (IADL's) and advanced activities of daily living (AADL's). BADL's are necessary to live in their own residence such as transferring, toileting, bathing, dressing, and feeding. IADS's are those activities necessary to maintain independence including shopping, driving, meal preparation, telephone operation, managing medications, doing laundry, and managing housework and home repairs. AADL's include societal, family, recreational, and occupational tasks. AADL's are sometimes assessed by quality of life instruments such as the Study Short Form 36, and Short-Form 12.

Polypharmacy and Pharmacodynamics. Older persons are at a higher risk of medication-related problems. During normal aging changes in pharmacokinetics and pharmacodynamics effect the properties of medications. As chronic diseases progress to end stage and co-morbidities increase, multiple prescribers engage in the care and can lead to unintentional drug interactions, overprescribing, and other challenges inherent to polypharmacy.

"Any symptom in an elderly patient should be considered a drug side effect until proved otherwise." (Gurwitz, et, al., 1995). As Gurwitz suggests in this quote, FIRST consider what you in your geriatric patient as a consequence of medication use. Medication side effects can range from sedation to renal impairment or a mechanical fall leading to hospitalization. Equally as important is to ask about other prescriber visits. Many geriatric patients see 3-5 specialists including cardiology, nephrology, rheumatology, oncology, dermatology, psychiatry and urology or gynecology to name a few. The more specialists a patient sees, the higher the risk of polypharmacy. Geriatric patients with 5 doctors had 42 prescriptions annually at risk for 16 errors (Rollason & Vogt, 2003).

Polypharmacy occurs when multiple medications are used for the same or similar conditions (duplicate therapy) or when a large number of medications are prescribed. Previously, a total of 9 medications indicated the benchmark defining polypharmacy and many providers continue to use the number of 9 to signal concern. The more medications employed the higher the risk of drug interactions and synergistic adverse effects. Each year more than 9 million adverse drug reactions occur in older Americans (Zhan &Bierman, 2001). In the geriatric population, 28% of hospitalizations were due to adverse reactions to medication with 11% related to non-compliance. Geriatric patients taking three or more chronic medications had a 33% risk of re-hospitalization within 6 months of discharge and 20% of those re-admissions were due to Medication-Related Problems (Rollason & Vogt, 2003).

According to the Center for Disease Control (2016)), 90.8% of those aged 65 and over, took a prescription drug in the past month. When the CDC compared 1988-94 to 2013-14, an increase of 17.2% was observed in adults aged 65 and over taking more than one prescription. The use of five or more prescriptions increased 28.4% in the same age group.

Health professions students should learn to suspect polypharmacy when the patient is needing refills of medications too quickly or when an agent prescribed for a temporary problem is refilled for too long a duration. For instance, antiemetic agents needed for longer than a couple of weeks should raise concern. The side effect profile of all medications prescribed must be carefully analyzed. The antiemetic may not be necessary if another drug causing nausea and vomiting is changed to an alternative with a better side effect profile. Students must learn to consider whether an additional medication is truly needed. If the treatment is for a side effect of another medication, changing the offending medication is likely a better option for the patient.

Pharmacodynamics. Pharmacodynamics describes the effect a drug has on the body. Pharmacokinetics indicate what the body does to the drug. Normal aging causes a decrease in the number of drug receptors as well as a change in sensitivity, resulting in changes in pharmacodynamics. Changes in homeostatic mechanisms such decreased baroreceptor sensitivity leads to very low blood pressure with the use of antihypertensive agents. Because of this change, many elders, particularly those over 90-years-old require lower doses of antihypertensive medications. In some instances, antihypertensives may be discontinued. Modest elevations in blood pressure may lead to increased brain perfusion resulting in improved cognition and decreased fall risk especially in persons over 90 years of age (Reinberg, 2017).

Age-related changes in the Central Nervous System (CNS) include a reduction in blood flow leading to decreased oxygenation. An increase in monoamine oxidase levels decreases norepinephrine and dopamine. Additionally, there is an increase in sensitivity to anticholinergic and sedative agents and increased permeability across the Blood Brain Barrier resulting in increased confusion and sedation. These pharmacodynamic changes contribute to higher fall risk and declines in mentation and overall function.

Avoiding Polypharmacy. To avoid polypharmacy, it is important to understand and recognize the side effects of prescribed medications and consider the risk versus benefit ratio of medication use for each individual patient.

Health professions students should pose the following questions:

- Is each medication necessary?
- Is any of the medication regimen contraindicated in the elderly?
- Are there any duplicate medications from the same drug class (I.e. Lorazepam for anxiety and Temazepam for sleep)?
- Is the patient taking the lowest effective dose?
- Can the medication regimen be simplified? Can any unnecessary medications be discontinued?

- Is the patient taking any similar nonprescription medications? Are there any potentially dangerous drug interactions? (Singh, 2010).

Experts indicate majority of clinical encounters result in one or more prescriptions. The *Assess-Review-Minimize-Optimize-Reassess* (ARMOR) tool may be applied to assess and ultimately avoid polypharmacy. ARMOR emphasizes quality of life as a key component in decision-making for medication changes (Kohll, 2010). The total number of medications are *ASSESSED* with attention to drugs with potential adverse outcomes. All medications are *REVIEW*ed for interactions, functional impacts, and risk to benefit ratio. During the *MINIMIZE* phase all non-essential medications are eliminated. The remaining drugs are assessed for duplication, renal and hepatic clearance, and target effects to *OPTIMIZE* the regimen. Lastly, vital signs, status of function, cognition, clinical conditions, and medication compliance are evaluated during the *REASSESS* phase.

Over 90-years old. It is estimated that persons over the age of 65 in the US will increase to over 2 billion by 2050. Persons aged 80 years and over will expand at the fastest rate (Ryan, O'Sullivan & Jackson, 2016). Currently, 12.6% of the US population is over 65 years old (1 in 8). By 2030, the geriatric population is estimated to climb to over 22% or1 in 5 (Mueller, Schur & O'Connell, 1997; Avorn,1990). It is essential that healthcare professionals obtain the skills to care for, prescribe, and supervise the use of medicines in this vulnerable group of patients.

One of the most concerning issues from a medication perspective is that clinical studies generally to not extend into the 80 to 90-year-old patient population. We don't truly know what medications do in this group nor do we know if medications need to be continued. Many intriguing, real-world circumstances are highly suitable to a geriatric IPE curriculum. Consider the case of the Type II Diabetic patient who is 95 years old: Does this patient still benefit from tight control of blood sugars or blood pressure? The treatment goal of Type II diabetes is to avoid long-term macro and microvascular complications such as retinopathy, renal, and cardiovascular changes. Teams of interprofessional students should ponder if, at 95 years of age, quality of life issues should become the focus of care over the physical issues? Should the patient be able to eat what they desire and is a hemoglobulin A1c of 8 or 9 acceptable for a 95-year-old patient? Are blood pressure medications or antilipemic agents needed at 95 years of age? Can the medication list be reduced to assist the patient with medication adherence, and will that result in a quality of life difference compared to a quantity of life with poorer quality? One of the last choices in life is to choose to eat or not eat. As healthcare professionals, should we encourage a patient to eat for quality of life?

Abuse. Awareness and prevention of elder abuse is a universal concern and responsibility. The conservative estimate of persons over the age of 60 who experience abuse in community settings was 1-in-6 or 15.7% (Yon, et al., 2017). Only 1-in-24 cases are thought to be reported. While an exact number is not known, anecdotal reports indicate that the incidence is much higher in institutional settings. Self-reports from staff in facilities in six countries revealed that 64.2% admitted having perpetrated some form of abuse in the past year (WHO, 2018). All health professions students benefit from learning the commonly occurring types of abuse, risk stratification of patients and caregivers, roles of the team members in responding to abuse, and the resources available to vulnerable seniors in need of protection. The ability to communicate with patients, clients and caregivers is crucial to the successful management of sensitive situations that are prone to emotional escalation, and legal and ethical liabilities. Crucial conversations and best practices in documentation are weighty topics well worth the IPE curriculum.

Advanced Directives. All geriatric team members must be adept at speaking to patients and families about end-of-life care and wishes. The documentation of Advance Directives are important elements that comprise important IPE learning activities. Every team member must respect the choices made by patients and surrogate decision makers. The IPE curriculum affords important opportunities to a) learn the concepts of beneficence, non-maleficence, advance care directives, and conservatorship, b) address personal bias in care and end-of-life choices, c) practice communication involving sensitive topics, and d) perform patient advocacy.

Mentation and cognition. The WHO (2019) reported the worldwide prevalence of dementia was 50 million with nearly 10 million new cases diagnosed each year. Dementia is a progressive syndrome that affects memory, orientation, thinking, learning, judgment, emotional control, social behavior, motivation, language, and movement. Dementia occurs in different forms and progresses through early, middle and late stages. Alzheimer type is the most common form of dementia at 60-70%. Other common types are Vascular, Lewy Body, and Frontal Lobe dementias. The clinical presentation of dementias in the moderate and severe stages is indistinct. Students should learn that taking a thorough history of the onset of dementia and the sequence of early changes is a valuable key to determining the dementia type. For example, Lewy Body Dementia (LBD) includes extrapyramidal signs similar with Parkinson's Disease (PD). The two may be distinguished by the fact that dementia is typically an early occurrence in LBD and a late occurrence in PD.

Persons with Mild Cognitive Deficit are often able to maintain a great deal of autonomy. Memory aids such as note keeping and reminders may be sufficient. With the onset of behavior changes, decreased judgement, safety issues, and loss of executive functions, ongoing care becomes multifaceted and persistent. Clinical cases concerning dementia are ripe for inclusion in geriatric IPE curricula due to the myriad domains of care involved. Family dynamics are magnified as challenges mount. Communication challenges within families and social groups become more significant. Family culture is essential to effectively managing the needs for caregiving, conservatorship, financial responsibility, etc. Behavior changes are especially challenging for families and care teams. Fear and agitation are common. Wandering, loss of spatial orientation leading to being lost even in familiar environments, and concepts of Sundowning and decreased night-time sleep are especially taxing for caregivers. Cognitive, mental, and emotional status have significant impacts on the needs of older adults.

The *Geriatric Depression Scale*, both the long and the short form, is widely utilized to recognize depression and to track the effects of interventions. The questions may be administered by anyone. Persons who are able may complete the questionnaire independently. A score of five or greater on the short form, or greater than 10 on the long form indicates clinical depression. The ability to attend to the test may be impacted by cognitive dysfunction but still renders a reliable result for persons who are able to grasp the questions.

When cognitive impairment is suspected, the *Mini-Cog* and the *Folstein Mini Mental Status Exam* (MMSE) are highly reliable assessments of cognition and memory. The Mini-Cog takes moments to complete and consists of two parts; a three-item recall test for memory, and a clock draw. The MMSE consists of 30 questions and takes approximately 15 minutes to complete. The tool measures registration, attention, calculation, recall, language, orientation, and the ability to follow simple commands. A score of 19-23 indicates mild impairment, 10-18 indicates moderate impairment, and less than 9 indicates severe cognitive impairment.

The *Global Deterioration Scale for the Assessment of Primary Degenerative Dementia* (GDS) provides a measure for staging the progression of dementia. Stages 1-3 are termed pre-dementia. Stages 4-7 describe the escalating effects of dementia ranging from mild to severe. The instrument utilizes common language and is suitable for non-clinicians making it a user-friendly tool for novice health professions students. The accurate descriptions of behavior in the various stages makes it a useful learning resource for students. It is important to note that the tools discussed do not diagnose the cause of the cognitive decline nor distinguish between types of dementia. Neither are they able to differentiate dementia from delirium.

P.K. Bevelle developed the *12-minute Experience of dementia.* The sensory alteration tool simulates age-related cognitive and physical changes. With a small investment programs can obtain the tools to provide students with the experience. Learners are provided a) goggles that simulate macular degeneration, b) gloves that mimic diminished dexterity and finger sensation, c) shoe inserts that simulate painful or difficult ambulation, and d) headphones that emit white noise to simulate reduced hearing and mental confusion. Upon receiving verbal instructions while wearing the gear, learners complete 5 simple daily tasks such as locating an item of clothing, putting dishes away, and other common activities (Clark, 2018).

Delirium. Delirium is marked by a sudden decline in mentation that is caused by a medical condition. It is common for untrained persons to mistake reversible conditions for progression of dementia, especially as dementia progresses. Cases of delirium are commonly due to new onset infections such as pneumonia, urinary tract infection in elders with dementia, and medication adverse effects, although many other conditions may cause the sudden decline (Hshieh, et al. 2014). All members of the care team must be proactive in responding to early suspicions of delirium from each professions' perspective. Therefore, IPE learning activities concerning delirium are especially appropriate to geriatric curricula.

Diminished capacity and competence. The determination of competence to manage one's own affairs is a very serious undertaking for geriatric care teams. Merriam-Webster defines competence as the state of having adequate skill and judgement for a specific duty. Competence is a legal provision that is tied to the execution of one's civil liberties. Capacity refers to an individual's mental or physical ability. The determination of competence/capacity based on medical conditions is usually the responsibility of the physician. Some states may permit Physician Assistants and Nurse Practitioners to determine competence in specific circumstances. The declaration of incompetence is the purview of the court.

Conservatorship implies the legal right and responsibility to make decisions and provide care for an elder who is no longer competent. Conservators may be appointed by the court. In many instances, conservatorship is determined by the individual before the onset of incapacity as in the case of *Advanced Directives* or the allocation of *Durable Power of Attorney*. Surrogate decision-makers are responsible for acting in the patient's best interest and deciding as the patient would if they were able (Cohen, et al. 2015). IPE cases and discussions of beneficence, non-maleficence, heroic measures, the living will, assisted suicide and others are all highly beneficial to health professions students from all disciplines. In addition to learning the role of each member of the treatment team, students benefit from understanding the roles of the patient, family, government, court, conservators, and surrogate decision makers.

Social and cultural considerations. The culturally sensitive geriatric team sees the older adult as a whole person comprised of physical, emotional, social and spiritual dimensions. Through the practice of person-centered care, continuity is preserved in the lives of elderly patients. Person-centered care engages health and social services as equal partners that combine to meet patient needs in real time. Consideration of persons desires, values, family circumstances, lifestyle, family and community roles are key factors in care decisions. Flexibility in prioritizing needs as they arise are hallmarks of culturally sensitive person-centered care (Gunn-Tove, 2015). Integrating an individual's spiritual practice serves to personalize the care and improve health outcomes. One's spiritual perspective is key to understanding how they approach loss, illness, disability, and mortality. True patient-centered care demands that health care professionals learn to understand and maximize the wishes of the patient whether one agrees with them or not. The care team must become familiar with a variety of faith traditions and adept at facilitating elders to participate as much as possible or desired (Lavretsky, 2010). Perhaps nowhere than during end-of-life care are geriatric teams more confronted with the needs of cultural sensitivity. Palliative care focuses on symptom control and comfort to maximize the quality of life. Team members must be aware that for some cultures discussing impending death is considered inappropriate. Others openly discuss concepts of an after-life and varying beliefs about transitioning to a spiritual realm. Certain African, Asian, Chinese, East Indian, Indonesian, Japanese, Native American, and Vietnamese families may request that a terminal diagnosis be withheld from the elderly patient. The goal is to diminish emotional stress and preserve hope. Traditional Taiwanese culture asserts that bad luck occurs if one speaks of impending death out loud. Persons from the Christian Scientist, Hindu, Jehovah's Witness, Mormon, Muslim and Seventh-day Adventist traditions may be opposed to some drugs and other measures that appear to hasten death. Persons who practice Buddhism may reject drugs that are thought to cloud the mind as the patient nears death (Givler & Maani-Fogeman, 2019).

Clinical and end-stage disease. End of life care includes the subdomains of symptom control, the so-called *good death*, after-care and bereavement. The hospice model of care encompasses the needs of family and loved ones to facilitate peace of mind and effective final communications with loved ones. A plethora of assessment tools are available for palliative care that can provide meaningful interprofessional learning experiences. The Agency for Healthcare Research and Quality Technical Brief Number 30 (2017) identified 152 palliative care assessment tools in eight domains. The tools encompass a) structure and process, b) physical, c) psychological and psychiatric, d) social aspects of care, e) spiritual, religious and existential, f) cultural, g) care at end of life, h) bereavement, and i) ethical and legal.

SUMMARY

The world of gerontology and geriatrics provides vast opportunities for interprofessional education and practice among healthcare disciplines:

- Curriculum designers are encouraged to carefully consider the comprehensive needs of elders before deciding against including a discipline. Non-traditional healthcare professions such as real estate, transportation, and financial management bring depth and breadth to the team as they ponder the daily lived experience and needs of older persons.

- Simulations, role play and other experiential activities provide learners the aging experience to better understand limitations and needs.
- Learners should assume professional roles on the team other than their own to gain a deeper understanding and appreciation of those professions.
- Standardized tools and assessments abound in geriatrics and provide framework for learning activities and objectives. They also serve to enforce the awareness and application of resources.
- IPE teams must obtain and model effective communication and team skills. Feedback should be timely, honest, relevant and constructive.
- Feedback should include acknowledgement of what students do well as well as specific and achievable objectives for areas needing improvement.
- Educators should remain alert to the needs of students who may experience difficulty as they engage in sensitive topics of aging, mortality, end-of-life care, loss, grief, family dynamics, and bereavement. Reflective exercises are important aspects of all geriatric curricula as learners grow professionally and personally throughout the process.
- As students grapple with the multifaced and complex issues inherent to geriatrics, educators should remain alert to combating frustration and the tendency to become overwhelmed. Learners must be reminded that they do not have to know everything; rather, they need to know where to locate resources to help address the elderly patients needs.
- In constructing cases, curriculum designers are cautioned to avoid overwhelming novice learners with complicated elements. During the early phases of education, it is best to include commonly occurring conditions and situations. As learners progress, the complexity of patient cases and problem lists may increase.
- Barriers to IPE in geriatrics are not unlike those of IPE in general. Issues of scheduling, budget, varying accreditation, professional bias, time, grading practices, faculty availability, and continuity of curriculum are common elements that often need to be readdressed from year-to-year.

A comprehensive list of pearls of geriatric interprofessional education are beyond the scope of a single book chapter. Perhaps the most fundamental element of geriatric IPE curricula is to ensure that learners understand that interprofessional practice is not an option to providing quality care to elders; it is essential.

REFERENCES

Agency for Healthcare Research and Quality. (2017). *Assessment tools for palliative care. Technical Brief Number 30.* Retrieved from https://effectivehealthcare.ahrq.gov/sites/default/files/pdf/palliative-care-tools_technical-brief-2017.pdf

American Geriatric Society. (2019). *Existing formal geriatric competencies and milestones*. Accessed June 13, 2019 from https://www.americangeriatrics.org/geriatrics-profession/core-competencies

Avorn, J. (1990). The elderly and drug policy: Coming of age. *Health Affairs*, *9*(3), 6–19. doi:10.1377/hlthaff.9.3.6 PMID:2121636

Capacity. (2019). In *Merriam-Webster.com*. Retrieved September 1, 2019 from https://www.merriam-webster.com/dictionary/capacity

Centers for Disease Control. (2016). *Health U.S. Chartbook on Long-term Trends Report 2016*, pg. 25. Retrieved from https://www.cdc.gov/nchs/data/hus/hus16.pdf

Clark, A. (2018). What does Alzheiumer's Disease feel like? *The Senior List*. Retrieved from https://www.theseniorlist.com/blog/patented-tool-provides-a-glimpse-into-the-world-of-alzheimers-disease/

Cohen, A. B., Wright, M. S., Cooney, L. Jr, & Fried, T. (2015). Guardianship and end-of-life decision making. *Journal of the American Medical Association. Internal Medicine (Tokyo, Japan)*, *175*(10), 1687–1691.

Competence. (2019). In *Merriam-Webster.com*. Retrieved September 1, 2019 from https://www.merriam-webster.com/dictionary/competence

Fisher, N. (2018). The history of hospice: A different kind of health care. *Forbes*. Retrieved from https://www.forbes.com/sites/nicolefisher/2018/06/22/the-history-of-hospice-a-different-kind-of-health-care/#7a072e70660c

Forciea, M. A. (2014). Geriatric Medicine: History of a young specialty. *American Medical Association Journal of Ethics*, *16*(5), 385–389. PMID:24847710

Givler, A., & Maani-Fogelman, P. A. (2019). The importance of cultural competence in pain and palliative care. *StatPearls, 5*(13). Retrieved from https://www.ncbi.nlm.nih.gov/books/NBK493154/

Gunn-Tove, M. (2015). A culturally sensitive approach to elderly care. *The Journal of Gerontology and Geriatric Research, 4*(241). Retrieved from https://www.omicsonline.org/open-access/a-culturallysensitive-approach-to-elderly-care-2167-7182-1000241.php?aid=64251

Hshieh, T., Inouye, T., & Inouye, S. (2014). Delirium. In Current Diagnosis and Treatment: Geriatrics (2nd ed.). Academic Press.

Keijsers, C.J.P.W., Dreher, R., Tanner, S., Forde-Johnston, C., Thompson, S. (2016). Interprofessional education in geriatric medicine. *Elsevier Masson SAS*. doi:10.1016/j.eurger.2016.01.011

Kohll, D. (2010). *Multiple Medication Dilemmas*. Retrieved from http://www.dorlandhealth.com

Lavretsky, H. (2010). Spirituality and aging. *Medscape. Aging Health*, *6*(6), 749–769. doi:10.2217/ahe.10.70

Mueller, C., Schur, C., & O'Connell, J. (1997). Prescription drug spending: The impact of age and chronic disease status. *American Journal of Public Health*, *87*(10), 1626–1629. doi:10.2105/AJPH.87.10.1626 PMID:9357343

Reinberg, S. (2017). High blood pressure may not be all bad in elderly. *WebMD*. Retrieved from https://www.webmd.com/hypertension-high-blood-pressure/news/20170117/high-blood-pressure-elderly-dementia#1

Rollason, V., & Vogt, N. (2003). Reduction of Polypharmacy in the Elderly. *Drugs & Aging*, *20*(11), 817–832. doi:10.2165/00002512-200320110-00003 PMID:12964888

Ryan, D. J., O'Sullivan, F., & Jackson, S. H. D. (2016). Clinical pharmacology: Prescribing medicines for older patients. *Medicine*, *44*(7), 433–437. doi:10.1016/j.mpmed.2016.04.005

Shah, K., & Villareal, D. T. (2017). Obesity. In H. M. Fillit, K. Rockwood, & J. Young (Eds.), *Brocklehurst's Textbook of Geriatric Medicine* (8th ed.). Elsevier.

Singh, U. (n.d.). *Department of Geriatrics*. Retrieved from https://www.healthplanofnevada.com

Tinnetti, M. E., Williams, T. F., & Mayewski, R. (1986). Fall Risk Assessment for elderly patients based on number of chronic disabilities. *The American Journal of Medicine*, *80*(3), 429–434. doi:10.1016/0002-9343(86)90717-5 PMID:3953620

Turk, M. A., & Nitu-Maquise, A. D. (2015). Rehabilitation team functioning. *Physical Medicine & Rehabilitation Knowledge*. https://now.aapmr.org/rehabilitation-team-functioning/

United States Census Bureau. (2017). *Population Projections*. Retrieved from https://www.census.gov/programs-surveys/popproj.html

United States Census Bureau. (2018). Older people projected to outnumber children for the first time in US history. *Newsroom*. Release number CB18-41. Retrieved from https://www.census.gov/newsroom/press-releases/2018/cb18-41-population-projections.html on September 18, 2019.

Walston, J. D. (2016). Common clinical sequelae of aging. In L. Goldman & A. Schafer (Eds.), *Goldman-Cecil Medicine* (25th ed.). Elsevier Saunders.

World Health Organization. (2010). Framework for action on interprofessional education and collaborative practice. Health Professions Network Nursing and Midwifery Office within the Department of Human Resources for Health.

World Health Organization. (2018). *Abuse Fact Sheet*. Retrieved from https://www.who.int/news-room/fact-sheets/detail/elder-abuse

World Health Organization. (2019). *Dementia Fact Sheet*. Retrieved from https://www.who.int/news-room/fact-sheets/detail/dementia

Yon, Y., Mikton, C. R., Gassoumis, Z. D., & Wilber, K. H. (2017). Elder abuse prevalence in community settings: A systematic review and meta-analysis. *The Lancet. Global Health*, *5*(2), e147–e156. Advance online publication. doi:10.1016/S2214-109X(17)30006-2 PMID:28104184

Zhan, C., Sangl, J., Bierman, A. S., Miller, M. R., Friedman, B., Wickizer, S. W., & Meyer, G. S. (2001). Potentially inappropriate medication use in the community-dwelling elderly. Findings from the 1996 medical expenditure panel survey. *Journal of the American Medical Association*, *286*(22), 2823–2829. doi:10.1001/jama.286.22.2823 PMID:11735757

Zoon, H. F. A., deGraf, C., & Boesveldt, S. (2016). Food odours direct specific appetite. *Foods, 5*(1). Retrieved from https://www.ncbi.nlm.nih.gov/pmc/articles/PMC5224573/

Chapter 8
Meeting the Learning Demands of a Dynamic Teaching Era:
The Challenge-Based Learning Strategy

Belinda del Carmen Carrión Chavarría
https://orcid.org/0000-0002-4245-1139
Escuela de Medicina y Ciencias de la Salud, Tecnologico de Monterrey, Mexico

Abigail Montserrat Molina Rodriguez
Escuela de Medicina y Ciencias de la Salud, Tecnologico de Monterrey, Mexico

Mildred Vanessa López Cabrera
https://orcid.org/0000-0002-6965-6636
Escuela de Medicina y Ciencias de la Salud, Tecnologico de Monterrey, Mexico

ABSTRACT

Teaching in the 21st century requires universities to offer educational programs based on skill development, student-centered settings, focus on the needs of the community, and context-rich experiences that prepare graduates for both local and international practice. Several educational strategies and trends have been designed and implemented to incorporate rapid sociocultural and care model transitions. This chapter focuses on the challenge-based learning (CBL) strategy application in medical education to foster a transformative learning experience in which the patient is the center of the educational process. Several examples of CBL are presented, and an analysis is performed of the benefits and difficulties for its implementation in medical education. In the end, there is a discussion about enabling resources and dynamics for excellence in medical education.

DOI: 10.4018/978-1-7998-3066-5.ch008

INTRODUCTION

In the present day, globalized society evolves exponentially linked to its knowledge-based economy. Every day there are new technological discoveries, challenges, and economic crises. Students and professionals realize that what they learned a year ago may now seem pointless. In an ever-changing society, professions need to meet demands that didn't exist before. Competition for both institutions and individuals is higher than ever (Yang et al., 2018)

Society is caught in the grip of this crisis, as it threatens the ability of new generations to evolve and therefore achieve success in work and life. The need for action is urgent to solve social, cultural, and economic challenges (Apple Inc, 2008). Particularly, education is faced with its own challenge because traditional teaching methods, like didactic teaching in the classroom, spoon-feeding approaches to teaching, big class sizes, and assessment via summative final examinations, are not enough. Those practices are even perceived as potentially inhibiting students' creativity and growth (Zhou, 2012).

For the advances to take place, creative thinking has become relevant across many areas of modern life, including education, medicine, and art. Evidence suggests that the skills of creative thinking can be learned and taught (Mahdi et al., 2015). In the XXI century, the main challenge for universities is not only to catch up with this evolution but to dream ahead and make an educational offer targeted for skill development, student-centered and focused on the needs of the community, to prepare their graduates for both local and international practice.

Health is a very dynamic pad where challenges and opportunities emerge daily due to indirect factors such as climate change, new disease vectors, and technology. This last one, technology is not just part of the doctors or healthcare team but also of providers and patients who are now equipped with wide access to information by the touch of a screen. Possible diagnoses and suspicious of complications are now available as information in daily life management. This constant access to information makes the need for users and students to be highly critical of the quality and the hidden interests of the information that is available for them (Chan, 2013).

Medical education is constantly in a process of redesign and change. The motivation to use non-traditional methodologies. The motivation to use non-traditional methodologies comes from the observation and experimentation of student behavior in traditional classes; there is a relationship between the type of stimulus received and the engagement of students during a lesson (Scheele et al., 2008). Medical schools have implemented major changes in educational strategies in the curriculum. Some examples offer patient-center education, simulation, challenge-based learning and others have been emerging as part of the new education agenda (Ozkan et al., 2006). In this environment, Challenge-based learning (CBL) has emerged as a leading strategy; it becomes an opportunity where teachers can guide their students across a medical challenge and encourages them to find a real solution. (Apple, 2008).

CBL as a teaching and learning method incorporates technology, teamwork, self-directed learning, peer learning, real-world problem solving, and reflective learning, which can extend from the classroom into the local community (Johnson and Adams, 2011). While in other methodologies the teacher usually proposes the content or problems associated with specific content, followed by practical activities that involve such content, CBL takes first the practical activity to then define the content that must be learned to solve the challenge. In CBL students are expected to ask questions, search the literature, conduct a preliminary survey, consult experts and try themselves hands-on activities (Yeng et al., 2018).

The objectives of this chapter are to: Describe the key elements to implement the Challenge Based Learning strategy, to analyze the benefits and difficulties of implementing Challenge Based Learning in medical education and to identify enabling resources within the own institution.

BACKGROUND

Challenge Based Learning (CBL) has emerged as a new approach to engage students in creative and innovative learning. Participants develop solutions that require an interdisciplinary and creative approach in which they acquire disciplinary and generic skills (Olivares et al., 2018). Generational changes have reached the classroom and clinical settings. Students now carry to class their computers and smartphones as tools for learning, as they used to take the stethoscope ten years ago (Johnson, Smith, Smythe & Varon, 2009).

For enterprises like Apple, CBL is an engaging, multidisciplinary approach, where students leverage the technology they use in their daily lives. The focus of their efforts is to solve complex and real-world problems in a safe environment of constant collaboration. This hands-on projects students work with other students, educators, governmental experts, and community leaders to develop a deeper knowledge of the subjects they are studying, to identify and solve challenges, make a difference in their community, and share their results with the world (Apple Inc, 2009).

CBL builds on the successes of problem-based learning models, where students engage in self-directed work scenarios based on real life. The teacher's primary role shifts from dispensing information to guiding the construction of knowledge by the students (New Media Consortium, 2011). CBL is a teaching and learning method that incorporates technology, teamwork, self-directed learning, peer learning, real-world problem solving, and reflective learning into its learning activities, which can extend from the classroom to the local community (Johnson et al., 2009).

CBL is the educational strategy that puts teachers, students, and the community together. They have the opportunity and the task to help each other while the educational process is there to learn to implement and solve real-life challenges. CBL is about giving the students the necessary abilities to confront the real world, to be prepared, and to start learning from the beginning that education is constant and the work of everyone (Olivares et al., 2018).

Since it's awareness, CBL has been applied in multiplied fields and disciplines, where it has become a part of the alternatives that universities have to implement in the curriculum. The approach to students is presented as a small full constructed problem, which usually consists of descriptions of sets of observable phenomena or events that need explanation.

Particularly in the field of computer science, learning has passed from traditional settings to innovation and integrative curriculums with CBL. Binder et al. (2017) studied an implementation for teaching software development on mobile devices. At the beginning of the semester, students were challenged to develop new applications for mobile devices. Faculty members received workshops and training to study the method and facilitate the activities. The implementation considered a population of four classes with a total of 110 students for a period of more than a year. The first task was for the students to select and integrate their working teams. An evaluation was carried out through questionnaires and semi-structured interviews. The authors concluded that CBL helps in understanding the problems in the deeper lever, and its solution motivated students more than traditional methods. Its contribution radicates in the confidence and safety that the participants report that they feel after being enrolled in a real challenge outside of school boundaries, but they could always go back and consult with their teachers and facilitators in the school (Binder et al., 2017).

In health education, CBL has many approaches, some oriented to the patient and others to public or global health. For some authors, the challenge usually consists of descriptions that take the form of a patient presenting a complaint supplemented with some critical signs and symptoms. For example, Yang et al. (2018) implemented a CBL approach to 48 undergraduate nurse students from a bilingual class. The students were presented initially with big ideas of real-world situations; they were asked to work together in small groups to identify the most challenging problems and present ideas to develop innovative solutions. The task was to formulate a plan for each solution and to carry out the actions to evaluate the outcome. A great part of this research was that they took their solutions to the real world. Some students started by interviewing overseas experts worked on the proposal, and implemented the technological solution in public parks, subways and schools. Their results showed that students could enhance their skills and engagement. According to the authors, CBL provides a good alternative to achieve an integrative training, characteristic of higher education.

For Olivares et al. (2018), CBL represented an opportunity to train medical students in creative and lateral thinking, as they were required to present wild and innovative proposals to tackle the sociocultural, scientific, and economic challenges of the XXI century. The "Semana i" or i-week in English is an implementation where the students worked one week in teams to present solutions to 10 health problems: cancer, diabetes, and mental health, to mention a few. More than 500 students were enrolled in the implementation of a private university; close to 62 faculty members and experts of the industry participated in the assessment of the development of skills. Their proposals were presented at the end of the week, in a poster session. Students had to argue the contributions to the real setting based on market research, extensive literature reviews, and validation with a panel of experts. The authors argue that this accompanied journey that students embark on could also help them discover a passion for learning and contributing to their community.

Another example is the one conducted by Eraña et al. (2019) with CSILab Crime Scene Investigation, were CBL was implemented as a pedagogical strategy. Students were faced with a week-long activity were they participated in multidisciplinary teams with experts to analyze different processes. It was concluded that although not every team was able to achieve the requirements for the solution, the students believe that CBL helped them recognize and understood the interventional areas and complex processes in just one week.

CBL has also been implemented across the medical curriculum through an integrated curriculum started since first-year courses, such as Biochemistry or Anatomy. Students are presented at the beginning with news related to the subjects to review, and the students must challenge themselves to propose a realistic solution. The purpose is to promote in the participants the importance of developing self-learning, teamwork, and reasoning skills across their education. Previously suggested readings were stated in our courses mainly from a classic medical textbook, and now we invite our students submerged in the technological world to search for information across different areas based on proper keyword or search. During this process, they must also learn to work in teams, correlate ideas and share information (Jaleel et al., 2001).

IMPLEMENTING CBL IN MEDICAL EDUCATION

In the implementation of CBL in medical education, four elements need to be considered for the experience to be successful: context-rich, extraordinary challenge, collaboration, and complex skills (Figure 1).

Figure 1. Elements of challenge-based learning in medical education

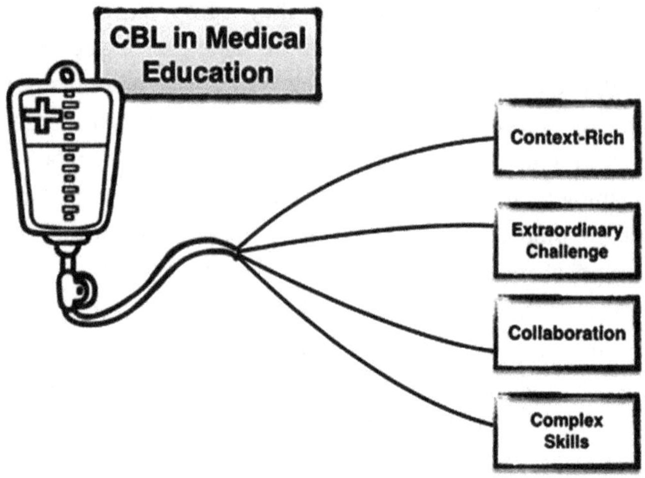

- The **context-rich** element refers to the design and engagement in a real scenario that integrates the expected learning outcomes related to a desired action from the student. For Eraña et al. (2019), this emerges from the requirement that students must design a proposal and implement it. The implementation itself carries a level of realism that provides the student with activities and reactions that can only emerge in a professional setting. This able the experience to draw attention, promote curiosity and engage the student. The scenario should also be wide enough to allow the student to be creative in his proposal, but also specific to be realizable. But above all, the context should be real and not hypothetical, so we move our students to what they might face as professionals. As Olivares et al. (2018) argue, some of these components are planned, and part of the educational experience, but others are part of a hidden curriculum that emerges accidentally and also becomes a valuable tool for character development.
- The **extraordinary challenge** element refers to involve students with situations where they are faced with a problem that needs great physical and mental effort in order to achieve a successful outcome. Most of the times, it can not be solved by a single individual, but actually requires the collaboration of multiple stakeholders from different regions. At the same time, it should give teachers and supervisors the ability to test their students' skills as the challenge proposal advances. When this medical professional in training reaches the work-based setting, they would have the responsibility of providing care to a patient. Therefore their life and their families' quality of life can be impacted. Dealing with sickness is an extraordinary challenge

faced on a daily basis by physicians and the healthcare team. Through formative settings, young professionals must understand that there is not just one solution and that every patient is a different situation. Even every patient of the same age and disease can manifest disease differently. These skills are applied in the medical field. For example, when a patient with pneumonia was the basal treatment indicated is amoxicillin, but in the case where the patient may be allergic or that the medication may not be reachable, our students must face the extraordinary challenge of proposing alternative solutions.

- The **collaboration** element refers to the need and the ability to work, share, and solve problems in teams. In a real-life working environment, professionals rarely handle patient care by themselves. Every professional starting from the lab technician until the medical specialists are essential to the patient. Health professionals must define their participation and duties and coordinate to successfully handle patient care, the opportunity of continuous feedback and peer interaction must not be dismissed. For Olivares et al. (2018) these teams also need to be multidisciplinary, with engagement not only of the healthcare team but also integrating engineers, lawyers, designers, and artists. The real contribution of CBL for collaboration would impact patient and doctor relationship, as students would consider the patient more than a subject of study, but a collaborator that has the same level of decision, and ultimate the final decision regarding treatment. By learning to communicate with the patient, either by asking simple questions to complete their medical history or by learning the difficult task to inform hard diagnosis and prognosis, collaboration proves to be a vital element.
- The **complex skills** element refers to the cognitive and behavioral processes that need to be developed to handle specific demands that surpass the resources of the individual (Folkman & Lazarus, 1980; Folkman, Lazarus, Dunkel-Schettler, DeLongis & Gruen, 1986). These strategies and behaviors are needed for students and educators alike to use at specific times when they face or cope with an event or situation that is adverse. Resources like resilience, hope, and empathy, restructure feelings of stress, denial, and conflict (Al-Sowygh, 2013).

The application of CBL has an inherent uncertainty factor provided by the human factor of the challenge itself. These skills are applied in the medical field, for example, when a medical emergency takes place, and the physician has to attend a delivery or a newborn presents complications. It can also be found in the safety of ambulatory care when gathering a medical history; patients do not share all the information, hide previous surgeries, or forget to mention medicines that they are taking. This uncertainty can definitely impact patient care and outcomes. Therefore it's an element that can not be taken lightly, and targeted strategies must be implemented

BASIS OF PARTNERED EDUCATION

The educational process has three elements: the institution, the student, and the educator (Harden and Laidlaw, 2017). It is important to consider the interrelation of the elements for the design and assessment of the educational experience as a whole. The achievement of educational outcomes depends on the understanding of the teaching-learning dynamic.

The Institution

The institution has the responsibility to foster an appropriate educational environment, and the platform in which it does is through the curriculum. The curriculum should encourage teamwork and collaboration, appropriate professional behavior, and creativity (Harden & Laidlaw, 2017). For Luna (2015), professionals need to develop disciplinary and transversal competencies, including collaborative work, ethics, problem-solving, and written or oral communication. The institution should support innovation, working alongside industry, support local and regional growth and jobs, and drive productivity (Olivares & Valdez, 2017; Universities UK, 2019). The physical proximity of teaching hospitals will become obsolete as the institutions will contain more self-learning facilities such as digital libraries, simulation laboratories, and teleconference installations. It will become a school without walls (Benor, 2014).

A medical school focused on excellence does not depend on the number of students enrolled in the program or the size of their building; it is determined by the long-term vision that does not follow trends, but actually sets them. The identity and culture of excellence sustain favorable results for several years. This is achieved daily in the classroom and clinic settings, and in the administrative offices that students do not see daily. These backstage activities that define and monitor planning, decision-making, and evaluate operations support the educational process as well (Stanika & Peter, 2018). The dynamics have interdisciplinary teamwork of finance, marketing and talent management departments that work seamlessly like a piece of well-keep machinery. The new information is integrated into the system and fuels informed decisions. The dark side of these processes, discussed in this chapter, emerges when the interaction of curriculum, students, and educators does not run smoothly. If there are gaps in coordination between processes or areas, innovation can be frustrated and lead to inefficiencies (López Cabrera & Valdez, 2019).

Partnership: Student and Educator

In order for CBL to be successful, a partnership must be established where the teacher-student has two-way communication based on trust, honesty, and confidence. The constructive feedback and respect for autonomy the teacher encourages this relationship will allow the challenge to motivate students to learn (Hesketh & Laidlaw, 2002).

This partnership might find reluctance from both parties. The teacher because they might feel that their role as a lecturer or expert is diminished (Harden, 1998). The student might not acknowledge the acquired competencies of becoming active in their own learning as their observations are from a novice perspective (DesLauriers et al., 2019).

Student

The increasing emphasis on student autonomy in medical education has moved the center of gravity away from the teacher and closer to the student (Harden, 1998). Students learn more when they are actively engaged in the classroom than they do in a passive lecture environment (DesLauriers et al., 2019) The student should be perceived as engaged in a cooperative enterprise focused on the production, dissemination, and application of knowledge (McCulloch, 2019). The partnership between teacher and student should be conceptualized as an arrangement and process in which both parts relate back and forth in a learning environment (McCulloch, 2019).

The partnership is established in a long-term relationship between professionalized providers and users, which is what happens between a student and his educator (McCulloch, 2019). On the basis of this perspective, both share the duties of providing the resources necessary to learn, participation in teaching as active learners, understanding on the process of learning, and advocate for institutional arrangements (McCulloch, 2019). Becoming an active learner engages the student to know what and why he is learning. This emphasizes the achievement of learning as a process and not as a product.

Educator

Harden and Laidlaw (2017) assure that educators have a high level of influence on the educational experience of the program as they define the scope of the learning objectives, and therefore impact the type of physicians that students will become.

A good educator can be defined as someone who helps the student to learn (Harden, 1998). Teaching is a complex task; faculty members need to be involved in the diverse roles of the medical educator must acquire (Montero et al., 2017). The demands in medical education have pushed the professor to become a full-around professional with a wide array of abilities starting from curriculum designer until a researcher. The traditional role of a lecturer has evolved to be part of a more dynamic intervention in the formation of a future health professional. This reflects the need to adopt several roles as well as acquire several skills that can nurture a learning environment where the student can observe him as a role model.

The basis of a modern education where there is a partnership with the student is based on communication. In this perspective comes constructive feedback that raises in the student self-awareness about their performance and leaves them to choose their actions (Hesketh & Laidlaw, 2002). Feedback should take the student to action into working areas that are still in progress and promote his/her particular capabilities (Hesketh & Laidlaw, 2002).

This versatile and dynamic modern role of a teacher arises the need for particular skills in them, such as: developing integral assessments, designing spiral curriculum maps, implementing blended learning programs and use of technological platforms (Harden & Lilley, 2018; Hesketh & Laidlaw, 2002). Harden and Lilley (2018) propose eight roles, such as facilitator/mentor, information provider/coach, professional, scholar/researcher, manager/leader, assessor/diagnostician, curriculum developer/implementer, and role model. In 2015 CanMeds Framework Project published by the Royal College of Physicians and Surgeons in Canadá proposed six roles of the medical educator (medical expert): being professional, communicator, collaborator, leader, health advocate, and scholar (Frank et al., 2015).

In Latin American, the teaching roles also are versatile, starting from teaching both in a classroom and bedside, doing research, and having administrative duties to attract income to the university as well as provide resources (Montero et al., 2017). Specifically in the Mexican Association of Medical Schools (AMFEM, for its initials in Spanish) they have proposed the following duties of the medical teacher as: design and development of teaching resources, coordination of education processes, professionalism promotion, design and application of evaluation instruments and involvement in scientific knowledge generation (Aguirre et al., 2012).

For certain in the future, medical education will have to teach the art and science of information management such as retrieval, assessment, and prioritization where loads of data are uploaded on the internet. On the other hand, it is expected they might address ethical and moral dilemmas and be able to handle emotional distress in their students (Benor, 2014).

ENABLING RESOURCES FOR CHALLENGED BASED LEARNING

The opportunity that CBL provides for students, educators, and universities to innovate, is achieved through the inclusion and adoption of enabling resources for learning (López Cabrera, Hernandez-Rangel, Mejía and Cerano, 2019). These resources represent alternative settings and formats in which action learning can be achieved and transferred to employability skills (Olivares, Adame, Treviño, López Cabrera, Turrubiates, 2019). Examples of these enabler resources are simulation-based education and educational technology.

Simulation-Based Education

This educational strategy started as a training resource for pilots through flight simulation activities (Bradley, 2006). The objective was to guarantee a considerable amount of flight-hours before any pilot would have the responsibility of flying an airplane. In 1934, after several planes crash, the United States' military bought simulators to train their pilots in complicated flight maneuvers and control panel indicators; only in World War I, this approach trained close to 500,000 pilots (Rosen, 2008). As new training needs were mapped, the technology and complexity of simulators had to evolve as well. Simulators were also developed to train workers in nuclear energy facilities on how to operate instruments and the procedures to be placed on an accident to safe keep the population.

The focus of simulation in these contexts was to guarantee the safety and health of human lives. In medical education, it is no different. In 1999, the Institute of Medicine (IOM) published a study about safety in the health system; they estimated that between 44,000 to 98,000 people died annually as a consequence of preventable medical errors in care (Kohn, Corrigan & Donaldson, 2000). On an operational level, this causes an economic burden of 17 to 29 billion dollars in yearly losses. But more importantly, on an ethical and moral level, the system needed to be fixed to improve the training of physicians and health personnel to provide the best care for patients and their families (Ziv, Wolpe, Small & Glick, 2003). Simulation solved the question of how to provide learning opportunities for professionals in training without exposing patients to risks or compromising their care (Olivares & Valdez, 2017).

Simulation in medicine started with the contributions of Asmund Laerdal, a toy manufacturer that worked with physicians to create the low-cost simulator of Resusci Anne; it was targeted to develop reanimation procedures skills (Bradley, 2006). In 1961, a transition was made to include more characteristics to resemble human interaction, such as cardiac and respiratory sounds (Olivares & Valdez, 2017). The developments made with the microchip and fast computer interphases contributed to creating sophisticated alternatives for highly-technical procedures (Stefanidis, Sevdalis, Paige, Zevin, Aggarwal, et al., 2015; Singh, Kaur & Trikha, 2012).

Traditionally, simulation in medical education recreates some of the components of the clinical encounter for training or assessment purposes (Gaba, 2004). Its purpose is to facilitate the transition from the trainer from novice to expert (Benner, 1982) through the development of critical thinking (Segura-Azuara, Valencia & López-Cabrera, 2018) and procedural skills (Tejos, Chahuán, Uslar, Inzunza, Villagrán et al., 2018), but it has also proven to ease emotional responses such as anxiety, in early patient encounters (Segura, Eraña, Luna-de-la-Garza, Castorena-Ibarra, and López Cabrera, 2019).

Some of the most used simulators include part-task trainers, virtual reality simulators, standardized patients, virtual patients, and full-body mannequins and robots. It is easily mistaken as a technology rather than an educational strategy, but its richness is the formulation of models to foster learning in a carefully designed experience (Jeffries, 2005; Stocker, Burmester & Allen, 2014; Walsh, 2013). Particularly in CBL, simulations are not on finding a diagnostic or perform impeccably a surgery knot; the focus is on context-rich and team-based approaches that formulate more questions on how to make care more efficient and human (Eraña-Rojas, López Cabrera, Ríos & Membrillo-Hernández, 2019).

The case about the benefits of simulation has been made, but it is important to mention as well that it requires an investment of both time and money. Although the first concern for many managers and administrators is how to provide a budget for these educational innovations, the resource that is often misestimated is time. Educators already have a tight schedule to follow to cover the content of the courses, and students have to optimize their time to fulfill their responsibilities. The preservation of time dedicated to providing feedback is imperative in this practice (Brukner, 1999; Hattie & Timperley, 2007). Several authors recommend a structured methodology known as debriefing (Maestre & Rudolph, 2015).

Educational Technology

In a context where technology is everywhere in daily activities, it is inconceivable to plan an educational curriculum or program that does not leverage it as an enabler for learning. Studies demonstrate that 98% of medical students use their laptops regularly, and 86% of smartphones as important tools for their learning (Johnson, Smith, Smythe & Varon, 2009).

The adoption of educational technology in institutions is an arduous process fueled by innovation processes that are focused on revolutionizing education so that it becomes more flexible, individualized, and collaborative (López Cabrera &

Valdez, 2019). A common mistake that is done is to be reactive to trends and hype of new products to guide the incorporation of resources. However, as no or last-minute planning of the economic impact is performed, this becomes an expensive way to develop innovation for medical schools. The reality is that when you are in that case, other schools, the ones that did think ahead of time, have already implemented pilot studies and are even presenting the results on educational conferences. But how do they do it?

It is not as complicated as it sounds; it requires a plan that integrates both short term and long term planning. The short term refers to the acquisition and maintenance of computer equipment for the library and faculty members (López Cabrera & Valdez, 2019). Examples of the long term refer to budget planning and faculty training in emergent technologies that are not yet widely implemented (López Cabrera, Herandez-Rangel, Mejía and Cerano, 2019).

The new technologies and trends that are being implemented are 360 videos, 3D printing, and Augmented (AR) and Virtual Reality (VR).

360 videos are stereoscopic and monoscopic representations of environments that capture setting from multiple perspectives (López Cabrera & Valdez, 2019). They provide an immersive video that can be a computer-generated image or recorded by a special arrangement of cameras that provide the viewer with depth perception. In medical education, they have used it for students to interact with human atlas and to understand medical imaging for specific procedures.

3D printing, also known as additive manufacturing, has its origins in creating rapid prototypes for production. This technology uses a computer-generated model to "print" layer by layer a physical three-dimensional object. In medical education, they have used it for teaching anatomy and surgical planning.

Augmented Reality is known as AR, describes a computer interaction that alters the perception of reality through the inclusion of computer-generated content (López Cabrera & Valdez, 2019). This simulation superimposes elements in real-time, and in medical education, it has been used for anatomy teaching and training of venipuncture for collection of blood specimens. Virtual Reality (VR) describes an alternative virtual world in which the user interacts through a set of goggles or headsets (López Cabrera, 2019). This immersion has been used in medical education as exposure therapy and for surgical training.

As students' acceptance of these teaching strategies increase (Tejos, Chahuán, Uslar, Inzunza, Villagrán et al., 2018), educators and universities are urged to revise their curriculum and educational programs to develop resources that aid in the achievement of educational objectives, and not the other way around (López Cabrera, Herandez-Rangel, Mejía and Cerano, 2019).

CONCLUSION

In this globalized society, the only constant changes, medical education is constantly evolving to meet these demands. Challenge Based Education provides a foundation for this change. CBL has emerged as one of the main factors of evolution in medical curriculum; students must be faced with different challenges, case scenarios, or simulated clinical patients, they constantly meet with different demands, learn to think creatively and work alongside the educator and classmates. Readers are encouraged to implementation of CBL considering the proposed key elements: rich-context, extraordinary challenge, collaboration, and complex skills. Designing an educational experience must consider educator, student, and institution, keeping a good interrelation of these components is vital for its success. Appropriate use of enabler resources, such as simulated based learning and technological learning leaves an open door for innovation.

The organizational philosophy and planning of the university would determine the preparedness they have for innovation. Schools with little organizational structure would not prioritize the need for innovation, and the lack of vision delay their competitiveness in an already saturated market (López Cabrera & Valdez, 2019). For Lewis (2006), the mission and vision of medical schools should worry less about achieving students' satisfaction through a survey, especially if it threatens the university's goal of making students into better people and professionals. But focus instead and reflect on how the delivered curriculum, the learned curriculum, and the hidden one impact on medical student's identity and the adoption of professionalism values (Harden & Laidlaw, 2017).

The stakeholders: students, educators, researchers, school administrators, politicians, and government officials, and the community should participate in setting and re-examining the purposes of the medical school. Aligning those objectives helps the learning community to start planning and implementing today the steps to achieve the goal of medical education: to prepare the next generation of health professionals to be the best version of themselves, preparing those that will provide the best care for the patients and their families.

REFERENCES

Aguirre, E., Castellanos, F., Galicia, H., González, A., Fabián, O., Ojeda, C., Sánchez, J., Servin, D., Vargas, R. C., & Vázquez, J. (2012). *Perfil por competencias docentes del profesor de medicina.* Asociación Mexicana de Facultades y Escuelas de Medicina.

Al-Sowygh, Z. H. (2013). Academic distress perceived stress and coping strategies among dental students in Saudi Arabia. *The Saudi Dental Journal, 25*(3), 97–105. doi:10.1016/j.sdentj.2013.05.002 PMID:24179318

Apple. (2010). *Challenge Based Learning: A Classroom Guide.* Apple Inc.

Benner, P. (1982). From novice to expert. *The American Journal of Nursing, 82*(3), 402–409. PMID:6917683

Benor, D. E. (2014). A New Paradigm Is Needed for Medical Education in the Mid-Twenty-First Century and Beyond: Are We Ready? *Rambam Maimonides Medical Journal, 5*(3), e0018. doi:10.5041/RMMJ.10152 PMID:25120918

Binder, F. V., Nichols, M., Reinehr, S. S., & Malucelli, A. (2017). Challenge Based Learning Applied to Mobile Software Development Teaching. *The 30th IEEE Conference on Software Engineering Education and Training*, 57-64.

Bradley, P. (2006). The history of simulation in medical education and possible future directions. *Medical Education, 40*(3), 254–262. doi:10.1111/j.1365-2929.2006.02394.x PMID:16483328

Brukner, H. (1999). Giving effective feedback to medical students: A workshop for faculty and house staff. *Medical Teacher, 21*(2), 161–166. doi:10.1080/01421599979798 PMID:21275731

Chan, C. Y. Z. (2013). Critical thinking and creativity in nursing: Learners' perspectives. *Nurse Education Today, 33*(5), 558–563. doi:10.1016/j.nedt.2012.09.007 PMID:23058105

Deslauriers, L., McCarty, L. S., Miller, K., Callaghan, K., & Kestin, G. (2019). Measuring actual learning versus the feeling of learning in response to being actively engaged in the classroom. *Proceedings of the National Academy of Sciences.* 10.1073/pnas.1821936116

Eraña Rojas, I. E., López Cabrera, M. V., Ríos, E., & Membrillo-Hernández, J. (2019). A challenge-based learning experience in forensic medicine. *Journal of Forensic and Legal Medicine, 68*, 101873. doi:10.1016/j.jflm.2019.101873 PMID:31627125

Folkman, S., & Lazarus, R. S. (1980). An Analysis of Coping in a Middle-Aged Community Sample. *Journal of Health and Social Behavior*, *21*(3), 219–239. doi:10.2307/2136617 PMID:7410799

Folkman, S., Lazarus, R. S., Dunkel-Schetter, C., DeLongis, A., & Gruen, R. J. (1986). Dynamics of a Stressful Encounter: Cognitive Appraisal, Coping, and Encounter Outcomes. *Journal of Personality and Social Psychology*, *50*(5), 992–1003. doi:10.1037/0022-3514.50.5.992 PMID:3712234

Frank, J. R., Snell, L., & Sherbino, J. (2015). *CanMEDS 2015: Physician Competency Framework*. Royal College of Physicians of Canada.

Gaba, D. M. (2004). The future vision of simulation in health care. *Quality & Safety in Health Care*, *13*(1), 2–10. doi:10.1136/qshc.2004.009878 PMID:15465951

Harden, R. M. (1998). AMEE guide No. 12: Multiprofessional education: Part 1- effective multiprofessional education: a three-dimensional perspective. *Medical Teacher*, *20*(5), 402–408. doi:10.1080/01421599880472

Harden, R. M., & Laidlaw, J. M. (2017). *Essential skills for a medical teacher*. Elsevier.

Harden, R. M., & Lilley, P. (2018). *The eight roles of the medical teacher*. Elsevier.

Hattie, J., & Timperley, H. (2007). The Power of Feedback. *Review of Educational Research*, *77*(1), 81–112. doi:10.3102/003465430298487

Hesketh, E. A., & Laidlaw, J. M. (2002). Developing the teaching instinct, 1: Feedback. *Medical Teacher*, *24*(3), 243–248. PMID:12098410

Jaleel, A., Rahman, M. A., & Huda, N. (2001). Problem-based learning in biochemistry at Ziauddin Medical University, Karachi, Pakistan. *Biochemistry and Molecular Biology Education*, *29*(2), 80–84. doi:10.1016/S1470-8175(01)00021-2

Johnson, L. F., Smith, R. S., Smythe, J. T., & Varon, R. K. (2009). *Challenge-Based Learning: An Approach for Our Time*. The New Media Consortium.

Johnsons, L., & Brown, S. (2011). *Challenge Based Learning: The Report from the Implementation Project*. The New Media Consortium.

Kohn, L. T., Corrigan, J. M., & Donaldson, M. S. (2000). *To Err is Human: Building a Safer Health System. Washington*. National Academies Press.

Lewis, H. (2006). *Excellence Without a Soul: How a Great University Forgot Education*. Public Affairs.

López Cabrera, M. V., Hernandez-Rangel, E., Mejía, G. P., & Cerano, J. L. (2019). Factors that enable the adoption of educational technology in medical schools. *Educación Médica, 20*(1), 3–9.

López Cabrera, M. V., & Valdez, J. E. (2019). Organizational philosophy and planning: the keys to the adoption of educational technology. In *Maria Clausen, A Closer Look at Educational Technology*. NOVA Science Publishers.

Maestre, J. M., & Rudolph, J. W. (2015). Theories and styles of debriefing:the good judgment method as a tool for formative assessment in healthcare. *Revista Espanola de Cardiologia, 68*, 282–287. doi:10.1016/j.recesp.2014.05.018 PMID:25239179

Mahdi, R., Sukarman, S. S., & Chan, M. K. Y. (2015). Fostering creativity through innovation engagement in science and technology education: Case study of Unversiti Teknologi MARA students. *Procedia: Social and Behavioral Sciences, 167*, 256–260. doi:10.1016/j.sbspro.2014.12.671

McCulloch, A. (2009). The student as co-producer: Learning from public administration about the student-university relationship. *Studies in Higher Education, 34*(2), 171–183. doi:10.1080/03075070802562857

Montero, L., Triviño, X., Dois, A., Sirhan, M., & Leiva, L. (2017). Percepción de los académicos del rol docente del médico. *Investigación en Educación Médica, 6*(23), 198–205. doi:10.1016/j.riem.2017.01.001

Olivares, S.L., Adame, E., Treviño, J., López Cabrera, M.V., & Turrubiates, M. (2019). *Action Learning: Challenges that impact employability skills.* Higher Education, Skills, and Work-Based Learning; Ahead-of-print.

Olivares, S. L., López Cabrera, M. V., & Valdez-García, J. E. (2018). Aprendizaje basado en retos: Una experiencia de innovación para enfrentar problemas de salud pública. *Educación Médica, 19*, 230–237. doi:10.1016/j.edumed.2017.10.001

Olivares, S. L., & Valdez, J. E. (2017). *Aprendizaje Centrado en el Paciente.* Editorial Médica Panamericana.

Ozkan, H., Degirmenci, B., Musal, B., Itil, O., Akalın, E., Kilinç, O., Ozkan, S., & Alici, E. (2006). Task-based learning program for clinical years of medical education. *Education for Health, 19*(1), 32–42. doi:10.1080/13576280500534826 PMID:16531300

Rosen, K. R. (2008). The history of medical simulation. *Journal of Critical Care, 23*(2), 157–166. doi:10.1016/j.jcrc.2007.12.004 PMID:18538206

Scheele, F., Teunissen, P., Luijk, S. V., Heineman, E., Fluit, L., Mulder, H., Meininger, A., Wijnen-Meijer, M., Glass, G., Sluiter, H., & Hummel, T. (2008). Introducing competency-based postgraduate medical education in the Netherlands. *Medical Teacher, 30*(3), 248–253. doi:10.1080/01421590801993022 PMID:18484450

Segura, N.A., Eraña, I.E., Luna-de-la-Garza, M.V., Castorena-Ibarra, J., López Cabrera, M.V. (2019). *Analysis of anxiety on early clinical encounters: Experiences using clinical simulation in undergraduate students*. Educación Médica. Transformar la educación para fortalecer los sistemas de salud.

Segura-Azuara, N. A., Valencia, J. L., & López Cabrera, M. V. (2018). Desarrollo del pensamiento crítico mediante simulación de alta fidelidad con estudiantes de medicina. In Ed Med, 7(28), 55-64.

Singh, P. M., Kaur, M., & Trikha, A. (2012). Virtual reality in anesthesia "simulation.". *Anesthesia, Essays and Researches, 6*(2), 134–139. doi:10.4103/0259-1162.108289 PMID:25885605

Stanika, N., & Peter, L. (2018). Community, strategic partner of the educational organization in the 21st Century. *International Conference of Knowledge-based Organization, 24*, 416-420.

Stefanidis, D., Sevdalis, N., Paige, J., Zevin, B., Aggarwal, R., Grantcharov, T., & Jones, D. (2015). Simulation in Surgery. *Annals of Surgery, 261*(5), 846–853. doi:10.1097/SLA.0000000000000826 PMID:25243562

Stocker, M., Burmester, M., & Allen, M. (2014). Optimization of simulated team training through the application of learning theories: A debate for a conceptual framework. *BMC Medical Education, 14*(1), 69–78. doi:10.1186/1472-6920-14-69 PMID:24694243

Tejos, R., Chahuán, J., Uslar, T., Inzunza, M., Villagrán, I., Riquelme, V., Padilla, O., Pizarro, M., Corvetto, M., Varas, J., & Riquelme, A. (2018). Simulated training program in abdominal paracentesis for undergraduate medical students. *Gastroenterologia y Hepatologia, 42*(4), 239–247. doi:10.1016/j.gastrohep.2018.10.001 PMID:30471721

Thorell, M., Fridorff-Jens, P. K., Lassen, P., Lange, T., & Kayser, L. (2015). Transforming students into digital academics: A challenge at both the individual and the institutional level. *BMC Medical Education, 15*(1), 48. doi:10.118612909-015-0330-5 PMID:25890174

Walsh, K. (2013). *Oxford Textbook of Medical Education*. Oxford University Press. doi:10.1093/med/9780199652679.001.0001

Willis, J. (1996). A flexible framework for task-based learning An overview of a task-based framework for language teaching. *Oxford Prabhu, 1987*, 52–62.

Yang, Z., Zhou, Y., Chung, J. W. Y., Tang, Q., Jiang, L., & Wong, T. K. S. (2018). Challenge Based Learning nurtures creative thinking: An evaluative study. *Nurse Education Today, 71*, 40–47. doi:10.1016/j.nedt.2018.09.004 PMID:30223169

Zhou, H. Y. (2012). The present situation of curriculum system and transformation of nursing education in China. *J. Qilu Nurs, 18*(15), 39–40.

Ziv, A., Wople, P. R., Small, S. D., & Glick, S. (2003). Simulation-based medical education: An ethical imperative. *Academic Medicine, 78*(8), 783–788. doi:10.1097/00001888-200308000-00006 PMID:12915366

ADDITIONAL READING

Deslauriers, L., McCarty, L. S., Miller, K., Callaghan, K., & Kestin, G. (2019). Measuring actual learning versus the feeling of learning in response to being actively engaged in the classroom. *Proceedings of the National Academy of Sciences*. 10.1073/pnas.1821936116

Eraña Rojas, I. E., López Cabrera, M. V., Ríos, E., & Membrillo-Hernández, J. (2019). A challenge-based learning experience in forensic medicine. *Journal of Forensic and Legal Medicine, 68*, 101873. doi:10.1016/j.jflm.2019.101873 PMID:31627125

Harden, R. M., & Lilley, P. (2018). *The eight roles of the medical teacher*. Elsevier.

López Cabrera, M. V., Hernandez-Rangel, E., Mejía, G. P., & Cerano, J. L. (2019). Factors that enable the adoption of educational technology in medical schools. *Educación Médica, 20*(1), 3–9.

Olivares, S. L., López Cabrera, M. V., & Valdez-García, J. E. (2018). Aprendizaje basado en retos: Una experiencia de innovación para enfrentar problemas de salud pública. *Educación Médica, 19*, 230–237. doi:10.1016/j.edumed.2017.10.001

Olivares, S. L., & Valdez, J. E. (2017). *Aprendizaje Centrado en el Paciente*. Editorial Médica Panamericana.

Rosen, K. R. (2008). The history of medical simulation. *Journal of Critical Care, 23*(2), 157–166. doi:10.1016/j.jcrc.2007.12.004 PMID:18538206

Segura, N.A., Eraña, I.E., Luna-de-la-Garza, M.V., Castorena-Ibarra, J., López Cabrera, M.V. (2019). *Analysis of anxiety on early clinical encounters: Experiences using clinical simulation in undergraduate students*. Educación Médica. Transformar la educación para fortalecer los sistemas de salud.

Walsh, K. (2013). *Oxford Textbook of Medical Education*. Oxford University Press. doi:10.1093/med/9780199652679.001.0001

Yang, Z., Zhou, Y., Chung, J. W. Y., Tang, Q., Jiang, L., & Wong, T. K. S. (2018). Challenge Based Learning nurtures creative thinking: An evaluative study. *Nurse Education Today*, *71*, 40–47. doi:10.1016/j.nedt.2018.09.004 PMID:30223169

KEY TERMS AND DEFINITIONS

Challenged-Based Learning: A pedagogical approach to education where students are faced with real-life problem scenarios and are expected to develop a creative and innovative solution.

Collaboration: CBL element involves the need and the ability to learn and practice working, sharing, and solving problems in pairs or teams.

Complex Skills: Cognitive and behavioral processes that need to be developed to handle specific demands that surpass the resources of the individual.

Context-Rich: A design and engagement in a real scenario that integrates the expected learning outcomes related to a desired action from the student.

Educator: A group of physicians, nurses, teachers, or co-workers involved in the education and improvement of an individual.

Extraordinary Challenge: Situation that needs a great physical and mental effort in order to achieve a successful outcome.

Medical Education: Curriculum that involves the subjects, challenges, and training to prepare a full license medical physician.

Simulation: Imitation of a medical escenario or patient case implemented to develop educational skills.

Tecnologico de Monterrey: Educational private non-for-profit institution located in Monterrey, Mexico, that has a completed medical curriculum for over 42 years.

Chapter 9
Using a Community-Based Collaborative Care Model as a Platform for Successful Interprofessional Education

Jannette Berkley-Patton
University of Missouri-Kansas City, USA

Carole Bowe Thompson
University of Missouri-Kansas City, USA

Katherine G. Ervie
University of Missouri-Kansas City, USA

Miranda Huffman
https://orcid.org/0000-0003-0446-7671
Meharry Medical College, USA

Nia R. Johnson
Saint Louis University, USA

ABSTRACT

Diabetes is a growing public health epidemic in the U.S. African Americans are particularly at-risk for diabetes with rates twice as high as whites. Health professionals are recommended to encourage their at-risk patients to participate in evidence-based lifestyle change programs, such as CDC's National Diabetes Prevention Program (DPP) and support their weight loss efforts. This chapter describes feasibility/ outcomes of a community-based collaborative care model used to implement a

DOI: 10.4018/978-1-7998-3066-5.ch009

weekly-group DPP facilitated by interprofessional teams of medical school students with three African American churches (N=72 participants; 93% overweight/obese). At 12-weeks, 30% of participants had lost at least 5 lbs.; among those attending at least nine sessions, 55% achieved at least 3% weight loss. Findings suggest interprofessional student teams can feasibly partner with churches to deliver the DPP and achieve weight-loss outcomes associated with reducing diabetes risk. Future research is needed to determine scalability/costs of using community-based collaborative care student models to address diabetes.

INTRODUCTION

Diabetes continues to be a major national health threat. National efforts to prevent diabetes have yielded lifestyle change programs (LCPs) that aim to reduce primary risks, including overweight/obesity (Ackermann & Marrero, 2007; Diabetes Prevention Research Group, 2002; 2004). The Diabetes Prevention Program (DPP) is a rigorously evaluated lifestyle intervention that has been proven to reduce or delay diabetes onset by up to 50 to 60% with diet changes, physical activity, and modest weight loss among at-risk individuals (Diabetes Prevention Research Group, 2002). National health organizations are making widespread attempts to disseminate evidence-based LCPs like the DPP to curb growing diabetes rates (e.g., CDC, 2018b). These dissemination efforts include educating health professionals on the importance of patient screening and referral to LCPs and partnering with patients in discussing their lifestyle change behaviors and outcomes. They also call for culturally-appropriate lifestyle change programs for high risk minority populations in community settings, recognizing most health settings do not provide these programs and offering LCPs in community settings may be less costly and more accessible (American Medical Association, 2019; CDC, 2018b). Accessibility of evidence-based LCPs could particularly be beneficial to African Americans communities where rates of diabetes tend to be disproportionately high and availability of LCPs are limited or nonexistent (CDC, 2017). Moreover, although reports on engaging health profession students to assist with diabetes prevention are rare (e.g., Gorrindo, Alon & Ladner, 2014), students' participation as health coaches in community-based LCPs could greatly assist national DPP dissemination efforts. This approach could also provide students with interprofessional opportunities to learn culturally competent ways to collaborate with underserved communities and partner with patients, particularly African Americans on their lifestyle change goals.

This chapter describes the planning, implementation, and outcomes of a pilot study used to test a community-based collaborative care model to disseminate the DPP using interprofessional teams of medical school students in partnership with the African American faith community. Specifically, the objectives of this chapter are first to provide background contextual information a multilevel religiously-tailored diabetes risk reduction intervention study (named *Project Faith Influencing Transformation [FIT]*) that included a weekly group-DPP component and was originally disseminated and tested in urban Kansas City (KC), Missouri African American churches. The second objective is to highlight the community-student engagement approach that was used to refine the Project FIT group DPP component for feasible implementation and impact as Project FIT 2.0 – a pilot study delivered by interprofessional teams of students serving as health coaches and paired with African American church health workers. The third objective is to describe how student teams and church health workers were trained and how they jointly implemented Project FIT 2.0 as a community-based collaborative care model in urban KC African American churches with volunteering adult participants. The fourth objective is to report on the feasibility and participant weight loss outcomes of the Project FIT 2.0 collaborative care model. The last objective is to provide a discussion of the findings in light of previous DPP research conducted in African American communities. The discussion also highlights future research and practice needed to further understand the impact, scalability, and sustainability of community-based collaborative care models to reduce the growing rates of diabetes.

BACKGROUND

The CDC estimates that 1 in 3 adults (about 86 million people) are living with pre-diabetes and 1 in 10 adults have been diagnosed with diabetes in the U.S. (Centers for Disease Control and Prevention [CDC], 2017; Lin et al., 2018). A primary clinical risk factor for pre-diabetes is overweight/obesity (American Diabetes Association [ADA], 2016), which is contributing to historically high rates of diabetes at a cost of $327 billion nationally in 2017 (ADA, 2018; Dall et al., 2009, 2011). African Americans are particularly burdened with diabetes, with rates twice as high as Whites (13% vs 7.5%; CDC, 2017). African Americans are also disproportionately burdened by diabetes complications including blindness, kidney disease, hospitalization, and lower-limb amputations (CDC, 2013a, 2017; Office of Minority Health, 2016). National studies indicate that nearly 60% of African Americans are obese/overweight, and rates continue to worsen – thereby further increasing risk for diabetes for many

African Americans (CDC, 2013b; Office of Minority Health, 2106). Increasingly, dissemination of evidence-based preventative lifestyle change programs (LCPs) has been recommended to reduce rising rates of chronic diseases, such diabetes, especially with high-risk populations (ADA, 2015; American Medical Association [AMA], 2019).

Recommendations from the CDC, ADA, and AMA include increasing patient screening/referrals to LCPs to promote weight loss and physical activity among overweight/obese and other at-risk individuals (CDC, 2018a; ADA, 2015, AMA, 2019). They also call for culturally-appropriate LCPs for high risk minority populations in community settings, recognizing most health settings do not provide these programs and offering them in community settings may be less costly and more accessible (ADA, 2015). Still, innovative strategies are needed to extend the reach of LCPs to underserved communities where accessible programs are limited and are often not sustained.

While traditional medical care has a role in addressing obesity/overweight and pre-diabetes, future health professionals also need to be familiar with LCPs as an effective tool to prevent onset of chronic diseases and their contributing health conditions, including obesity (e.g., AMA, 2019). Health professionals must also be able to provide culturally competent care and have knowledge about social determinants of health to deliver care to diverse populations (Liaison Committee on Medical Education [LCME], 2019). In addition, they must be able to deliver care in interprofessional practice, which requires excellent communication skills and teamwork. Accreditation requirements require students to have opportunities for service learning and interprofessional educational experiences to promote the development of these competencies (LCME, 2019). Health professional student-led LCPs can address two key issues: providing novel educational, service learning experiences for students on collaborative, interprofessional teams and increasing access to sustainable LCPs for underserved populations.

The Diabetes Prevention Program (DPP): An Evidence-based Lifestyle Change Program

The DPP is an evidence-based lifestyle change intervention that has been proven to reduce DM incidence by 58% with clinically meaningful weight loss (a modest 5%) and 150 minutes per week of physical activity among overweight/obese adults with pre-diabetes (Diabetes Prevention Research Group, 2002, 2004). More recent studies have found that even a 3% weight loss can significantly reduce diabetes and other chronic disease risks (e.g., Wilkinson et al., 2019). The DPP consists of 16 core sessions topics (e.g., healthy eating, physical activity, coping strategies, stress management) delivered over 6 months and 6 maintenance sessions over the following

6 months, for a total of 22 sessions. In each session, coaches record participants' weight and review their food and exercise logs. Coaches also monitor participants' progress on self-defined goals. The original DPP trial used highly skilled coaches (e.g., psychologists, nutritionists) to deliver the DPP. To improve dissemination, the DPP has been adapted for several settings (e.g., community hospitals, clinics, YMCA's, churches) and a variety of coaches (e.g., nutritionists, psychologist, diabetes educators, lay health workers) have been trained to facilitate the program (e.g., Ackermann & Marrero, 2007; Adams, Hebert, McVey, & Williams, 2016; Berkley-Patton et al., 2018; Brunisholz et al., 2017; Sattin et al., 2016). The DPP has now been widely disseminated by the CDC as the National DPP using the *PreventT2* curriculum (Nhim et al., 2019).

Despite these dissemination efforts, the DPP has yielded few benefits for African Americans for various reasons, including limited cultural tailoring and access. Studies report that high program costs and almost no availability of DPP classes in African American communities contribute to limited DPP access for many African Americans (e.g., Gary-Webb et al., 2018; Jiang et al., 2015; Li et al., 2015). To address these issues, the current study's researchers (first and second authors) developed and implemented a culturally-tailored, multilevel diabetes risk reduction program (Project Faith Influencing Transformation [FIT]) for the Black Church context – an institution that has extended reach, influence, and an emphasis on health in African American communities (Pew Research Center, 2015; Taylor, Chatters, & Levin, 2004). Project FIT was delivered by trained church members and the YMCA. The first iteration of Project FIT was funded by the National Institute of Minority Health and Health Disparities. To sustain Project FIT and expand its reach for increased dissemination and accessibility in low-resource African American communities, an interdisciplinary team of the researchers and faculty subsequently trained medical (MD) and physician assistant (PA) students from the School of Medicine (SOM) at the University of Missouri Kansas City (UMKC) to work on interprofessional teams alongside church members to provide free DPP classes throughout urban Kansas City African American faith communities.

This chapter describes: a) the contextual background of Project FIT, b) student and community engagement to inform adaptation of Project FIT to a community-based collaborative care model, and c) methods to test the feasibility and impact of the community collaborative-care model using interprofessional student-church member teams and a pretest-posttest, no control group research design.

Project FIT Contextual Background

Project FIT was initially developed as a multilevel diabetes risk reduction intervention, with the added benefit of having potential to also reduce cardiovascular disease risks, in African American churches (Berkley-Patton et al., 2018a). The project was developed using a community-based participatory research approach, whereby the KC FAITH Initiative Community Action Board, which consists of representatives from faith, health, community, and academic organizations came together to plan the intervention based on findings from a health needs assessment conducted across the Kansas City urban metropolitan area in 11 African American churches with 449 church and community members (Berkley-Patton et al., 2018b). Findings identified diabetes and heart disease as the top priority health issues that needed to be addressed in African American faith communities. The needs assessment also identified top feasible and important strategies to include (e.g., health screenings, nutrition education, physical activity, weight loss programs). The resulting intervention included a religiously-tailored Project FIT tool kit with materials/activities (e.g., sermon guides, responsive reading, diabetes risk checklist, commitment cards) for trained church leaders to deliver to all church members and community members served through multilevel church outlets (e.g., individual, peer-to-peer, ministry groups, church services) at 6 participating churches (N=352; Berkley-Patton et al., 2018a). The churches were randomized to Project FIT or standard education (comparison arm). Health screenings (e.g., weight, blood pressure, blood glucose) were conducted at baseline and again at 8 months to track outcomes (Bauer, Berkley-Patton, Bowe-Thompson, & Christensen, K., 2018; Bowe Thompson et al., 2015). Persons with diabetes and cardiovascular disease risk factors were immediately referred to and enrolled in their church's DPP for intervention churches or a 6-week health education program for comparison churches. The DPP arm of Project FIT was implemented at the group level in partnership with the YMCA whose certified diabetes educators facilitated DPP classes at the cost of $449 per DPP participant, which was covered by the grant and free to participants.

Findings from this study indicated that Project FIT significantly increased likelihood of 5-pound weight loss compared to controls, and average overall weight loss in the Project FIT intervention arm was 0.5 pounds (inclusive of all participants with two datapoints, regardless of whether they attended any of their DPP classes; Berkley-Patton et al., 2018a). Project FIT DPP arm participants attending 4 or more sessions lost about 4% on average of their initial body weight in 2 of the 3 intervention churches. The post-debriefing found that church and community members were highly satisfied with the project and wanted it to continue. The KC FAITH CAB also encouraged adapting and sustaining Project FIT for low-cost, long-term sustainability and community-wide impact.

A Community-Based Participatory Approach to Adapt FIT to a Collaborative Care Model

Because a highly engaged CBPR approach was used to develop the Project FIT intervention with faith, health, and community leaders, inclusion of students in a similar process was considered to be highly important. Therefore, the authors met with classes of MD and PA students along with a class of nursing students to discuss how students could be trained as health coaches in order to offer the program to more churches in underserved KC urban areas. Students in these classes advised on the importance of making clear the benefits that could be gained from serving as student health coaches (e.g., unique training experience, opportunities for research experiences for their CV). They also commented that students would be interested in contributing to improving community health and in working on interprofessional teams as health coaches. However, they believed that not all students would readily be willing to give up being in the clinical environment and that shared time between clinical experiences and the community would be the best approach.

Feedback about the proposed Project FIT 2.0 program was also sought by the research team in ongoing discussions with the KC FAITH Initiative CAB. The CAB's input included the need for church leaders/members to assist with the delivery of DPP classes in partnership with the students to make the classes more acceptable to members. They also believed it was important to continue to distribute Project FIT materials in the DPP classes and more broadly throughout participating churches, regardless if members participated in the DPP. In doing so, they believed the pastor needed to remain highly committed to the program and promote Project FIT with members. The CAB also advised the research team to include physical activity – a component that was prioritized but was not included in the original Project FIT study due to limited resources and capacity. Lastly, the CAB believed including students would be a much-wanted addition to help sustain Project FIT in underserved African American communities. The resulting methods in testing the feasibility and outcomes of the community-based collaborative care pilot study, Project FIT 2.0, based on student and community input are described below.

METHODS

Setting, Participants, and Procedures

Participating Churches

Churches from the original Project FIT that expressed interest in sustaining the program were recruited for the Project FIT 2.0 pilot study. All participating churches were in low-resource areas of urban KC, MO (within 5 miles of UMKC SOM) and met church-selection criteria. This criteria consisted of having: a) a minimum of 100 active adult church members ages 18 and higher who regularly attended Sunday service(s) or were active in the church outreach ministry (e.g., food/clothing pantry, social services, daycare), b) a commitment from the senior pastor to fully implement group study activities and promote all study events, c) a commitment from at least 2 church members willing to coordinate study activities, participate in study trainings, facilitate the DPP classes with students, and report implementation data monthly, and d) willingness to host 2 health screening events along with 2 survey assessments. All participating churches received $500 for delivering study activities including hosting the DPP and $500 in stipends to be divided equally among their CHWs, for a total of $1,000.

Participants

Participants were recruited from participating churches using several strategies, which included announcements made by the research team in Sunday morning and midweek bible study services, announcements in church bulletins, flyers, and posters that provided study information. Interested church and community members were screened to determine study eligibility, which included a) self-identify as African American; b) aged 18 to 80; c) willingness to participate in 2 surveys and 2 health screening events during and after church services (once at baseline and again about 3 months later); d) regularly attended the participating church (at least once a month) or used the church's outreach services (e.g., daycare services, food programs) at least 4 times/year; e) willingness to participate in a 12-week Project FIT 2.0 weight loss program with low-impact exercise; f) physically able to participate in low-impact exercise, like a walking group; g) able to complete surveys independently (without assistance), and h) want to lose 5 or more pounds. Interested members were excluded if they were: pregnant or wanted to get pregnant over the next year and/or had a blood pressure result from the church-based health screening >160/100 (an unsafe blood pressure level to participate).

Procedures

Upon meeting study eligibility and providing informed consent, participants completed a baseline survey that collected information on demographics, lifestyle behaviors, psychosocial measures, and a health screening (e.g., weight/height for BMI, blood pressure), which took approximately 30 to 60 minutes to complete. They completed a similar survey and health screening at 3 months, which was after the completion of their 12th DPP class. Additionally, beginning with the first class session, participants' attendance and weight were recorded at the beginning of each of the 12 class sessions. Participants received $30 for completing the baseline and $30 for completing the 3-month survey/health screening. Additionally, student attendance at their designated sessions was tracked. Study procedures were approved by the UMKC Institutional Review Board.

Data Analysis

For the current study, weekly weight information from weeks 1 through 12 was used for the 60 participants who had at least two weights recorded to calculate weight loss. Student and participant DPP class attendance was also tracked. Categorical variables were summarized using frequencies and compared using chi-square tests. Continuous variables were summarized using mean and standard deviation and compared using Student's t-tests.

Description of the Community-based Collaborative Care Model

An interdisciplinary faculty team of SOM researchers and faculty from Family Medicine, the PA Program, and the Biomedical and Health Informatics Department finalized the design of the collaborative care model based on student and KC FAITH CAB input and implemented the model with students and church members. Here, the authors describe how student teams and church members were trained to serve as health coaches, their joint implementation of Project FIT 2.0, and joint debriefing and celebration activities, as shown in Figure 1.

Training

Student Training

Students' training took place over an entire Fall semester with 2 hours per week over 12 weeks in the SOM. At the start of the training, about 2 students from each program (MD and PA) were grouped to form interprofessional teams made up of

Figure 1. Project FIT 2.0 Community-based Collaborative Care Model Delivered by Interprofessional Student and Church Member Teams

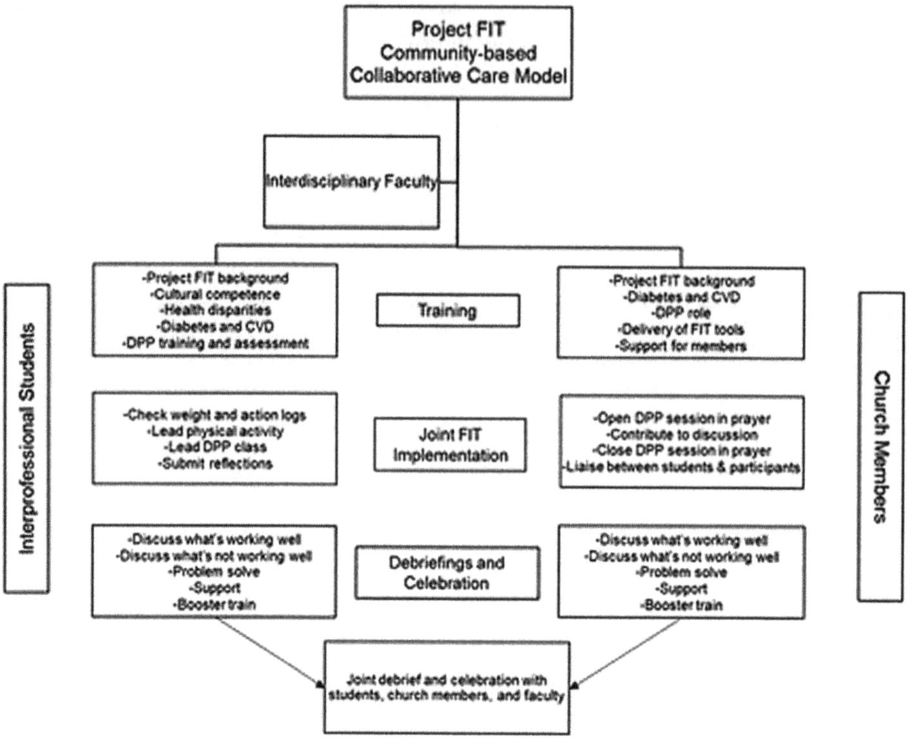

4 to 5 students. The training consisted of a review of the original DPP study and Project FIT (e.g., community-engaged processes used, the needs assessment survey, the role of the KC FAITH Initiative, Project FIT implementation and evaluation by church leaders/members), study outcomes, and lessons learned. Students' were made aware of the engagement of other students on the design of Project FIT 2.0 and their expressed potential benefits (e.g., student opportunities to participate in research) and pitfalls (e.g., reduced student clinical training time). The training also included a session on cultural competency which focused on African American culture in general and topics on cultural privilege, biases, and humility. To provide deeper insight into African American church culture, a local African American pastor presented a lecture on the history, role, and influence of the church in African American communities. The pastor also reviewed common Christian church tenets and activities that could influence health beliefs and behaviors among African Americans and the importance of respectful attire, communication, and demeanor in the church settings. To enhance students' active listening and communication

skills, a lecture on motivational interviewing was delivered by an expert in this area who also oversaw students' one-on-one role playing to support participants' health behavior change goals in a non-judgmental, autonomous manner. The training also included sessions on diabetes and heart disease, with a focus on related health disparities among African American populations. A class session was used to discuss low-impact exercises and review exercise resources (e.g., online videos, apps) to prepare students to lead exercise in their DPP classes. Lastly, the DPP training materials were reviewed extensively, and students completed mock DPP sessions in their assigned interprofessional teams, which included taking turns role modeling facilitators and acting as participants.

The CDC's National Diabetes Prevention Program *Prevent T2* curriculum (CDC, 2018b) was used and adapted for Project FIT 2.0 to be the length of a semester with 12 sessions. In reducing the number of *Prevent T2* class sessions from 22 to 12, several sessions included two topic areas (e.g., *Get active to prevent T2/Track your activity, Get support/Cope with triggers;* see the *Prevent T2: A Proven Program to Prevent or Delay Type 2 Diabetes* curriculum for topic areas and content; CDC, 2018b). Students also learned how to review participant food/activity/goal setting logs, conduct weigh-ins and blood pressure checks, and download participant data from these activities to an online database program accessed via a website link.

Church Health Worker (CHW) Training

Each church appointed at least 2 church members to serve as CHWs who liaised between the SOM research team and faculty and received training in their role as Project FIT 2.0 health workers. Although they did not receive intensive training in facilitation of the DPP, they did receive a review on the DPP, the original Project FIT (see above), and the Project FIT 2.0 DPP manual. Additionally, their specific roles in working with students to implement FIT 2.0 were reviewed and included discussion on: the flow of the sessions; scriptures to be read (or they could select relevant scriptures) during the class; contributions to discussions that focused on African American culture regarding lifestyle behaviors, values, traditions; securing someone from the church to provide security; identifying appropriate class and exercise space along with space to store materials; and checking on/supporting participants during the week. Original Project FIT materials were also reviewed (e.g., sermons guide, responsive reading, church bulletins, risk checklists) and provided to CHWs to distribute in the FIT 2.0 DPP classes.

Joint Implementation

All Project FIT 2.0 DPP classes were held in the evenings from 6:00pm to 7:30pm in the following Spring semester. Each CHW was instructed to talk with their pastor and/or church leadership team to select the day of their session (any day between Monday and Thursday). Students then used the churches' identified days to select the day of the week that worked best with their schedule and were placed in teams accordingly, as described above. Project FIT 2.0 was launched after all baseline data were collected with assistance from the MD and PA students. Prior to the start of each session, CHWs would bring the scale and class materials to their church's designated class space and arrange the room for the session. Upon arrival, students would calibrate their class scale and briefly review roles (e.g., who will conduct weigh-ins, log review, lead DPP session, lead exercise), which were assigned and agreed upon by the student team in the prior week. Students took turns each week in conducting weigh-ins and log checks, and downloading this data to university study firewalled, password-protected online database. Next, CHWs would open each class session by leading prayer and reading the assigned scripture. Then, 2 students would serve as the lead coaches for the 45-minute DPP session and 2 to 3 students would serve as lead coaches for the 30-minute exercise session on a rotating basis. CHWs contributed to class discussions, particularly on issues participants brought up that were deep in African American cultural and/or church meaning (e.g., how to improve the nutritional content of cultural foods, how faith and prayer can assist in changing health behaviors). At the end of each class, CHWs closed the session with prayer and stored the class materials. Students submitted their weekly reflections via a weblink to the project online database.

Debriefings and Celebration

Four class sessions at the university were set aside throughout the Spring semester to serve as debriefing sessions with the student coaches. In these sessions, students discussed what was working well and not so well in their role as facilitators and solved emerging problems (e.g., how to get late-arrival participants' weight recorded and action logs reviewed without class disruption; Huffman et al., under review). They also talked about the functioning of their team (e.g., class preparation, implementation, data collection) and working collaboratively with the CHW. Moreover, faculty and research team members attended all Project FIT 2.0 classes and used a checklist to ensure students and CHWs completed their assigned tasks. In the class debriefing sessions, faculty provided constructive feedback (e.g., respectfully ask other participants to contribute to the discussion when a dominant participant overtakes the conversation, double-check weight entries) to students based on their

Table 1. Project FIT 2.0 Participant Characteristics (N=72)

Characteristics	Overall N (%)
Age (years)	
18-49	11 (15.3)
50-64	30 (41.7)
65-80	16 (22.2)
Missing	15 (20.8)
Sex	
Male	15 (20.8)
Female	43 (59.7)
Missing	14 (19.4)
Marital Status	
Never married	13 (18.1)
Married/partnered	19 (26.4)
Divorced/separated	22 (30.6)
Widowed	4 (5.6)
Education	
Less than high school	1 (1.4)
High school/GED	8 (11.1)
Some college	20 (27.8)
4 year college	29 (40.3)
Insurance	
Medicare	6 (8.3)
Medicaid	2 (2.8)
Private insurance	40 (55.6)
Other insurance	4 (5.6)
No insurance	6 (8.3)
Living Situation	
Own home	40 (55.6)
Rents	9 (12.5)
Other living situation or homeless	9 (12.5)
Household Monthly Income	
$0-1,000	3 (4.2)
$1,001-2,000	9 (12.5)
$2,001-3,000	13 (18.1)
$3,001 or more	25 (34.7)
Missing/refused	22 (30.6)
Body Mass Index (kg/m^2)	
Normal (18-24.9)	5 (6.9)
Overweight (25-29.9)	14 (19.4)
Obese (30 or higher)	53 (73.6)

observation notes and checklists. Similarly, the research team members provided observational feedback to CHWs immediately after class sessions (e.g., contribute more to the conversation when cultural topics arise, let students know if you'll be late in opening the church). At the end of the semester and after all posttest data had been collected, a large celebration dinner was held for students and CHWs to share stories, fellowship, and receive and discuss preliminary findings. Additionally, Project FIT 2.0 progress and findings were regularly shared in the KC FAITH CAB meetings.

RESULTS

Of the 3 participating churches, all were Christian, bible-based churches (2 Baptist churches and 1 Church of God in Christ) with membership sizes that ranged from 250 to 750 members (about 400 members on average). The churches were located 2 to 4 miles from the UMKC SOM (3 miles on average).

Overall, 72 church and community members were recruited from the 3 participating churches (about 25 participants per class) and completed baseline surveys. Of these 60 (83%) completed the 3-month survey. Among participants, 64% were aged 50 and older, and most were female (60%), as shown in Table 1. Over 90% of participants were overweight or obese.

Weight loss was assessed overall and on number of sessions attended at 1-month and at 3 months. Results indicated overall weight loss averaged 1.72 pounds at the 12-week weigh-in, and nearly 30% of participants lost at least 5 pounds, as shown in Table 2. However, only 50% attended 4 or more sessions. Overall, 28% lost at least 3% of their initial body weight; 8% achieved 5% weight loss. At 1-month,

Table 2. Project FIT Weight Change by Number of Project FIT 2.0 Sessions Attended (N=60)

Weight Loss	Overall	At 1-Month			At 3 Months		
		£ 3 Sessions	4 Sessions	*p*	£ 8 Sessions	^{3} 9 Sessions	*p*
	N=60	N=29	N=31		N=40	N=20	
Weight loss (pounds; mean, SD)	-1.72 (6.4)	-0.30 (6.2)	-3.06 (6.4)	.095	0.22 (5.9)	-5.62 (5.6)	.001
5 pounds, %	28.3	20.7	35.5	.210	17.5	50.0	.008
3 percent, %	20.0	13.8	25.8	.252	12.5	35.0	.041
5 percent, %	8.3	3.4	12.9	.192	2.5	20.0	.021

participants who attended all 4 sessions lost more pounds (-3.06 versus -0.30) and achieved greater percentages of weight loss than those who attended 3 or fewer sessions (n.s.). At 3 months, participants who attended 9 or more sessions lost significantly more pounds than those attending 8 or fewer sessions (-5.62 versus +0.22; p=.001). Also, among participants who attend 9 or more sessions, 55% lost at least 3% body weight; 20% of those who attended 9 or more sessions achieved 5% weight loss at 3 months.

Additionally, among all students and all class sessions conducted across the 3 participating churches, only 1 no-show was detected, resulting in a nearly 100% perfect student attendance overall. The only classes that were cancelled were due to weather and on 1 occasion when a CHW did not show up for class, and therefore the church was locked, which prohibited the opportunity to hold the class.

DISCUSSION

To the authors' knowledge, this is the first study to report on the feasibility and impact of engaging interprofessional teams of students paired with CHWs in African American church settings to implement a collaborative care model with the goal of assisting a community sample in their weight loss efforts. This approach is novel in that it increases access to the DPP for underserved, low-resource African American urban communities while providing a novel educational experience for health professional students. Equally novel, interprofessional teams of students worked collaboratively with trained CHWs to deliver the Project FIT 2.0 DPP intervention. The nearly 100% perfect attendance achieved by student coaches in their DPP classes indicates that students were highly committed to the program, and that this approach is highly feasible for implementation and has high potential for feasible sustainability.

Additionally, in partnering with the urban faith community, the feasible reach of the collaborative care diabetes prevention model with African Americans at risk for diabetes was demonstrated. Although participants had to want to lose 5 pounds to enroll in the Project FIT 2.0 study (a selection criterion), over 90% of the participants were either overweight or obese. These findings suggest that there is great need to promote lifestyle changes and weight loss in underserved communities to prevent not only diabetes, but other chronic diseases, such as cardiovascular diseases and some cancers. Many university medical schools may be ideally located in urban areas and have the faculty and student capital needed to respond to this health priority by making evidence-based LCPs, such as the DPP, readily accessible in trusted community settings. However, this approach should be used only after respectful collaborative approaches that fully-engage community and university partners have been conducted (e.g., see Berkley-Patton et al., 2018b).

Most importantly, this study's findings indicated that, on average, participants lost weight, with an average weight loss of nearly 2 pounds. While this may be a small amount, average weight loss in the current study was more than the average weight loss found in the original Project FIT intervention (Berkley-Patton, 2018a). This average included all participants with two weight datapoints, and included many participants who attended very few class sessions. Past studies have found even less weight loss among African American participants in church-based obesity prevention and diabetes prevention studies (e.g., Boltri et al., 2011; Davis-Smith, 2007, Dodani & Fields, 2010). Therefore, the current pilot study findings suggest that collaborative interprofessional student-CHW teams may do just as well or better than other health coaches who have delivered similar types of interventions (Kumanyika, Whitt-Glover & Haire-Joshu, 2014). Also, similar to past DPP studies, increased attendance in the current study yielded improved weight loss outcomes (e.g., Eaglehouse, 2017). Of note, 55% of participants attending nine or more class sessions achieved a 3% weight loss. This is important, since recent studies have found that a 3% weight loss can robustly result in improvements in health conditions associated with metabolic syndrome, including high blood pressure, cholesterol, and blood glucose (e.g., Wilkinson et al., 2019). Future research is needed to determine the impact of this lower weight loss threshold with community samples of African Americans. Moreover, future research is needed to identify strategies to improve attendance, especially with underserved populations who may have other basic needs that may need to be addressed (e.g., transportation, access to affordable healthy foods, childcare) to improve DPP session attendance rates and further improve weight loss outcomes.

Lastly, the community-based collaborative care model may have several benefits for students in medical and other health profession education programs. It addresses several health education program standards, including providing students with skills in preventative health practices, cultural competency, communication, and community-based collaborative care to address health disparities (LCME, 2019). The model also provided intensive service-learning opportunities that were new to the medical school. Additionally, by assisting with the study, students learned skills in translational research, particularly in implementing an adapted evidence-based DPP in faith-based settings with African American populations. They were also provided opportunities to share their experiences as health coaches and problem solve with their fellow classmates and, at the end of the program, with church-community members. Future research is needed to determine if students trained with these experiences as health coaches and translational research early in their training as future health professionals more readily demonstrate their learned skills in their future clinical practice careers compared to those who have not received such training and experience.

From using a community-based approach, the collaborative care model may also have several community benefits. Interprofessional teams of students paired with community partners may be a low-cost delivery method to extend reach of evidence-based LCPs to underserved persons who may not otherwise have opportunities to participate. Including interprofessional teams in medical education continues to be a key area of curricula development and advancement (Mann et al., 2014). Positive feedback from participants in debriefing sessions suggested high feasibility and acceptability of universities partnering with community-based organizations in non-medical settings. For this study, churches were selected as a trusted setting with an extensive presence in African American communities, which may assist in increasing the accessibility of LCPs with African Americans. Still, future research is needed on whether training church members more intensely in the DPP together with students will further impact weight loss outcomes. Future research is also needed on how student coaches can be teamed with community members in non-church settings to reach underserved populations that may not want to participate in a culturally and religiously tailored DPP class. Furthermore, the community-based approach may be more low-cost than providing the DPP in medical settings, and therefore may increase sustainability of such programs. There is much to learn about the cost effectiveness of using trained interprofessional student-community member teams to deliver the DPP in community-based settings and the potential of this approach – if widely disseminated, to have an impact on population health, especially in underserved communities. Further research is also needed on how interprofessional teams of students-CHWs can provide other needed health services with underserved populations, such as diabetes and high blood pressure management programs, using community-based collaborative care models.

Despite its potential benefits for community participants and students, this community-based collaborative care study had several limitations. Participant satisfaction with the project was collected in posttest study debriefings and were not more rigorously collected on posttest surveys. However, this information has been collected from participants in more recent phases of Project FIT with cohorts of interprofessional student-CHW teams with nearly 90% of participants reporting being highly satisfied that student coaches created a comfortable learning environment, were well-organized and well-prepared, used appropriate teaching strategies, and were motivational and encouraging. These more recent findings indicate the acceptability of students in the role of community-based health coaches. Additionally, the most recent cohort of nearly 70 students served 17 churches, with five churches on a waitlist, which suggests that interest and demand for this community-based collaborative DPP model is seen as beneficial to the African American faith community. Also as a limitation, the current study was a pilot and therefore was not fully powered and did not employ a control group with church randomization, which limits determination of its efficacy. However, the pilot findings suggest movement in the right direction for weight loss and, as was mentioned earlier, produced overall findings in line with or better than the original Project FIT 2.0 DPP and other church-based studies with reported weight loss outcomes (Berkley-Patton et al., Dodani et al., Boltri et al.). Lastly, the Project FIT 2.0 DPP did not include the 6 maintenance sessions that are included in CDC's *Prevent T2* curriculum (CDC, 2018b). Students only facilitated the 16 core DPP topics since the number of in-class DPP sessions (some sessions covered 2 topics) was time-limited to 12 weeks in order to have access to students and provide course credit during the span of an average semester. Future practice is needed on testing delivery of the 6 maintenance sessions, which typically occur over 6 months, using a hybrid of online and in-class sessions facilitated by students and/or CHWs.

Since the completion of this study, the replicable community-based collaborative care model has been tested with 2 more cohorts of students and has expanded to also include pharmacy and psychology students (for course credit), and volunteer MD and PA students who have now served over 25 urban churches in low-resource African American communities. These accomplishments suggest the potential increased capacity to provide health systems with future health professionals who have skills in cultural competency, communication, preventative health, and interprofessional practice gained from their service learning experiences. These future professionals will also have skills to encourage their patients to participate in LCPs and be able to support their efforts to engage in healthy behaviors. These accomplishments also suggest the potential reach and sustainability of collaborative care models in underserved community-based settings to improve population health, particularly with a focus on health disparities and chronic diseases. such as diabetes.

FUTURE RESEARCH DIRECTIONS

This study is one of the first to provide participant health outcomes from the use of interprofessional teams of students serving as health coaches to deliver the DPP, a LCP that could have several health benefits beyond diabetes prevention, including reducing risk for cardiovascular diseases, improving sleep, and improving stress management. Notably, students did so in low-resource, underserved communities with a non-traditional health partner – African American churches. Future research is needed to determine if the community-based collaborative care model used in this study could have further application in addressing other health issues that burden underserved populations, such as diabetes management, pain management, and mental health issues, in partnership with trusted institutions like churches.

Additionally, students worked one-on-one with Project FIT 2.0 DPP participants in reviewing their action, food, and physical activity logs weekly. This critical component of the group-format DPP allowed for individual participant attention and aligns with providing patient-centered care regarding issues and successes identified by the participant. These weekly, highly personal interactions also provided students with opportunities to improve their communication skills with participants and to partner with participants in problem-solving and establishing new weekly health goals. Students were able to discuss these participant-centered interactions and get feedback from their peers and faculty in the four debriefing sessions held during their university class. Still, future research is needed to understand whether the quality and content of these interactions, and the impact of the amount of time spent could be predictive of notable weekly participant behavior change and weight loss successes. Also, future research is needed to determine if further student training in motivational interviewing skills could further impact weight loss among participants. Past studies have shown that motivational interviewing can be a powerful behavioral change strategy for weight loss (e.g., Carels et al., 2007), and there is a growing trend to include motivational interviewing training in medical education programs (Kaltman & Tankersley, 2019).

Furthermore, implementation of the community-based collaborative care model was carried out with course credit for students who worked alongside volunteering CHWs who received a small stipend to jointly delivery the DPP over the span of a semester. Future research is needed to determine the success of this model on participant weight loss if students and CHWs were to deliver the full 22 core and maintenance DPP sessions over the CDC-recommended 12-month period. Future practice would also possibly be needed to identify appropriate 12-month for-credit medical education courses that could feasibly align with collaborative care interprofessional models – possibly inclusive of other health profession programs (e.g., nursing, pharmacy) – to provide the entire year-long DPP in community settings.

Future practice is also needed to determine mechanisms for university third-party payment models from potential DPP reimbursements from the Centers for Medicare & Medicaid Services (CMS) when DPP Medicare/Medicaid participants complete the 12-month DPP. The CMS DPP proposed rule for a supplier performance-based payment structure aims to tie DPP suppliers' payments to Medicare/Medicaid participants' achieving designated DPP attendance and weight loss goals.

CONCLUSION

This chapter described a community-based collaborative care model that engaged interprofessional teams of students paired with CHWs to deliver the evidence-based weekly-group DPP over 3 months in African American churches. The findings from this pilot study strongly suggest that this approach is highly feasible with interprofessional teams of students serving as health coaches and with dependable commitment from the students. This approach could greatly increase capacity to widely disseminate the DPP free-of-charge in underserved African American communities, settings where the DPP is scarcely available. The findings also suggest that this model of DPP delivery has potential to achieve clinically meaningful weight loss among African Americans, a population at high risk for diabetes. Future studies are needed to explore scalable/sustainable approaches for community-based collaborative care models that engage students in assisting with DPP dissemination in partnership with underserved communities that are disproportionately burdened with diabetes.

ACKNOWLEDGMENT

The authors would like to thank the participating churches and their church health workers for their unwavering commitment to this project. The authors would also like to thank the first cohort of Project FIT students for being willing to serve as health coaches in this first examination of the described community-based collaborative care model. Additionally, we'd like to thank Alex Bauer and Kelsey Christensen for their incredible work as clinical health psychology doctoral students assisting with this project and Jenifer Allsworth for providing the statistical analysis. This research was supported with resources from the University of Missouri-Kansas City.

REFERENCES

Ackermann, R. T., & Marrero, D. G. (2007). Adapting the Diabetes Prevention Program lifestyle intervention for delivery in the community: The YMCA model. *The Diabetes Educator, 33*(1), 74–65. doi:10.1177/0145721706297743 PMID:17272794

Adams, R., Hebert, C. J., McVey, L., & Williams, R. (2016). Implementation of the YMCA Diabetes Prevention Program throughout an Integrated Health System: A Translational Study. *The Permanente Journal, 20*(4), 82–86. doi:10.7812/TPP/15-241 PMID:27828773

American Diabetes Association. (2015). Standards of Medical Care in Diabetes—2015: Summary of Revisions. *Diabetes Care*, *38*(Suppl. 1), S4. doi:10.2337/dc15-S003

American Diabetes Association. (2016). Classification and diagnosis of diabetes. Sec. 2. In Standards of Medical Care in Diabetes. *Diabetes Care*, *39*(Suppl. 1), S13–S22. doi:10.2337/dc16-S005 PMID:27555625

American Diabetes Association. (2018). Economic costs of diabetes in the U.S. in 2017. *Diabetes Care*, *41*(5), 917–928. doi:10.2337/dci18-0007 PMID:29567642

American Medical Association. (2019). *Prevent Diabetes STAT*. Retrieved from http://www.ama-assn.org/sub/prevent-diabetes-stat/

Bauer, A., Berkley-Patton, J., Bowe-Thompson, C., & Christensen, K. (2018). Predictors and missed opportunities for blood glucose screening among African Americans: Implications for church-based populations. *Journal of Health Disparities Research and Practice*, *12*(2), 4.

Berkley-Patton, J., Bowe Thompson, C., Bauer, A., Berman, M., Bradley-Ewing, A., & … . (2018a). Using faith community engagement to increase reach and impact of a diabetes/CVD health promotion intervention in African American churches. *Annals of Behavioral Medicine*, *52*(Suppl 1), S2.

Berkley-Patton, J., Bowe Thompson, C., Bradley-Ewing, A., Berman, M., Booker, A., & … . (2018b). Identifying health conditions, priorities, and relevant multilevel health promotion intervention strategies in African American churches: A faith community health needs assessment. *Evaluation and Program Planning*, *31*(67), 19–28. doi:10.1016/j.evalprogplan.2017.10.012 PMID:29156312

Boltri, J. M., Davis-Smith, M., Okosun, I. S., Seale, J. P., & Foster, B. (2011). Translation of the National Institutes of Health Diabetes Prevention Program in African American churches. *Journal of the National Medical Association*, *103*(3), 194–202. doi:10.1016/S0027-9684(15)30301-1 PMID:21671523

Bowe Thompson, C., Ruhland Petty, T., Berkley-Patton, J., & Berman, M., C., Booker, A., et al. (2015, November). *Project FIT (Faith Influencing Transformation): The Good, the Bad, and the Ugly of Sunday Morning Health Screenings in African American Churches*. Paper presented at the 143rd Annual Meeting and Scientific Session of the American Public Health Association, Chicago, IL.

Brunisholz, K. D., Kim, J., Savitz, L. A., Hashibe, M., Gren, L. H., Hamilton, S., Huynh, K., & Joy, E. A. (2017). A formative evaluation of a diabetes prevention program using the RE-AIM framework in a learning health care system, Utah, 2013-2015. *Preventing Chronic Disease*, *14*(E58), 160556. doi:10.5888/pcd14.160556 PMID:28727546

Carels, R. A., Darby, L., Cacciapaglia, H. M., Konrad, K., Coit, C., Harper, J., Kaplar, M. E., Young, K., Baylen, C. A., & Versland, A. (2007). Using motivational interviewing as a supplement to obesity treatment: A stepped-care approach. *Health Psychology*, *26*(3), 369–374. doi:10.1037/0278-6133.26.3.369 PMID:17500624

Centers for Disease Control and Prevention. (2013a). CDC health disparities and inequalities report – United States 2011. Diabetes— United States, 2006 and 2010. *Morbidity and Mortality Weekly Report*, *62*(Suppl 3), 99–104.

Centers for Disease Control and Prevention. (2013b). CDC health disparities and inequalities report – United States 2011. Obesity— United States, 1999–2010. *Morbidity and Mortality Weekly Report*, *62*(Suppl 3), 120–128.

Centers for Disease Control and Prevention. (2017). *National diabetes statistics report: estimates of diabetes and its burden in the United States, 2017*. Atlanta, GA: U.S. Department of Health and Human Services, Centers for Disease Control and Prevention. Retrieved from https://www.cdc.gov/diabetes/data/statistics/statistics-report.html

Centers for Disease Control and Prevention. (2018a). *Screen & Refer Patients to a Lifestyle Change Program*. Retrieved from https://www.cdc.gov/diabetes/prevention/why-refer.html

Centers for Disease Control and Prevention. (2018b). *National Diabetes Prevention Program. Curricula and Handouts*. Retrieved from https://www.cdc.gov/diabetes/prevention/resources/curriculum.html

Dall, T. M., Mann, S. E., Zhang, S., Quick, W. W., Seifert, R. F., Martin, J., Huang, E. A., & Zhang, S. (2009). Distinguishing the economic costs associated with type 1 and type 2 diabetes. *Population Health Management*, *12*(2), 103–110. doi:10.1089/pop.2009.12203 PMID:19361253

Dall, T. M., Roary, M., Yang, W., Zhang, S., Chen, Y. J., & … . (2011). Health care use and costs for participants in a diabetes disease management program, United States, 2007-2008. *Preventing Chronic Disease*, *8*(3), A53. PMID:21477493

Davis-Smith, M. (2007). Implementing a diabetes prevention program in a rural African-American church. *Journal of the National Medical Association*, *99*, 440–446. PMID:17444435

Diabetes Prevention Program Research Group. (2002). Reduction in the incidence of Type 2 diabetes with lifestyle intervention or metformin. *The New England Journal of Medicine*, *346*(6), 393–403. doi:10.1056/NEJMoa012512 PMID:11832527

Diabetes Prevention Program Research Group. (2004). Achieving weight and activity goals among Diabetes Prevention Program Lifestyle participants. *Obesity Research*, *12*(9), 1426–1434. doi:10.1038/oby.2004.179 PMID:15483207

Dodani, S., & Fields, J. Z. (2010). Implementation of the Fit Body and Soul, a church-based life style program for diabetes prevention in high risk African Americans: A feasibility study. *The Diabetes Educator*, *36*(3), 465–472. doi:10.1177/0145721710366756 PMID:20508263

Eaglehouse, Y. L., Venditti, E. M., Kramer, M. K., Arena, V. C., Vanderwood, K. K., Rockette-Wagner, B., & Kriska, A. M. (2017). Factors related to lifestyle goal achievement in a diabetes prevention program dissemination study. *Translational Behavioral Medicine*, *7*(4), 873–880. doi:10.100713142-017-0494-0 PMID:28397158

Gary-Webb, T. L., Walker, E. A., Realmuto, L., Kamler, A., Lukin, J., Tyson, W., Carrasquillo, O., & Weiss, L. (2018). Translation of the National Diabetes Prevention Program to engage men in disadvantaged neighborhoods in New York City: A description of Power Up for Health. *American Journal of Men's Health*, *12*(4), 998–1006. doi:10.1177/1557988318758788 PMID:29540131

Gorrindo, P., Alon, P., & Ladner, T. (2014). Medical students as health educators at a student-run free clinic: Improving the clinical outcomes of diabetic patients. *Academic Medicine*, *89*(4), 625–631. doi:10.1097/ACM.0000000000000164 PMID:24556762

Huffman, M., Bowe Thompson, C., Lister, S., Johnson, N., Ervie, K., & .... (Manuscript submitted for publication). Can health professional students help fight the diabetes epidemic? A report on an interprofessional service-learning opportunity in African American churches. *Journal of Interprofessional Care*.

Jiang, L., Manson, S. M., Dill, E. J., Beals, J., Johnson, A., Huang, H., Acton, K. J., & Roubideaux, Y. (2015). Participant and site characteristics related to participant retention in a diabetes prevention translational project. *Prevention science. The Official Journal of the Society for Prevention Research*, *16*(1), 41–52. doi:10.100711121-013-0451-1 PMID:24384689

Kaltman, S., & Tankersley, A. (2019). Teaching motivational interviewing to medical students: A systematic review. *Academic Medicine*. Advance online publication. doi:10.1097/ACM.0000000000003011 PMID:31577585

Kumanyika, S. K., Whitt-Glover, M. C., & Haire-Joshu, D. (2014). What works for obesity prevention and treatment in black Americans? Research directions. *Obesity Reviews*, *15*, 204–212. doi:10.1111/obr.12213 PMID:25196414

Li, R., Qu, S., Zhang, P., Chattopadhyay, S., Gregg, E. W., Albright, A., Hopkins, D., & Pronk, N. P. (2015). Economic evaluation of combined diet and physical activity promotion rograms to prevent type 2 diabetes among persons at increased risk: A systematic review for the Community Preventive Services Task Force. *Annals of Internal Medicine*, *163*(6), 452–460. doi:10.7326/M15-0469 PMID:26167962

Liaison Committee on Medical Education. (2019). *Functions and Structure of a Medical School. Standards for Accreditation of Medical Education Programs Leading to the MD Degree*. Association of American Medical Colleges and American Medical.

Lin, J., Thompson, T. J., Cheng, Y. J., Zhuo, X., Zhang, P., Gregg, E., & Rolka, D. B. (2018). Projection of the future diabetes burden in the United States through 2060. *Population Health Metrics*, *16*(1), 9. doi:10.118612963-018-0166-4 PMID:29903012

Mann, K. V., Mcfetridge-Durdle, J., Martin-Misener, R., Clovis, J., Rowe, R., Beanlands, H., & Sarria, M. (2009). Interprofessional education for students of the health professions: The "Seamless Care" model. *Journal of Interprofessional Care*, *23*(3), 224–233. doi:10.1080/13561820802697735 PMID:19387906

Nhim, K., Gruss, S. M., Porterfield, D. S., Jacobs, S., Elkins, W., Luman, E. T., Van Aacken, S., Schumacher, P., & Albright, A. (2019). Using a RE-AIM framework to identify promising practices in National Diabetes Prevention Program implementation. *Implementation Science; IS*, *14*(1), 81. doi:10.118613012-019-0928-9 PMID:31412894

Office of Minority Health. (2016). *Diabetes and African Americans*. Retrieved from http://minorityhealth.hhs.gov/omh/browse.aspx?lvl=4&lvlID=18

Pew Research Center. (2015). *America's Changing Religious Landscape*. Retrieved from https://www.pewforum.org/files/2015/05/RLS-05-08-full-report.pdf

Sattin, R. W., Williams, L. B., Dias, J., Garvin, J. T., Marion, L., Joshua, T. V., Kriska, A., Kramer, M. K., & Venkat Narayan, K. M. (2016). Community trial of a faith-based lifestyle intervention to prevent diabetes among African-Americans. *Journal of Community Health*, *41*(1), 87–96. doi:10.100710900-015-0071-8 PMID:26215167

Taylor, R. J., Chatters, L. M., & Levin, J. (2004). *Religion in the lives of African Americans: social, psychological, and health perspectives*. Sage.

Wilkinson, M. J., Manoogian, E., Zadourian, A., Lo, H., Fakhouri, S., Shoghi, A., Wang, X., Fleischer, J. G., Navlakha, S., Panda, S., & Taub, P. R. (2020). Ten-hour time-restricted eating reduces weight, blood pressure, and atherogenic lipids in patients with metabolic syndrome. *Cell Metabolism*, *31*(1), 1–13. doi:10.1016/j.cmet.2019.11.004 PMID:31813824

ADDITIONAL READING

Albright, A., & Gregg, E. W. (2013). Preventing type 2 diabetes in communities across the US: The National Diabetes Prevention Program. *American Journal of Preventive Medicine*, *44*(4), S346–S351. doi:10.1016/j.amepre.2012.12.009 PMID:23498297

Arvey, S. R., & Fernandez, M. E. (2012). Identifying the core elements of effective community health worker programs: A research agenda. *American Journal of Public Health*, *102*(9), 1633–1637. doi:10.2105/AJPH.2012.300649 PMID:22813092

D'amour, D., & Oandasan, I. (2005). Interprofessionality as the field of interprofessional practice and interprofessional education: An emerging concept. *Journal of Interprofessional Care*, *19*(sup1, S1), 8–20. doi:10.1080/13561820500081604 PMID:16096142

Fisher, K., Dill, M., & Orlowski, J. (2018). Analysis in Brief. Growth in Medical School Enrollment and Clerkship sites available. *Association of American Medical Colleges, 18*(3), 1-3.

Lancaster, K. J., Carter-Edwards, L., Grilo, S., Shen, C., & Schoenthaler, A. M. (2014). Obesity interventions in African American faith-based organizations: A systematic review. *Obesity Reviews*, *15*(4), 159–176. doi:10.1111/obr.12207 PMID:25196412

Resnicow, K., Baranowski, T., Ahluwalia, J. S., & Braithwaite, R. L. (1999). Cultural sensitivity in public health: Defined and demystified. *Ethnicity & Disease*, *9*(1), 10–21. PMID:10355471

Stewart, T., & Wubbena, A. C. (2015). A systematic review of service-learning in medical education: 1998–2012. *Teaching and Learning in Medicine*, *27*(2), 115–122. doi:10.1080/10401334.2015.1011647 PMID:25893932

Tuomilehto, J., Lindstrom, J., Eriksson, J., Valle, T. T., Hämäläinen, H., Ilanne-Parikka, P., Keinänen-Kiukaanniemi, S., Laakso, M., Louheranta, A., Rastas, M., Salminen, V., Aunola, S., Cepaitis, Z., Moltchanov, V., Hakumäki, M., Mannelin, M., Martikkala, V., Sundvall, J., & Uusitupa, M. (2001). Finnish Diabetes Prevention Study Group. Prevention of type 2 diabetes mellitus by changes in lifestyle among subjects with impaired glucose tolerance. *The New England Journal of Medicine*, *344*(18), 1343–1350. doi:10.1056/NEJM200105033441801 PMID:11333990

KEY TERMS AND DEFINITIONS

Collaborative Care: A strategy used to provide health care services and support in partnership directly with patients and/or with community and health organizations that are providing services and care with the patient.

Community-Based Participatory Research: An approach to conducting health science research that starts with the community identifying the priority health issues to be addressed and engages the community in all phases of research from conceptualizing the research agenda to research planning, implementation, evaluation and dissemination of findings, with the ultimate goal to reduce health disparities.

Cultural Competence: The ability to understand patient needs and provide quality care in a manner acceptable to the patient regardless of their ethnicity, race, gender, religious and/or other personal characteristics or beliefs.

Interprofessional Student Teams: A group of students from different professional backgrounds that come together to provide care or supportive services to patients, clients, or communities.

Lifestyle Change Programs: Programs that provide information, skills, and support to help persons engage in health promotion behaviors including physical activity, healthy nutritional intake, stress management, and connecting with others to reduce risk for and/or manage chronic diseases and increase longevity.

National Diabetes Prevention Program (DPP): A CDC evidence-based program that has been proven to significantly reduce risk for onset of diabetes through modest weight loss and physical activity.

Service Learning: Activities that engage students in service that benefits the community or persons external to the university while providing students with opportunities for personal reflection and experiential learning that aligns with curriculum objectives.

Chapter 10
The Physician Assistant Profession:
Collaboration Through Interprofessional Education

Katherine G. Ervie
University of Missouri-Kansas City School of Medicine, USA

Julie Wright Banderas
https://orcid.org/0000-0001-7085-304X
University of Missouri-Kansas City School of Medicine, USA

ABSTRACT

In the United States, quality healthcare is an expectation. The accepted healthcare delivery approach relies on interprofessional, collaborative, and person-centered teams. As a result, health professions education must implement education and training to graduate a healthcare workforce that is competent in interprofessional collaboration. Physician assistants (PA) have an important role in the healthcare team. The purpose of this chapter is to provide a historical background to the interprofessional collaborative healthcare team, the formation of interprofessional education (IPE) competencies and partnerships, and the valued role of physician assistants. The need for evidence-based results to guide IPE curricular decisions for PA programs and characteristics of published IPE activities involving PA students are summarized. Potential barriers to successful interprofessional education and resolutions to those challenges are discussed.

DOI: 10.4018/978-1-7998-3066-5.ch010

INTRODUCTION

An interprofessional and collaborative health care workforce has been a proposed strategy to improve problems faced by global health systems for many years. Two motivators for interprofessional practice are the shortage of health professionals and patient safety. Despite the longstanding incentives and frequent endorsements, U.S. health systems have been slow to develop or require prototypical models of interprofessional and collaborative patient care. Interprofessional education (IPE), however, has become a widely adopted approach by the majority of health education and training programs. IPE is a path to graduate competent health care professionals, who enter the workforce prepared to function collaboratively and as an effective member of the interprofessional care team.

BACKGROUND

The concerns over medical errors and patient safety are longstanding and well described. Numerous federal and private agencies, professional organizations, and educational associations have been committed to the exploration of root causes and feasible solutions for decades. A guided look at selected reports and projects underscores the changing knowledge, involved participants, and terminology over time and shows the evolution toward today's favored interprofessional, collaborative, and person-centered approach to health care delivery.

One of the first national groups dedicated to improving patient safety and health care outcomes was the Institute for Healthcare Improvement (IHI), which began in 1986 as a part of the National Demonstration Project on Quality Improvement in Health Care. The IHI developed an Interdisciplinary Professional Education Collaborative in 1994, "with the aim of making quality improvement a standard component in the education of health professionals in all disciplines" and began the Health Professions Education Collaborative in 2003 as a part of a unifying movement around improving health care for all. (Institute for Healthcare Improvement, n.d.) For over thirty years, the IHI has partnered with diverse organizations and global communities to study and demonstrate successful and reproducible health care models for improved patient safety. Through sustained innovation, the IHI has been at the forefront of studying techniques to reduce errors, for example leading the move from team-based care to testing interprofessional collaborations. In 2007, the IHI launched the Triple Aim initiative, to provide a universal and actionable framework for optimizing health, care, and cost. The Triple Aim is representative of the many IHI sustained global training programs and tools, which are adaptable across government agencies, clinical health systems, and health professions education

("Institute for Healthcare Improvement," n.d.). In the last decade, the IHI's patient safety focus has transitioned from patient-centered care to improved global health care systems and outcomes for a community and the individual.

The Committee on the Quality of Health Care in America was established in 1998 by the Institute of Medicine, now known as the National Academy of Medicine. The purpose of the committee was to develop strategies for improvements in health care. The committee's first focus was on patient safety and medical errors as described in the influential report, *To Err is Human: Building a Safer Health System.* This report is frequently cited to draw attention to patient safety, and the need to improve patient health outcomes. The authors of *To Err is Human* used medical error data reported about New York, Colorado and Utah hospitalized patient cohorts to estimate the possible prevalence among all U.S. hospital admissions in 1997. The extrapolated national rate of preventable fatal in-patient medical errors impressively exceeded the eighth leading cause of death in 1997 (Institute of Medicine (US) Committee on Quality of Health Care in America, 2000). The committee investigated many conditions and contributing factors reported in the literature to create medical errors and provided related recommendations to improve patient safety. Failures of teamwork and interprofessional communication were two identified causes. Borrowing from the aviation industry, the committee recommended strategies to "promote effective team functioning" highlighting concepts of teamwork, team training, and patient involvement. (Institute of Medicine (US) Committee on Quality of Health Care in America, 2000, p. 173). Another important recommendation included in this report was to advise Congress to create a Center for Patient Safety within the Agency for Healthcare Research and Quality (AHRQ). The AHRQ is a primary resource for improving the safety of health care in the U.S., by providing education and training, implementation tools, and funding for demonstration projects. (Agency for Healthcare Research and Quality, n.d.)

The follow-up report in 2001 from the Committee on the Quality of Health Care in America, *Crossing the Quality Chasm: A New Health System for the 21st Century*, provided detailed plans for implementation in practice. Specific approaches for patient centered care are described in multiple recommendations and interprofessional collaborative care terminology was introduced as "cooperation among clinicians." (Institute of Medicine, 2001, p. 62). It is also in this report that the committee proposed methods for preparing the health care workforce for patient-centered and interprofessional collaborative care through restructuring clinical education and provision of retooling opportunities for those in practice. Although somewhat focused on medicine, there was a recommendation for a multidisciplinary summit of the health professions to address curricular change and suggestions for training in the groups that would work together to provide collaborative care. A next step for this committee was to convene a summit with health professions educators and students. The committee proposed a set of five core competencies that all clinicians entering the workforce should possess to improve the quality of patient care and meet patient needs. These competencies include providing patient centered care, working in interdisciplinary teams, employing evidence based practice, applying quality improvement and utilizing informatics. (Institute of Medicine, 2001). The summit participants were tasked with developing strategies to integrate these competencies in health professions curricula. Key recommendations were put forth in the resulting report, *Health Professions Education: A Bridge to Quality*, that formed the basis for interprofessional education. Key concepts included use of common language, coordination of accrediting bodies for health professions, and identification of ideal training models (Institute of Medicine, 2003).

In 2009 the first six national education associations of schools of health professions formed a collaborative, the Interprofessional Education Collaborative (IPEC). In 2011, the Physician Assistant Education Association (PAEA) signed on as one of the supporting organizations and was officially included as an IPEC institutional member in 2016. Initially the IPEC studied the national and international interprofessional education landscape to develop the IPEC core competencies and presented four general interprofessional collaborative practice competency domain categories. In 2016, the IPEC board reorganized the four competencies into a singular domain of interprofessional collaboration, to encompass the four original proposed domains. (Interprofessional Education Collaborative, 2016). These four competencies include values and ethics for IPE, roles and responsibilities, interprofessional communication, and teams and teamwork. These competencies and the respective sub-competencies are to be used to guide the design and assessment of contemporary IPE curricula.

The IPEC mission underscores the link between IPE and practice The IPEC mission is, “IPEC, working in collaboration with academic institutions, will promote, encourage, and support efforts to prepare future health professionals so that they enter the workforce ready for interprofessional collaborative practice that helps ensure the health of individuals and populations”. (Vision & Mission, 2019). A prepared and effective workforce must take into account the availability of workforce team members. Trends in oversupply and shortages of healthcare professionals shift over years and vary by profession. Whether there are physician shortages is debated and varies by discipline and timing. There is, however, an increasing number of non-physician health professionals entering the workforce including physician assistants.

THE PHYSICIAN ASSISTANT PROFESSION

The Physician Assistant profession developed from a long history of non-physician providers used to provide healthcare services. Historic precedents include the feldshers in Russia, barefoot doctors in China and the Frontier Nursing Services in the mountains of Kentucky. Even from our military history in the 1930s, former military corpsmen received on-the-job training in the federal prison system to extend the services of prison physicians. During World War II, the U.S. Coast Guard trained over 600 purser mates to provide healthcare on merchant ships (Timeline, n.d.).

In the 1950s, the idea began to take shape of a physician extender that could perform tasks that had previously been performed by physicians and expand the capabilities of a primary care physician, especially in medically underserved areas. With the identification by the U.S. Surgeon General in 1959 of a medical personnel shortage, Dr. Charles Husdon proposed the PA concept utilizing military trained personnel to the American Medical Association. Private physicians began to develop their own trained assistants which sometimes led to debate of the legality of physicians to delegate duties to an assistant. In the late 1950s, Dr. Eugene Stead first proposed a training program to extend the duties of nurses but faced opposition by the National League of Nursing. Dr. Stead responded to this opposition by enrolling four ex-Navy corpsman as the first class of PA students in 1965 at Duke University.

The birth of the PA profession occurred during a time of transformation in the U.S. With the growth of medical specialities, advancing medical technology and increasing hospital services, physicians began to choose the practice of specialty medicine over primary care. Fewer generalist physicians were being trained and lacked in numbers to replace retiring family medicine physicians. The shortage was noted especially in the small towns and rural areas. The White House conference on Health in 1965 raised the issue of physician shortages and began the exploration of healthcare professions that might offset this shortage (Timeline, n.d.).

During this time, the call to address social inequities including the increasing poverty, racial and gender divide grew. In 1964, The Civil Rights Act outlawed discrimination against African Americans, including racial segregation. It removed socioeconomic barriers to voter registration and ended racial segregation in schools, workplace and facilities that serve the public including hospitals and clinics. Soon after, in 1965, Medicare and Medicaid were passed by the United States Congress which expanded the need for basic medical services for the elderly and poor.

With the increase in patient numbers coupled with a shortage of primary care physicians, additional healthcare providers were needed. A highly trained and combat tested workforce was identified in the military corpsman returning from duty in the Vietnam war. During their service they had worked on medical teams composed of physicians, nurses, medics, and corpsman. On return to civilian life, the corpsman was the only team member without an identified role in the current healthcare system. The ability to provide a civilian occupation for returning veterans held great political appeal. Capitalizing upon the experience and training of the corpsman created a new training pool to meet healthcare demands and did not draw from other established professions, such as nursing, which could create new workforce gaps.

The educational model developed by Dr. Eugene Stead for the new profession was based on his fast-track training of physicians during World War II at Emory University. He knew from his experience with the highly trained military personnel, that the educational period could be shorter than that for traditional medical students. Dr. Stead proposed that the close supervision by their physician employers would ensure competence and further development of needed skills in practice (Hooker, Cawley & Everett, 2017). All pioneer PA programs were based on this medical model that provided students an education and orientation similar to the physicians with whom they would work.

The development of the PA profession and education model was the first time that knowledge previously reserved for physicians was being shared. PAs were now capable of carrying out those responsibilities that had in the past lived in the domain of a physician. The supervisory relationship between the PA and the physician provided the PA with ongoing oversight and opportunity to develop their skills as needed in specific practice settings. The legal relationship of the PA to the physician was unique in the healthcare system. Although recent guidelines have been proposed by the American Academy of Physician Assistants (AAPA) to eliminate the legal and administrative ties between a PA and a specific physician, the collaborative nature of the PA-physician relationship remains unchanged (Optimal Team Practice, n.d.).

As the PA profession and number of educational programs grew, the American Medical Association in 1971, recognized the PA profession and provided guidance and resources to develop a national certification process, accreditation of educational programs, and codification of practice laws. The profession continued to gain support and in 1978 was recognized by the Institute of Medicine report titled *Manpower Policy for Primary Health Care* as bringing value to the practice of primary care (Institute of Medicine, 1978). At the time, there was a projected increase in physician supply, but the report cited that even with this projected physician surplus, PAs still played an important role in the delivery of care.

Despite support for the profession, PA education programs were negatively impacted as a result of a second national report by the Graduate Medical Education National Advisory Committee (GMENAC) in 1981. The GMENAC committee, organized by the U.S. Secretary of Health Education and Welfare, was charged to examine the physician supply issue. The advisory committee projected an oversupply of physicians and made recommendations to reduce medical school enrollment, limit the use of foreign-trained physicians, and review the need to train non-physician providers (Graduate Medical Education National Advisory Committee, 1981). This report resulted in the significant reduction of federal funding for PA education programs. Today, with a retrospective viewpoint of the unforeseen healthcare impact of HIV and chronic health conditions, increasing use of physician services, and graduate medical education training hour regulation, the question remains if the committee identified a true physician surplus versus one of maldistribution.

Even with a setback in funding dollars for training programs, PAs continued to be trained and utilized in primary care. However, the clinical versatility of PAs broadened and PAs were hired to work in a variety of specialties and practice settings to meet healthcare demands. The passage of the Omnibus Budget Reconciliation Act of 1986 expanded Medicare reimbursement policies for PA services providing legitimacy of PA services in medical care delivery. The passage of the Affordable Care Act in 2010 created new models for health care and recognized the PA profession as a vital component to its success. Although the demand for PAs and the acceptance of their role in healthcare has grown, the recognition of the cost-effectiveness of PA utilization in healthcare delivery has had significant impact in promoting the profession.

Current PA education continues to be rooted in its history of a medical model and provides a broad, generalist education. Although discussion continues at a national organization level, the current terminal degree for the profession is a master's level degree. To practice as a PA, a graduate must graduate from an Accreditation Review Commission on Education for the Physician Assistant (ARC-PA) accredited PA program, pass the Physician Assistant National Certification Exam administered by the National Commission on Certification of Physician Assistants (NCCPA), and be licensed by the state in which they practice. Although PAs practice in every state and in every medical setting and speciality, specific scope of practice is determined at the state level.

In 2011, the American Academy of Family Physicians (AAFP) in conjunction with the American Academy of Physician Assistants (AAPA) published a joint policy statement recognizing that "family physicians and PAs working together in a team-oriented practice, such as the patient-centered medical home, is a proven model for delivery of high-quality, cost effective patient care" and call for policies and regulations "that recognize that PAs function as primary care providers in the patient-centered medical home as part of a multidisciplinary, physician-directed clinical team" (Rathfon & Jones, 2011, p. 1). In order to achieve this goal however, the two organizations identified the need for increased interprofessional education opportunities for PAs, medical students, and residents in their training.

For the model of interprofessional practice to be successful, students must be exposed to the concept of interprofessional education during their training. The Physician Assistant Education Association (PAEA) published the *Core*

Competencies for New Physician Assistant Graduates and identified interprofessional collaborative practice and leadership as a core competency (Physician Assistant Education Association, 2019). These PAEA competencies incorporated the IPEC defined competencies for interprofessional collaborative practice and those of interprofessional education including values and ethics for interprofessional practice, team and teamwork, roles and responsibility and interprofessional communication. Providing opportunity for students to develop skills in communication, respect, humility, professionalism, collaboration, self-awareness and trust, is vital to building a person-centered healthcare team.

Accreditation agencies across healthcare professions have responded to this need by including specific accreditation standards to ensure interprofessional education and the necessary skills are included in the curriculum. In the Accreditation Standards for Physician Assistant Education fifth edition, standard B2.10 states that "The curriculum must prepare students to work collaboratively in interprofessional patient centered teams. Instruction must include content on the roles and responsibilities of various health care professionals, emphasize the team approach to patient centered care beyond the traditional physician-PA team approach, and include application of these principles in interprofessional teams" (Accreditation Review Commission on Education for the Physician Assistant, Inc., 2019, p. 15).

The PAEA and Society of Teachers of Family Medicine (STFM) published a position paper titled *Educating Primary Care Teams for the Future: Family Medicine and Physician Assistant Interprofessional Education* in 2012 which recognized "future primary care workforce needs are best met through the training and deployment of integrated teams of health professionals who provide and coordinate care with a patient-centered model" (p. 34). A second position statement recommended "the development and integration of new interprofessional curricula for medical and physician assistant (PA) students and family medicine residents" (p. 34). The authors identify the patient-centered medical home (PCMH) as a framework to achieve more effective, safe, timely, efficient, equitable, and patient-centered health care. Within the PCMH model, recommendations are made for advancing educational collaboration to expand the availability of primary care teams who have trained and will practice together in future PCMH. This joint position paper promotes the PA as ideally suited to play a major role in medical homes due to their generalist education and collaborative approach to practice. PAs can help with critical issues around access, coordination of care, quality improvement, and patient self-management support.

The position paper authored by PAEA and STFM cites five trends supporting the need for interprofessional education. The first is the push for patient safety brought to attention by the *IOM To Err is Human.* One of the outcomes of this report was the implementation of duty hour restrictions for medical residents which lead to greater employment opportunities for PAs to address gaps in patient coverage. A second trend comes from financial restraints imposed on educational institutions with decreased federal funding. Educational institutions face the challenge on how to increase class sizes but maintain educational quality and decrease costs. As institutions are forced to search for innovative ways to educate, they must also strive to incorporate IPE. Educating learners from different health professions provides an opportunity to develop teamwork and communication skills to promote patient safety. In an effort to maximize resources, educational institutions recognize that training learners on fundamental concepts in combined classroom and clinical settings not only maximize resources but provides opportunities to become familiar with collaborative team practice.

A fourth trend is the increased use of ambulatory care settings utilized for clinical education. Increasing numbers of learners across professions results in competing needs for clinical training sites staffed by community providers and faculty. The challenge to recruit and retain quality training sites in sufficient numbers must be considered in how students are educated. A final trend is the move toward competency-based education and assessment. First adapted in 2002 by the Accreditation Council on Graduate Medical Education (ACGME), the focus on defined outcomes and demonstrated abilities of trainees/graduates is now emphasized in medical and PA student education. Faculty must ensure that trainees have the knowledge, skills, and abilities required to perform their expected professional role. Implementation of interprofessional education has the potential to ascertain that all trainees have the abilities to obtain the expected IPEC competencies for team-based collaborative care.

REVIEW OF IPE INVOLVING PHYSICIAN ASSISTANT STUDENTS

The evidence linking IPE directly to improved patient outcomes is lacking. However, the proposed connections between IPE, interprofessional collaborative practice, and improved patient safety and health care outcomes are well reasoned. Prompted by accreditation requirements and collaborative statements from professional organizations such as the PAEA and STFM, IPE is being broadly adopted. Robust investigation of the IPE interventions that are being implemented is needed. Ideally, studies will be designed to make comparisons using a common set of IPE outcomes, such as the IPEC competencies, and validated measures. There is a need for evidence-based results to guide IPE curricular decisions for physician assistant programs. A PubMed search, which was limited to English-language articles published from January 2012 to October 2019, yielded 24 publications that described implementation and evaluation of IPE activities that involved physician assistant students; two of the 24 publications evaluated the same IPE curriculum by different methods. Characteristics of the published reports are summarized in Table 1.

The most commonly used definition of interprofessional education is "when students from two or more professions learn about, from, and with each other to enable effective collaboration and improve health outcomes." (World Health Organization, 2010, p. 7). Physician assistant students have been reported to participate in IPE activities with a broad range of learners including family medicine residents and students from dental, medicine, music therapy, nursing, nutritional sciences, occupational therapy, pharmacy, physical therapy, public health, social work, and speech and language pathology disciplines. The published projects involved from one to ten other professions with PA students.

The described IPE activities varied in format, setting, and duration. Some were implemented as required coursework, while others were voluntary experiences and elective courses. Both one time events and longitudinal curricula were described. Many involved students brought together to complete multiple learning activities that used combinations of large and small IPE group discussion sessions. Patient case discussions were a common method for creating a healthcare experience. Six projects described the use of small group contextual case simulations or simulated patients. Online collaboration and pre-work were frequently utilized. Two studies described IPE delivered within a basic science course (i.e., cadaver anatomy and graduate physiology) in a classroom setting. Nine projects included patient interaction and clinic-based components. These nine IPE activities were typically voluntary and involved small numbers of students. Four were paired with service learning clinical experiences (i.e., mission trip, community outreach prevention event, student run free health clinic). There were two studies that did not study implementation of an IPE activity, but instead surveyed PA students about interprofessional experiences gained throughout their clinical curriculum.

The IPE learning outcomes and competencies that were used in these studies, varied according to the educational setting, the involved interprofessional partners, and timing in the students' curricula. For most activities the educators developed both IPE competencies and contextual medical knowledge or patient care related competencies. With the exception of the earliest reports, most activities were designed using the IPEC competencies; competencies related to roles/responsibilities and teams/teamwork were most frequently evaluated. Few described competencies that could be closely linked to changes in practice, such as collaborative decision making and problem solving. Assessment tools included various combinations of standardized survey questionnaires, author designed surveys, faculty observations, student reflection papers, and focus group methods. The majority of outcomes relied on student reported ratings and reflections. Frequently, surveys were administered as pre and post IPE event measures and the overall total group change and change between and within learner disciplines were analyzed. Changes in student perceptions, attitude, and knowledge regarding IPE competencies were the most frequently measured outcomes. Behavior change or clinical impact were rarely measured.

Unfortunately, IPE research is frequently implemented without rigorous study design. Many of the studies include small groups of students and are not powered to find significant differences. Additionally, most investigators report early results following the initial implementation of IPE activities. There is a lack of long-term followup to evaluate sustained changes in outcomes or later appreciation for IPE. Use of pre and post surveys measuring confidence and attitudes are often limited by very high pre-test scores at the start of an intervention, thus limiting opportunities for change post test. (Seif et al., 2014). This phenomenon has been proposed to be a common occurrence with two standardised surveys used in IPE education research, the Interdisciplinary Education Perception Scale (Seif et al., 2014) and the Readiness for Interprofessional Learning Scale (RIPLS). (Mahler, Berger, & Reeves, 2015). Mahler, Berger and Reeves (2015) describe additional issues with the RIPLS that are likely issues across other IPE standardized scales. Although some IPE standardized tools have been validated, too frequently in IPE research, they are implemented and results reported without conducting psychometric analysis of the results in the new study population. Additionally, researchers often adapt validated scales by rearranging items and relabeling subscales to match evolving IPE terminology. In these cases, the reported results are not clearly defined or validated. Many of the identified studies involving PA students were designed to address specific barriers to IPE, but when implemented identified new challenges.

IPE IMPLEMENTATION CHALLENGES AND RESOLUTIONS

Despite the agreement among healthcare systems, educators, professional organizations and accreditation agencies regarding the importance of including IPE in the curriculum, challenges with implementation exist. " Multidisciplinary training is difficult to implement because of professional boundaries, the traditional hierarchical structure of health care, clinical specialization, faculty experience and educational isolation" (Crossing the Quality Chasm, 2001, p. 210-211). Lawlis, Anson and Greenfield (2014) identified the barriers and enablers of interprofessional education through the involvement of three primary stakeholder levels: government and professional, institutional, and individual. Five key fundamental elements that are critical to achieve sustainable IPE education were identified across stakeholder levels. These elements can either inhibit or enhance the sustained efforts of IPE and include: 1. Government funding; 2. Institutional funding; 3. Faculty development programs; 4. Institutional organizational structure to support the embedding IPE into curricula; 5. Commitment across disciplines to be involved in IPE (Lawlis, Anson & Greenfield, 2014).

In traditional health education programs, learning often occurs in silos. Unfortunately, this model may inhibit learners from being aware of the educational process and roles and responsibilities of other health professions learners. Whereas, learners may be familiar with traditional models of education and practice for a profession but not be aware of the evolving roles that may be occurring in the profession to meet population needs. Exposing learners to current roles and responsibilities of the different health care professions must occur in order to understand the scope of practice of future colleagues. However, preferred activities combine these interprofessional collaborative competencies with a relevant clinical scenario. Students may not be as invested in IPE formats that rely primarily on lectures and contrived patient cases. Active learning formats and online technologies are positively accepted by students. Small group simulation which promote student decision making and portray life-like scenarios are preferred. (Hale & DiLollo, 2016; Shrader, Kern, Zoller, & Blue, 2013). The use of simulation as a case-based learning activity to achieve IPE objectives is difficult to accomplish because of the number of events that must be scheduled and limited availability of faculty and facilities. Computer-based virtual patient cases, however, have been shown to overcome these barriers. (Shoemaker, Platko, Cleghorn, & Booth, 2014).

How to accomplish the task of including multiple health professions in an IPE activity can be challenging. The number of learners in some large group IPE activities is daunting and exceed 400 to 500 students when many health professions are included. Adequate number of faculty facilitators, physical space, and sustainability are issues to address. Already full curricula make scheduling difficult across multiple programs. Many times there may be different ideas on what is the best way to include IPE in the curriculum. Although accreditation standards exist, many are left to interpretation, on the meaning of compliance or needs may be different between programs. Reviews of the literature demonstrate differences across studies of key performance measures to determine success of IPE implementation. For example, some measure changes in attitude while others evaluate faculty buy-in to determine successful implementation (Lawlis). Curricula that incorporate assignments where students collaborate in the care of a real or simulated patient allow the opportunity to measure changes in multiple outcomes including confidence, attitudes, and behavior, in addition to IP related competencies and patient quality outcomes. (Shoemaker 2014, Seif 2014, Hale 2016)

Faculty themselves may not be familiar with teaching IPE concepts. They may be asked to undertake additional IPE tasks in addition to a full teaching load. Faculty development initiatives have been identified as necessary to address barriers to IPE and facilitating culture change across faculty, institutions, and professions

Table 1. Characteristics of published interprofessional education activities involving physician assistant students[a]

Source	IPE Curriculum Format	Outcomes Evaluated	Assessment Measures	Included Professions	Student Sample Size[b]
Bridgeman, M. B., Rusay, M., Afran, J., Yeh, D. S., & Sturgill, M. G. (2018)	Required, medication errors prevention case based workshop	Student pre/post attitudes toward IPE and interprofessional patient care	Modified version of the Attitudes Towards Health Care Teams Scale	P, M, PA	375
Buff, S. M., Jenkins, K., Kern, D., Worrall, C., Howell, D., Martin, K., & Blue, A. (2015)	Elective, interprofessional service learning experience including online education, team learning, and community activities	Student post experience survey to evaluate student appreciation and knowledge of their own and other professions, interaction with other professional students, and student teamwork skills	Author designed student instrument, with items rated on a 5 point Likert scale	biomedical science, dietetics, health administration, M, N, P, PT, PA	230
Buhse, M., & Della Ratta, C. (2017)	Team-based learning (TBL) implemented in an interprofessional classroom setting to teach chronic illness concepts, three 6 hour sessions	Students rated IPEC core competencies overall team effectiveness after TBL activity, Faculty debriefing following TBL activity	TBL iRAT (individual readiness assessment test) and tRAT (team RAT) scores, author designed survey to evaluate IPEC competencies	N, PA, PH	120
Cohen, E. V., Hagestuen, R., González-Ramos, G., Cohen, H. W., Bassich, C., Book, E., & Morgan, J. C. (2016)	Elective, multi-day training on best practices of Parkinson disease (PD) and key elements for integrated team-based care	Student pre/post and 6 month follow-up ratings of perceived knowledge about PD, team-based care, role of other disciplines and attitudes toward health care teams. Students completed faculty created PD knowledge test at the end of training	Attitudes Toward Health Care Teams Scale	health care practitioners and students: M, MT, N, PA, PT, OT, SLP, SW	1468 trainees and 100 controls
Edwards, S., Molina, P. E., McDonough, K. H., Mercante, D. E., & Gunaldo, T. P. (2018)	Embedded IPE exercise in required didactic curriculum; graduate-level human physiology course, female athlete case assignment	Student pre/post ratings for IPEC learning outcomes with focus on roles/responsibilities and teams and teamwork	Author designed instrument	PT, PA, other graduate studies	71
Hale, L. S., & DiLollo, A. (2016)	Required, graduate-level course, combined short-term activities and longer duration activities, faculty members trained in IHI TeamSTEPPS (Team Strategies and Tools to Enhance Performance and Patient Safety) facilitation	Students completed pre/post surveys that assessed confidence with IPEC core competencies: roles and responsibilities, interprofessional communication, teams and teamwork, & values/ethics and functional skills in evidence based practice	Author designed student instrument, with items rated on a 5 point Likert scale	PA, SLP, audiology, aging studies students	278
Kayingo, G., Kidd, V. D., Gilani, O., & Warner, M. L. (2015)	Convenience sample from PA students who had completed at least 4 weeks in a required primary care rotation	Student reported characteristics of their primary rotations, the composition of care teams, type of teaching, satisfaction, the roles of PA students as they rotate, and influence on interest in primary care practice	Author designed instrument	PA, other	179
Kraft, S., Wise, H. H., Jacques, P. F., & Burik, J. K. (2013)	Embedded in required didactic curriculum, single small group simulation of the patient/ family-centered care experience of team-based discharge planning	Student pre/post surveys to gather student perceptions how IPE contributed to student learning about discharge planning, IP collaboration, and the development of caring/compassionate attitudes	Author designed student instrument, with items rated on a 5 point Likert scale, plus one open-ended question about the strengths and weakness of DPS post IPE	OT, PA, PT	172

continued on following page

Table 1. Continued

Source	IPE Curriculum Format	Outcomes Evaluated	Assessment Measures	Included Professions	Student Sample Size[b]
Lie, D. A., Forest, C. P., Walsh, A., Banzali, Y., & Lohenry, K. (2016)	Purposive sample of student volunteers who had participated in an IP student run clinic	Author led focus groups to capture student perceptions what learning occurs in IP student run clinic setting and how learning occurs	Author designed prepared script with semi-structured, open-ended questions.	M, OT, PT, PA	50
Lie, D.A., Walsh, A., Segal-Gidan, F., Banzali, Y., & Lohenry, K. (2013)	Elective, longitudinal 8 months geriatrics IPE curriculum that consisted of three 4-hour classroom based sessions and one IP team geriatric patient interaction	Author led focus groups to capture PA student opinions about relevance of IPE in curriculum and perceptions about effective delivery methods	Author designed prepared script with semi-structured, open-ended questions.	M, OT, P, PT, PA	evaluation limited to 12 participating PA students and 10 controls
McBride, J. M., & Drake, R. L. (2015)	Required IP cadaver anatomy course, course set up included PA student pre-reading, morning didactic section, afternoon laboratory prosections presented by medical students	Post course surveys to gather student rated value of the IPE experience and student rated usefulness of medical student demonstration component of the course	Author designed instrument	M, PA	30 M student demonstrators and 50 PA students
Smithburger, P. L., Kane-Gill, S. L., Kloet, M. A., Lohr, B., & Seybert, A. L. (2013)	Elective, four simulated case activities involving medical scenarios hypertensive crisis and sepsis	Faculty observation rating of student communication and teamwork skills. Student rated acceptance and impression of the use of simulation in an IP environment	Communication and Teamwork Skills Assessment Survey (CATS) and author created student 8 item survey	M, N, P, PA, SW	8 (feasibility project)
Pippitt, K., Moloney-Johns, A., Jalilibahabadi, S., & Gren, L. H. (2015)	Convenience sample from PA students who had completed required clinical experience, 3 to 8 paired student clinical rotation experiences over 2 years	Student pre and post rated attitude regarding roles, benefits of IPE, and impact of IPE on patient care. Separate debriefing sessions at the end of IPE with students and faculty	Assumed author designed attitude assessment survey with unknown number of items rated on a 5-point Likert scale. Open ended debriefing questions analyzed for themes.	M, PA	20 (feasibility project)
Sonney, J., Willgerodt, M., Lindhorst, T., & Brock, D. (2018)	Elective, single event, case video vignette portraying possible child mistreatment	Trainee and facilitator quantitative and qualitative surveys to evaluate progress toward learning objectives. IPE outcomes included team roles and communication	Not described	N, PA, SW, family medicine residents	69
Noonan, C. D., Scow, S., Sheagley, B.A., & Bunn, J. (2018)	Elective, interprofessional service learning experience focused on PT impact on pain management in a rural international patient population	Students and preceptors completed survey following completion of service learning experience to assess perceptions regarding how addition of ideation of pain management	Author designed survey	M, P, PT, PA	16
Palmer, R., & Stilp, C. (2017)	Convenience sample from Combined Medical-Physician Assistant Student Rural Rotation (Med-PARR) pilot program that addresses the challenges of placing two clinical learners concurrently in a rural clinical location	Student self- reported IP goals at the beginning of the IPE experience. Student self -reflection on goals at the end of rotation	Author designed instrument	M, PA	not reported

continued on following page

Table 1. Continued

Source	IPE Curriculum Format	Outcomes Evaluated	Assessment Measures	Included Professions	Student Sample Size[b]
Phillips, W. R., & Keys, T. (2018)	Elective, 12 week non-graded one credit hour classroom course in primary care	Student post experience course evaluation and rating of course influence on interest in primary care career	Author designed instrument	D, N, P, PA	84
Reeves, S. A., Denault, D., Huntington, J. T., Ogrinc, G., Southard, D. R., & Vebell, R. (2017)	Required simulation-based, patient safety-focused learning session	Student post-session assessment of session quality and perceived effectiveness. One-year post-session student survey for rating and commenting about use or observed communication skills in clinical setting	Author designed instrument	N, M, PA	254
Seif, G., Coker-Bolt, P., Kraft, S., Gonsalves, W., Simpson, K., & Johnson, E. (2014)	Elective, participation in a student run free clinic, interprofessional service learning course with course objectives focused on service learning and clinical skills	Pre/post student questionnaire to assess interprofessional teams and readiness for IPE experiences (teamwork and collaboration, professional identity, roles & responsibilities; Pre/post student rated perceptions of actual cooperation and understanding others' values; Pre/post student rated perceptions of teaching methods on their clinical reflection and reasoning	Interdisciplinary Education Perception Scale (IEPS), Readiness for Interprofessional Learning Scale (RIPLS), Self-Assessment of Clinical Reflection and Reasoning (SACRR)	M, OT, P, PT, PA	232 total, 100 participated in both the service learning course and student run free clinic
Segal-Gidan, F., Walsh, A., Lie, D., Fung, C. C., & Lohenry, K. (2014)	Elective, longitudinal 8 months geriatrics IPE curriculum that consisted of three 4-hour classroom based sessions and one IP team geriatric patient interaction	Student pre/post survey rating perceptions about IPE experiences; student reflection post-event	Readiness for Interprofessional Learning Survey (RIPLS)	M, OT, P, PT, PA	evaluation limited to 50 participating PA students and 38 controls
Shoemaker, M. J., Platko, C. M., Cleghorn, S. M., & Booth, A. (2014)	Required IPE activity, virtual patient simulation of a patient with diabetes mellitus and peripheral neuropathy	Student submission of written patient treatment plan and responses to reflective questions regarding benefits of collaboration, understand approach of other professionals, and relevance for future practice	Author designed instrument	OT, PT, PA	100
Shrader, S., Kern, D., Zoller, J., & Blue, A. (2013)	Required, interprofessional high fidelity simulation of a hospitalized patient	At baseline, students rated perception of interdisciplinary education. IP teams submitted a patient clinical outcomes checklist, which was scored by faculty. Trained faculty rated the teams and teamwork	Interdisciplinary Education Perception Scale (IEPS), author designed clinical outcomes score (COS), author modification of the TeamSTEPPS team performance observation tool to create a teamwork score (TWS)	M, P, PA	120
Sullivan, K., Charrette, A., Massey, C., Bartlett, D., Walker, C., Bond, I., & Fong, J. J. (2015)	Elective, pre-event IPE session and participation in a local community prevention event	Student pre/post survey rating perceptions about IPE experiences; student reflection post-event	Readiness for Interprofessional Learning Scale (RIPLS)	N, P, PA, PT	63

continued on following page

Table 1. Continued

Source	IPE Curriculum Format	Outcomes Evaluated	Assessment Measures	Included Professions	Student Sample Size[b]
Thompson, B. M., Bratzler, D. W., Fisher, M. J., Torres, A., Faculty, E., & Sparks, R. A. (2016)	Elective, longitudinal classroom and clinic based IPE experience delivered through a course that included interactive classroom based learning and IP clinical sessions	Student pre/mid/and post ratings regarding interprofessional attributed and readiness for IPE Student depictions of IP team relationships and communication for patient care at pre/mid/post time points	Readiness for Interprofessional Learning Scale (RIPLS), TeamSTEPPS Teamwork Attitudes Questionnaire (T-TAQ), adaptation of life circle diagramming technique	D, M, N, OT, P, PH, PT, PA, SLP, SW, nutritional sciences	80

a=From a PubMed search, which was limited to English-language articles published from January 2012 to October 2019

b=Sample may be the total number of IPE participants or the number of participants included in data analysis.

D = dental, M = medical, IP = interprofessional, IPE = interprofessional education, MT = music therapy, N= nursing, OT = occupational therapy, P = pharmacy, PT = physical therapy, PA = physician assistant, PH = public health, SLP = speech language pathology, SW = social work

(Lawlis, Anson & Greenfield, 2014). Moreover, support from administration and program directors across professional programs is imperative for the success of an IPE curriculum.

CONCLUSION

Historically, there have been few randomized and/or controlled studies to evaluate IPE modalities. However, knowing the limitations of currently published IPE research, it is reasonable to draw ideas from what is available. As IPE formats are modified or new approaches are introduced adequate evaluation should be incorporated as they are implemented. Looking forward, contemporary IPE will need to address the IPEC competencies. Immediate next steps in IPE is to increase the connection with clinical practice. IPE will ideally catch up and integrate aspects of high quality care for everyone, incorporate the patient and family, and reach populations under adversity. The PA profession's identity is grounded in team-based care. PAs have worked in collaboration with their physician, patients, and other colleagues since the profession began. PAs are well-positioned to coordinate care across health professions and specialties.

REFERENCES

Accreditation Review Commission on Education for the Physician Assistant, Inc. (2019). *Accreditation Standards for Physician Assistant Education*. Retrieved from http://www.arc-pa.org/wp-content/uploads/2018/06/Standards-4th-Ed-March-2018.pdf

Agency for Healthcare Research and Quality (AHRQ). (n.d.). Retrieved December 11, 2019, from https://www.ahrq.gov/

Bridgeman, M. B., Rusay, M., Afran, J., Yeh, D. S., & Sturgill, M. G. (2018). Impact of an interprofessional medication error workshop on healthcare student perceptions. *Currents in Pharmacy Teaching & Learning*, *10*(7), 975–981. doi:10.1016/j.cptl.2018.04.013 PMID:30236436

Buff, S. M., Jenkins, K., Kern, D., Worrall, C., Howell, D., Martin, K., & Blue, A. (2015). Interprofessional service-learning in a community setting: Findings from a pilot study. *Journal of Interprofessional Care*, *29*(2), 159–161. doi:10.3109/13561820.2014.934956 PMID:25003549

Buhse, M., & Della Ratta, C. (2017). Enhancing Interprofessional Education with Team-Based Learning. *Nurse Educator*, *42*(5), 240–244. doi:10.1097/NNE.0000000000000370 PMID:28252549

Cohen, E. V., Hagestuen, R., González-Ramos, G., Cohen, H. W., Bassich, C., Book, E., Bradley, K. P., Carter, J. H., Di Minno, M., Gardner, J., Giroux, M., González, M. J., Holten, S., Joseph, R., Kornegay, D. D., Simpson, P. A., Tomaino, C. M., Vandendolder, R. P., Walde-Douglas, M., ... Morgan, J. C. (2016). Interprofessional education increases knowledge, promotes team building, and changes practice in the care of Parkinson's disease. *Parkinsonism & Related Disorders*, *22*, 21–27. doi:10.1016/j.parkreldis.2015.11.001 PMID:26620547

Educating primary care teams for the future: family medicine and physician assistant interprofessional education. (2012). *The Journal of Physician Assistant Education: The Official Journal Of The Physician Assistant Education Association*, *23*(3), 33–41. Retrieved from http://search.ebscohost.com.proxy.library.umkc.edu/login.aspx?direct=true&db=cmedm&AN=23072069&site=eds-live&scope=site

Edwards, S., Molina, P. E., McDonough, K. H., Mercante, D. E., & Gunaldo, T. P. (2018). The potential of interprofessional education to translate physiology curricula effectively into future team-based healthcare. *Advances in Physiology Education*, *42*(2), 354–359. doi:10.1152/advan.00183.2017 PMID:29761708

Hale, L. S., & DiLollo, A. (2016). Immersive Interprofessional Education Using an Evidence-Based Practice Course. *The Journal of Physician Assistant Education: the Official Journal of the Physician Assistant Education Association*, *27*(3), 117–125. doi:10.1097/JPA.0000000000000083 PMID:27548762

Hooker, R. S., Cawley, J. F., & Everett, C. M. (2017). *Physician Assistants: Policy and practice* (4th ed.). F. A. Davis Company.

Institute for Healthcare Improvement. (n.d.). *The IHI Triple Aim*. Retrieved from http://www.ihi.org:80/Engage/Initiatives/TripleAim/Pages/default.aspx

Institute of Medicine. (1978). *A Manpower Policy for Primary Health Care: Report of a Study*. The National Academies Press., doi:10.17226/9932

Institute of Medicine. (2001). *Crossing the Quality Chasm: A New Health System for the 21st Century*. The National Academies Press. doi:10.17226/10027

Institute of Medicine. (2003). *Health Professions Education: A Bridge to Quality*. The National Academies Press. doi:10.17226/10681

Institute of Medicine (US) Committee on Quality of Health Care in America. (2000). *To Err is Human: Building a Safer Health System* (L. T. Kohn, J. M. Corrigan, & M. S. Donaldson, Eds.). Retrieved from https://www.ncbi.nlm.nih.gov/books/NBK225182/

Interprofessional Education Collaborative. (2016). *Core Competencies for Interprofessional Collaborative Practice: 2016 Update*. http://bit.ly/2zLEARR

Kayingo, G., Kidd, V. D., Gilani, O., & Warner, M. L. (2015). Primary Care Teams, Composition, Roles, and Satisfaction of PA Students During Primary Care Rotations. *The Journal of Physician Assistant Education: the Official Journal of the Physician Assistant Education Association*, *26*(2), 88–93. doi:10.1097/JPA.0000000000000022 PMID:26211031

Kraft, S., Wise, H. H., Jacques, P. F., & Burik, J. K. (2013). Discharge Planning Simulation: Training the Interprofessional Team for the Future Workplace. *Journal of Allied Health, 42*(3), 175–181.

Lie, D. A., Forest, C. P., Walsh, A., Banzali, Y., & Lohenry, K. (2016). What and how do students learn in an interprofessional student-run clinic? An educational framework for team-based care. *Medical Education Online*, *21*(1), 31900. doi:10.3402/meo.v21.31900 PMID:27499364

Lie, D. A., Walsh, A., Segal-Gidan, F., Banzali, Y., & Lohenry, K. (2013). Physician Assistant Students' Views Regarding Interprofessional Education: A Focus Group Study. *The Journal of Physician Assistant Education: the Official Journal of the Physician Assistant Education Association, 24*(1), 35–41. Advance online publication. doi:10.1097/01367895-201324010-00005 PMID:23858824

Mahler, C., Berger, S., & Reeves, S. (2015). The Readiness for Interprofessional Learning Scale (RIPLS): A problematic evaluative scale for the interprofessional field. *Journal of Interprofessional Care, 29*(4), 289–291. doi:10.3109/13561820.2015.1059652 PMID:26176984

McBride, J. M., & Drake, R. L. (2015). Student perceptions of an interprofessional educational experience: The importance of goal articulation. *Anatomical Sciences Education, 8*(4), 381–385. doi:10.1002/ase.1547 PMID:26040781

Noonan, C. D., Scow, S., Sheagley, B. A., & Bunn, J. (2018). Shifting Perspectives on Pain Management after an Interprofessional International Service Learning Experience: A Qualitative Assessment of Pilot Data. *Journal of Interprofessional Care, 32*(5), 645–647. https://doi-org.proxy.library.umkc.edu/10.1080/13561820.2018.1471053. doi:10.1080/13561820.2018.1471053 PMID:29741408

Optimal Team Practice. (n.d.). *Learn More About OTP*. Retrieved December 11, 2019, from AAPA website: https://www.aapa.org/advocacy-central/optimal-team-practice/

Palmer, R., & Stilp, C. (2017). Learning by Doing: The MD-PA Interprofessional Education Rural Rotation. *Rural and Remote Health, 17*(1). Advance online publication. doi:10.22605/RRH4167 PMID:28328232

Phillips, W. R., & Keys, T. (2018). Interprofessional Primary Care Course Curriculum and Evaluation. *Family Medicine, 50*(3), 217–222. doi:10.22454/FamMed.2018.998057 PMID:29537465

Physician Assistant Education Association. (2019). *Core Competencies for New Physician Assistant Graduates*. Retrieved from https://paealearning.org/wp-content/uploads/2018/10/Core-Competencies-for-New-PA-Graduates_FINAL_061918.pdf

Pippitt, K., Moloney-Johns, A., Jalilibahabadi, S., & Gren, L. H. (2015). Collaboration Versus Competition: An Interprofessional Education Experience. *Family Medicine, 47*(4). PMID:25853601

Rathfon, E., & Jones, G. (2011). *Family Physicians and Physician Assistants: Team-Based Family Medicine. A Joint Policy Statement of the American Academy of Family Physicians and American Academy of Physician Assistants.* Retrieved from: https://www.aafp.org/about/policies/all/fp-pa.html

Reeves, S. A., Denault, D., Huntington, J. T., Ogrinc, G., Southard, D. R., & Vebell, R. (2017). Learning to Overcome Hierarchical Pressures to Achieve Safer Patient Care: An Interprofessional Simulation for Nursing, Medical, and Physician Assistant Students. *Nurse Educator*, *42*, S27–S31. doi:10.1097/NNE.0000000000000427 PMID:28832459

Segal-Gidan, F., Walsh, A., Lie, D., Fung, C. C., & Lohenry, K. (2014). Knowledge and Attitude Change in Physician Assistant Students After an Interprofessional Geriatric Care Experience: A Mixed Methods Study. *The Journal of Physician Assistant Education: the Official Journal of the Physician Assistant Education Association*, *25*(2), 25–30. doi:10.1097/01367895-201425020-00006 PMID:25016910

Seif, G., Coker-Bolt, P., Kraft, S., Gonsalves, W., Simpson, K., & Johnson, E. (2014). The development of clinical reasoning and interprofessional behaviors: Service-learning at a student-run free clinic. *Journal of Interprofessional Care*, *28*(6), 559–564. doi:10.3109/13561820.2014.921899 PMID:24865993

Shoemaker, M. J., Platko, C. M., Cleghorn, S. M., & Booth, A. (2014). Virtual patient care: An interprofessional education approach for physician assistant, physical therapy and occupational therapy students. *Journal of Interprofessional Care*, *28*(4), 365–367. doi:10.3109/13561820.2014.891978 PMID:24593330

Shrader, S., Kern, D., Zoller, J., & Blue, A. (2013). Interprofessional Teamwork Skills as Predictors of Clinical Outcomes in a Simulated Healthcare Setting. *Journal of Allied Health, 42*(1), e1-6.

Smithburger, P. L., Kane-Gill, S. L., Kloet, M. A., Lohr, B., & Seybert, A. L. (2013). Advancing interprofessional education through the use of high fidelity human patient simulators. *Pharmacy Practice*, *11*(2), 61–65. doi:10.4321/S1886-36552013000200001 PMID:24155851

Sonney, J., Willgerodt, M., Lindhorst, T., & Brock, D. (2018, January). Elizabeth: Typical or Troubled Teen? A Training Case for Health Professionals to Recognize and Report Child Maltreatment. *MedEdPORTAL : The Journal of Teaching and Learning Resources*, *14*(1), mep_2374-8265.10712. Advance online publication. doi:10.15766/mep_2374-8265.10712 PMID:30800912

Sullivan, K., Charrette, A., Massey, C., Bartlett, D., Walker, C., Bond, I., & Fong, J. J. (2015). Interprofessional education with a community fall prevention event. *Journal of Interprofessional Care*, *29*(4), 374–376. doi:10.3109/13561820.2014.969834 PMID:25317499

Thompson, B. M., Bratzler, D. W., Fisher, M. J., Torres, A., Faculty, E., & Sparks, R. A. (2016). Working together: Using a unique approach to evaluate an interactive and clinic-based longitudinal interprofessional education experience with 13 professions. *Journal of Interprofessional Care*, *30*(6), 754–761. doi:10.1080/13561820.2016.1227962 PMID:27797628

Timeline. (n.d.a). Retrieved December 11, 2019, from Institute for Healthcare Improvement website: http://www.ihi.org/about/Documents/IHI_Timeline_2018.pdf

Timeline. (n.d.b). Retrieved December 11, 2019, from Physician Assistant History Society website: https://pahx.org/timeline/

Report of the Graduate Medical Education National Advisory Committee to the Secretary, Department of Health and Human Services electronic resource. (1981). Hyattsville, MD: U.S. Dept. of Health and Human Services, Public Health Service, Health Resources Administration, Office of Graduate Medical Education; For sale by the Supt. of Docs., G.P.O. Retrieved from http://search.ebscohost.com.proxy.library.umkc.edu/login.aspx?direct=true&db=edsgpr&AN=edsgpr.ocn690419361&site=eds-live&scope=site

Vision & Mission. (n.d.). Retrieved from IPEC Interprofessional Education Collaborative website: http://ipecollaborative.org/vision---mission.html

World Health Organization. (2010). *Framework for action on interprofessional education and collaborative practice*. Retrieved from: https://apps.who.int/iris/bitstream/10665/70185/1/WHO_HRH_HPN_10.3_eng.pdf?ua=1

Chapter 11
Interprofessional Eye Care: A Vision That Really Works

Corey W. Waldman
University of Texas-San Antonio School of Medicine, USA

Elizabeth Hoppe
College of Optometry, Western University of Health Sciences, USA

Ida Chung
College of Optometry, Western University of Health Sciences, USA

D. Joshua Cameron
College of Optometry, Western University of Health Sciences, USA

Naveen K. Yadav
College of Optometry, Western University of Health Sciences, USA

Christine T. Pham
College of Optometry, Western University of Health Sciences, USA

Stephanie Bowlin
Western University of Health Sciences, USA

ABSTRACT

Doctors of Optometry and optometric students, interns, and residents are valuable members of the interprofessional team. Including both primary eye care and more specialized optometric care that can encompass elements of secondary and tertiary care in the collaborative care of patients ensures a holistic, whole-body approach to wellness and supports patients' quality of life. Doctors of Optometry play a vital role in ensuring optimal health throughout the lifespan, and in particular, for people with chronic conditions and complex health concerns. The authors explore examples of how optometrists participate in the healthcare team and describe how optometrists can make an impact for patients across the life span.

DOI: 10.4018/978-1-7998-3066-5.ch011

INTRODUCTION

Doctors of Optometry and optometric students, interns, and residents are valuable members of the interprofessional team. Including both primary eye care and more specialized optometric care, that can encompass elements of secondary and tertiary care, in the collaborative care of patients ensures a holistic, whole-body approach to wellness and supports patients' quality of life. Doctors of Optometry play a vital role in ensuring optimal health throughout the lifespan, and in particular, for people with chronic conditions and complex health concerns.

The American Optometric Association emphasizes the role of optometrists as independent primary health care professionals. The full definition of the profession with examples of the scope of practice and professional role is provided in Figure 1 (American Optometric Association).

Figure 1. Definition of Doctors of Optometry from the American Optometric Association

Doctors of Optometry (O.D.s/optometrists) are the independent primary health care professionals for the eye (American Optometric Association). Optometrists examine, diagnose, treat, and manage diseases, injuries, and disorders of the visual system, the eye, and associated structures as well as identify related systemic conditions affecting the eye.

- **Doctors of Optometry prescribe medications, low vision rehabilitation, vision therapy, spectacle lenses, contact lenses, and perform certain surgical procedures.**
- **Optometrists counsel their patients regarding surgical and non-surgical options that meet their visual needs related to their occupations, avocations, and lifestyle.**
- **An optometrist has completed pre-professional undergraduate education in a college or university and four years of professional education at a college of optometry, leading to the doctor of optometry (O.D.) degree. Some optometrists complete an optional residency in a specific area of practice.**
- **Optometrists are eye health care professionals state-licensed to diagnose and treat diseases and disorders of the eye and visual system.**

-Approved by the AOA Board of Trustees, June 2012

The National Academies of Practice expands on this definition to further elaborate how Doctors of Optometry are integrated within communities and different practice settings. This longer description, shown in Figure 2 (National Academies of Practice), also serves to highlight both the types of services and the kinds of patients for which Doctors of Optometry can be expected to serve as members of the care team.

Schools and Colleges of Optometry have been incorporating and assessing interprofessional education and collaborative clinical practice as well as the impact of integrating optometric education resources with other health professionals

Figure 2. Definition of Doctors of Optometry from the National Academies of Practice

Doctors of Optometry (O.D.s/Optometrists) are primary health care professionals (National Academies of Practice). As licensed, independent health care professionals, Doctors of Optometry play a primary and integral role in inter-disciplinary health care by examining, diagnosing, treating, and managing diseases, injuries, and disorders of the visual system, the eye, and associated structures. Doctors of Optometry are involved in the coordination of care of associated systemic diseases and zoonotic diseases and serve a sentinel role in the identification of ocular side effects of systemic medications. Doctors of Optometry are defined as physicians under Medicare, and are an essential part of the national health care delivery system providing direct patient access to health care in nearly 6,500 communities across the country. In 3,500 of these communities, Doctors of Optometry are the only providers of vision and eye health care services.

Doctors of Optometry:

- **Practice in many different healthcare settings that include private and group practice, within hospitals, Accountable Care Organizations, Federally Qualified Health Centers, School Based Health Centers, Rural Health Clinics, Certified Nursing Facilities, Rehabilitation Facilities, U.S. Armed Forces, Veterans Health Administration, Indian Health Service, Civil Service, and other settings**
- **Assist with improving overall population health and quality of life through prevention and early diagnosis of vision and eye health problems and prevention of chronic disease**
- **Detect systemic diseases through identification of associated eye findings during a comprehensive face-to-face eye examination. There are over 275 systemic conditions with ocular involvement**
- **Participate in Physician Quality Reporting System (PQRS) and Merit-Based Incentive Payment System (MIPS) and other quality initiatives to improve patient outcomes and wellness by enhanced disease prevention and patient education for behaviors that have been linked to systemic diseases with known vision and eye findings including but, not limited to hypertension, obesity, diabetes, smoking, and UV exposure.**
- **Are essential to the implementation of the comprehensive pediatric vision care benefit mandated by the Affordable Care Act and attending regulations**
- **Coordinate the vision, eye health, and wellness of their patients with fellow Optometrists and other health care providers**
- **Offer services to assist individuals with functional vision problems, traumatic brain injury, visual impairment and blindness. Treatments may include vision therapy or tools to address functional vision problems or vision rehabilitation for those with vision impairment with the goal to optimize vision and maintain independence and quality of life**
- **Provide a continuum of patient-centered care for people of all ages focused on prevention, health maintenance, acute care, chronic care, habilitation, and/or rehabilitation, with special emphasis on minimizing life-long impacts and the burden of visual impairment on at-risk populations that include aging adults and the very old, as well as infants and children.**

(Aravamudhan, Vitek, & Casser, 2015; Christian, MacIver, & Alfieri, 2015; McLeod & Bush, 2015; Sanchez-Diaz et al., 2015; Yumori et al., 2015).

Post-graduate optometric residency training has also proven to be an optimal setting for incorporating IPE into health professional education (Dowd & Smith, 2015). In addition to the formal didactic and clinical curricula, there are many opportunities to incorporate IPE and collaborative practice in the co-curriculum. Doctors of optometry and optometric students have found value in collaborating as a member of the health care team during international medical mission trips (Nehmad, Reynolds, & Anderson-Worts, 2015).

The Association of Schools and Colleges of Optometry (ASCO) is an institutional member of the Interprofessional Education Collaborative (IPEC), and in February of 2016 ASCO hosted its own Interprofessional Education and Collaborative Practice Summit, bringing together faculty members and administrators from optometric institutions, professional organizations, and partners from a number of other disciplines. The importance of interprofessional education in optometric education is exemplified in ASCO's "Attributes of Graduates of the Schools and Colleges of Optometry" report. The expected competencies are shown in Figure 3 (Association of Schools and Colleges of Optometry).

Figure 3. Interprofessional Attributes of Graduates (Association of Schools and Colleges of Optometry)

- **have the ability to appropriately use all resources, including the use of ancillary personnel, intra- and interprofessional collaboration, co-management, and referral, in ensuring the best quality patient care;**
- **manage their practices in a manner that is appropriate within the health care delivery system and that promotes patient access to eye and vision care;**
- **have the ability to recognize personal limitations regarding optimal patient care and to work with the broader health care community in providing the best care possible;**
- **have a commitment to work as an integral member of the larger interprofessional health care team to improve patient care outcomes;**
- **have the ability to recognize and initiate the coordination of patient care requiring advanced medical, systemic, interprofessional, or specialty care;**
- **have the ability to work in cooperation with those who receive care, those who provide care, and others who contribute to or support the delivery of prevention and health services**

On every level, from associations and organizations, to schools and colleges, and in the community, optometrists have embraced the opportunity to engage in interprofessional education and collaborative practice. Roles, responsibilities, and opportunities for engagement continue to evolve with many opportunities yet unexplored.

In the next sections of this chapter we will explore examples of how optometrists participate in the health care team and describe how optometrists can make an impact for patients across the life span. We will explore the various factors that can affect the visual system and provide an overview of the role of healthy eyes and a healthy visual system across the lifespan. We will provide examples of collaboration and opportunities for full engagement and we will share case examples in which optometric services can be incorporated to maximize patient outcomes and well-being. Table 1 provides an overview of the service needs and interprofessional care team members for various age groups across the life span.

PEDIATRICS

Table 1. Timeline: Vision Care Across the Life Span

Patient Age Group	Service Needs	Interprofessional Care Team Members
Pediatric 0-5 6-17	Early diagnosis and treatment of ocular developmental abnormalities. At least one comprehensive eye exam before entering formal schooling. Correcting vision errors that impact learning: 1) visual input problems 2) visual processing problems	Pediatricians, School Nurses and Teachers, Parents, Pediatric ophthalmologists
Adult Primary Care 18-39 40-64	Correcting refractive errors. Treating eye injuries and screen-related visual problems. Early detection of sight threatening disorders. Management of presbyopia. Treatment of age-related eye diseases and systemic and chronic health conditions that impact vision.	Family medicine, Internists, Nurse Practitioners, Ophthalmologists, Physician Assistants, Pharmacists
Geriatric 65+	Age-related vision changes and diseases. Maintenance of quality of life.	Geriatricians, Physical therapists, Occupational therapists, Social workers

Introduction

Vision health in the pediatric population is a significant public health concern. One in five preschool children are estimated to have eye or vision problems, and one in four school-aged child wears correction for refractive errors (American Optometric Association, 2017). Early treatment is important for prevention of permanent vision loss or blindness. The opportunity to influence vision development early is a driving force to have effective and efficient models of eye care delivery, starting in infancy. The American Optometric Association has developed evidence-based guideline for the eye and vision care of the pediatric patient (American Optometric Association, 2017) These guidelines define the eye care and services for pediatric patients and includes a comprehensive list of references.

Types of Services Provided

Infants

At six months the developing infant has reached a number of critical developmental milestones, making this the appropriate age for the first comprehensive eye exam by an eye doctor. Within the first 6 months of life, rapid changes occur in the visual system including developing visual acuity, focusing, binocular function, and eye tracking. Early diagnosis and treatment are critical to avoid vision loss during this critical phase of development and prevent negative long-term effects (American Optometric Association, 2017) One of the primary goals of examining young children is to detect amblyopia (lazy eye) and initiate treatment with lenses, drops, surgery or therapy as early as possible to prevent permanent decrease in vision. A comprehensive eye evaluation includes evaluation of significant refractive errors such as hyperopia, astigmatism or myopia, eye muscle alignment, and eye diseases with a dilated fundus exam.

InfantSEE®, a national public health initiative, provides a free onetime assessment of a well-baby eye check (InfantSEE). The InfantSEE® program has had more than 150,000 assessments reported, 13,700 identified with cause for concern, 18,000 eye and vision conditions identified (InfantSEE).

Preschoolers

After the initial eye exam before the age of 1 year, the recommended eye exam frequency is at 3 years of age and then 5 years of age. However, the CDC reports fewer than 15% of preschool children receive an eye exam and less than 22% have a vision screening for distance visual acuity (Centers for Disease Control and Prevention). Uncorrected refractive errors have been associated with delays in development of cognitive ability and motor skill with detrimental effect on vision development, learning, school success, and socialization (Roch-Levecq, Brody, Thomas, & Brown, 2008). The reality is that many eye and vision problems are asymptomatic in this age range; therefore, it is important that preschool children receive an eye examination (U.S. Preventive Services Task Force, 2011).

School-Age

Vision may change frequently during the school years. The most common problems are due to the development and progression of refractive errors. Myopia (nearsightedness) generally occurs in children during their early school years and increases in magnitude as they get older. In school-aged children, the prevalence of myopia is increasing. It is estimated that more than 33% of 12 to 17 year olds are myopic, and these numbers are increasing (World Health Organization, 2015).

There are two main types of vision problems in children that impact learning. They are input and output visual issues. Input problems prevent a clear retinal image or a single image. These include refractive errors, strabismus, eye misalignments, focusing problems, eye movement problems, or eye disease. Input problems result in decreased efficiency with reading. Output problems are visual processing issues. It is the way in which the brain processes the information that it receives from the eyes. Visual processing skills include laterality/directionality, figure-ground, sequencing of visual information. Problems manifest themselves as spelling, learning to read, and difficulty with math. Vision problems resulting in significant interference in student academic success was evident back in 1999 when the national PTA adopted a resolution on learning-related vision problems education and evaluation, stating that vision tests for learning related visual skills are necessary for success in the classroom, and may be a possible missing link struggling students (National PTA, 2005; Remick, 2018).

Intraprofessional Collaboration Model of Eye Care

Pediatric eye care is provided by opticians, optometrists and pediatric ophthalmologists. These eye care professionals collaborate closely with many other professionals, particularly with pediatricians, school nurses and teachers in the care of pediatric patients.

Pediatricians

Pediatricians are the gate keepers of children's health and naturally for well-child visits which may include an eye health screening. The American Academy of Ophthalmology and the American Academy of Pediatrics recommend vision screenings at various stages of vision development (Donahue et al., 2016). Pediatricians provide infant vision screenings, called the red reflex test, to ensure light is passing into the eye and no scar, opacity or tumor is present. Although a vision screening can reveal a possible vision problem, it can't diagnose it. If potential eye problems are detected a referral is made to have the child examined by a trained optometrist or pediatric ophthalmologist.

Pediatrician offices can partner with eye doctor offices to educate parents on the importance of a well-baby eye check up to encourage early detection and treatment of visually debilitating eye problems (InfantSEE).

School-Based Vision Program

School nurses are the most likely to perform vision screenings in school-age children. The National Association of School Nurses talks about the 12 components of a strong vision health system of care ranging from the role of parent education, to early detection, to systemized follow up for potential eye and vision problems, to agencies serving as resources for families, to effective communication and adherence to treatment (National Association of School Nurses, 2017). The heart of an effective system communication and collaboration among all providers, resulting in the provision of care and continuity of care (Hartmann, Block, Wallace, National Expert Panel to the National Center for Children's, & Eye, 2015). Detection is ineffective if it is not diagnosed. Diagnosis is ineffective if treatment is not delivered. Treatment is not effective if adherence is absent. The longevity of successful treatment outcomes is long-term management (Marsh-Tootle, Russ, Repka, & National Expert Panel to the National Center for Children's Vision Eye, 2015). Eye doctors can work with school nurses and families increasing the number of children who receive care. A study in San Jose, CA comparing utilization of full-time nurses found increased greater follow up rates of 96-98% as compared to 41-67% in schools with part-time nurses (Rodriguez, Srivastava, & Landau, 2018). Nurses are critical team members in providing care coordination for school-aged children who are in need of vision care.

Teachers

Teachers can play a significant role in identifying vision related learning problems. A child with undiagnosed vision problems may struggle to learn in the classroom where much of information is through the visual system. An undiagnosed vision problem may also lead to a misdiagnosis of Attention Deficit/Hyperactivity Disorder (ADHD) or dyslexia. A study showed a child with a diagnosis of ADHD is three times more likely to have a binocular vision problem impacting near work including reading efficiency, called convergence insufficiency (Granet, Gomi, Ventura, & Miller-Scholte, 2005). Treatment of convergence insufficiency with therapy has been associated with reduction in the frequency of adverse academic behaviors. (Borsting et al., 2012).

Teachers can be trained to improve their ability to detect children with vision problems in the classroom. In a study by Krumholtz, he demonstrated the effectiveness of a teacher training to help identify children with vision problems (Krumholtz, 2004). Teachers are the gateway to parents, who are the guardians to children accessing the vision care needed.

Models of Care

The Oyler School OneSight Vision Center is a model of collaboration. In Ohio it is estimated that only one in seven kindergartners has an eye exam prior to entering school. To address this issue, a team of public-private partners has come together to create the OneSight Vision Center at Oyler SchoolOneSight, the first of its kind self-sustaining vision center in the U.S. Full-service include comprehensive eye exams, glasses, fittings, adjustments, medical eye care and vision therapy.

Partners include:

- Cincinnati Health Department will run the OneSight Vision Center daily operations
- Oyler School donated space and ongoing maintenance for the vision center
- Ohio Optometric Association and American Optometric Association provided expertise, guidance and funding
- Cincinnati Eye Institute (CEI) and The CEI Foundation provided expertise, guidance and funding
- Growing Well Cincinnati and Cincinnati Public Schools provided guidance, support and counsel
- OneSight, a leading global vision care charity sponsored by Luxottica, provided all exam equipment, eyewear, operational expertise and start-up funding to support Vision Center staff

Children examined in the school-based eye clinic were more likely to have an Individualized Educational Plan (IEP) or a suspected vision-related problem, including a higher prevalence of hyperopia, astigmatism, exophoria, and reduced convergence (Lasher, 2015).

Realeyes is a creative funding program administered by the Ohio Department of Health Funding. Individuals completing vehicle registration/renewal at the Ohio Bureau of motor vehicles can elect to contribute to fund by donating $1 to educate young Ohioans of the importance of vision health and eye safety. The Realeyes program has reached more than 1.1 million school children in over 46,000 classrooms in all of Ohio's 88 counties since its inception in the year 2000 (American Optometric Association).

ADULT / PRIMARY CARE

Introduction

According to the American Optometric Association, adult primary eye is an evaluation of eye health, vision, and ocular manifestation of systemic diseases in patients age 18 years or older (American Optometric Association, 2015). It is estimated that more than 3 million Americans age 40 years or older are either legally blind or have a vision impairment (American Optometric Association, 2015). This number is expected to expand in 30 years due to aging of the United states population and the increase in diabetes or other chronic diseases (American Optometric Association, 2015). Eye and vision disorders in an adult population have broad effects in health care due to their potentials to impact activities of daily living. It is vital to create best practices for patient-centered care with a team of health care professionals. Interprofessional collaboration is an active and interactive process that requires 2 or more professions to work together to improve quality of care.

Types of Services

18-39 Years of Age

In the past, vision problems in young adults were largely due to refractive errors or eye injuries (American Optometric Association, 2015). More recently, young adults are becoming more symptomatic for eye strain and headaches from computer related visual problems (J. Long & Helland, 2012). With an increase in computer use, handheld devices, and visual displays in vehicles, this population is greatly exposed to harmful blue light (Lawrenson, Hull, & Downie, 2017). Blue light is a short wavelength that can cause phototoxic retinal damage, eyestrain, and disruption of sleep wake cycles (Lawrenson et al., 2017). In addition, frequent computer and handheld device use can also cause dry eye syndrome from reduced blink rate (Jaiswal et al., 2019). Visual demands of the workplace and in school brings about the need for regular eye care. The treatment options for refractive error are eyeglasses or contact lenses. Treatment for eyestrain in young adults can be eye glasses or vision therapy.

Though prevalence of ocular disease is relatively low, many eye diseases can initially develop without signs or symptoms (American Optometric Association, 2015). Among the many diseases, glaucoma may begin to appear in young adults.

Diabetes also affects young adults and is the leading cause of blindness among working age Americans (American Optometric Association, 2015). To ensure early detection of any sight threatening disorders, periodic examinations are needed. It is recommended for a low risk young adult to have a comprehensive eye and vision exam at least every 2 years (American Optometric Association, 2015).

40-64 Years of Age

At the age of 40, patients start to experience the onset of presbyopia. Presbyopia is an age-related visual condition that results from a decline in accommodation and focus (American Optometric Association, 2015). The progression of presbyopia continues causing periodic changes in power of near optical correction (American Optometric Association, 2015). Individuals within this group are also at higher risk for age related eye disease including dry eye syndrome, cataracts, glaucoma, and age-related macular degeneration (American Optometric Association, 2015). As the patient ages, there are a variety of chronic disease that have ocular manifestations. Examples of systemic diseases with ocular manifestations includes diabetes mellitus, hypertension, autoimmune disorders, inflammatory disorders and neurological disorders. Individuals who are at risk for developing eye and vison problems due to a systemic disease should have yearly eye and vision examinations.

Professional Collaboration

An adult comprehensive eye care team is with the involvement of optometrist, ophthalmologist, and primary care physicians, pharmacists. The team works together to develop strategies to enhance patient care. The collaboration between professions is based on an integration of knowledge and expertise of each professional.

Ophthalmology

Ophthalmologists provide surgical and nonsurgical services for patients. This profession is further divided into subspecialties: general ophthalmology, glaucoma, cornea, retina and vitreous, oculoplastics, ocular oncology, ocular pathology, pediatrics/strabismus, uveitis, and neuro-ophthalmology. It is common to co-manage adult patients between optometry and ophthalmology depending on the nature of the ocular disease. In particular, post-operative care of cataract, refractive, and glaucoma surgical patients may be co-managed by ophthalmologists and optometrists. Also, optometrists may assist the ophthalmologist in the medical management of glaucoma patients as well. Optometrists often prove helpful to the cornea specialist in prescribing contact lenses for patients which corneal pathology such as keratoconus (Hodge et al., 2015). Optometrists may also be helpful in performing refractions and prescribing glasses or contacts for patients managed medically and surgically by ophthalmologists for conditions such as diplopia, pathologic myopia, or presbyopia. For patients suffering from severe visual dysfunction from diseases such as glaucoma, diabetic retinopathy, or macular degeneration, a referral to an optometrist specializing in low vision examinations and treatments is an essential part of their care (Hodge et al., 2015; Murphy, 2013 November 15; Yeu, Donnenfeld, & Chang, 2018 February 21).

Primary Care Physicians (Including Medical Doctors and Mid-Level Nurse Practitioners and Physician Assistants)

Primary care physicians are crucial in the management of chronic systemic disease like diabetes mellitus and hypertension. In order to reduce the risk of visual impairments, it is important for primary care physicians to regulate patient's glycemic, blood pressure, and lipid control (Hendrick, 2015). Studies have shown that diabetic management is critical to reduce the progression of diabetic retinopathy (Hendrick, 2015). Primary care physicians are also a gateway to other professionals such as rheumatology, endocrinology, cardiology, and neurology. Outlined by the American Optometric Association, diabetics are to have an eye exam yearly.

Clinical Pharmacy

Clinical pharmacy is an important element of the healthcare team and promotes patient care by interacting with the physician and patient (Francis & Abraham, 2014). They can educate patients by providing information about the usage of drugs and medical devices (Francis & Abraham, 2014). Specifically, clinical pharmacists can help improve compliance in diabetics. Programs with clinical pharmacy diabetic education proved beneficial in reducing mean FBS and HbA1c significantly (Francis & Abraham, 2014). They counsel patients regarding proper usage of insulin pens, administration of insulin injection, dietary restrictions, lifestyle modifications and importance of regular checkup (Francis & Abraham, 2014). More diabetic patients are being referred to optometrist or ophthalmologist by clinical pharmacy. Likewise, optometrist or ophthalmologist consult with clinical pharmacy for medication compliance.

Geriatrics

65 Years of Age and Older

The occurrence of visual impairment in this group increases rapidly with age. Reduced vision in the geriatric population can adversely affect their activities of daily living and independence (American Optometric Association, 2015). Common visual impairment within this group is refractive error, age related cataracts, age related macular degeneration or other ocular manifestation of chronic systemic diseases. Maintaining good vision may play a role in preventing falls. Vision problems like reduced visual field, contrast sensitivity, depth perception and visual acuity have been linked to the risk of falls (American Optometric Association, 2015). A lack of diagnosis or treatment in vision problem in the elderly may contribute to cognitive decline leading to depression (American Optometric Association, 2015). It is recommended in this age group to have an eye examination yearly. Treatment options for refractive error are eye glasses. Conditions glaucoma, age related macular degeneration, or chronic systemic conditions affecting the eye can be co-managed with ophthalmology.

Professional Collaboration

The professional collaboration in geriatrics is similar to the adult healthcare team. In addition to a healthcare team mentioned in adult care, social workers, occupational therapists and physical therapists are also needed.

Social Workers

Once a patient is seen by an optometrist, patients are often referred to the social worker to address a wide range of psychosocial needs (D. D. Long & Rosen, 2017). Concepts include coping with a diagnosis, employment challenges, anxiety about performing activities of daily living, learning to deal with vision loss, and loss of independence (D. D. Long & Rosen, 2017). Long, D. et al discusses a framework where social workers facilitate 3 different vision related groups. 1.) survivors of brain injury and stroke 2.) vision impairment and low vision 3.) understanding of and coping with visual impairment to family members of patients (D. D. Long & Rosen, 2017).

Occupational/Physical Therapists

Occupational and physical therapy is concerned with a patient's ability to participate in activities of daily living including self-care (Fishman Hellerstein, 1999). Occupational therapy, physical therapy, and optometry have been sharing professional concepts and working closely for many years. Optometry emphasizes the role of vision and occupational/ physical therapy focuses primarily on the individual's movement and balance abilities with vision being the most important sensory system (Fishman Hellerstein, 1999). Although therapy can be utilized at any age, it is very important within the geriatric population as the risk for falls increases. Occupational therapy provides an individual with ways to adapt to and prevent injury around their home (Fishman Hellerstein, 1999). They can make recommendations from lighting improvements to assistive devices to contrast techniques. Physical therapy helps with issues related to balance, gait training, or fall risk. They make a home visit to assess overall safety and suggest ways to adapt to specific needs (Fishman Hellerstein, 1999). The greatest advantage of this collaboration is to provide appropriate treatment with patients with special needs with visual dysfunction.

CARE FOR SPECIAL PATIENTS/SPECIAL POPULATIONS

Introduction

Children and adults with special healthcare needs are defined by the Maternal and Child Health Bureau as those who have one or more chronic physical, developmental, behavioral, or emotional conditions and who also require health and related services of a type and amount beyond that required generally (Maternal and Child Health Bureau). The idea of an interprofessional team approach is crucial in the care of patients with special needs. For eye care, these special needs patients include but are not limited to those with genetic origins (Down Syndrome, Fragile X Syndrome), neurologic origins (Cerebral Palsy, Intellectual disability, autism, attention deficit hyperactivity disorder), or acquired (brain injury, learning disabilities). For the multidisciplinary team, the question is not *if* but *who*. In addition to optometrists, occupational therapists, speech and language pathologists, physical therapists, psychologists, physicians, educators, and parents are all vital team contributors to a coordinated and collaborative effort to provide care.

Optometrists provide rehabilitative services in the treatment of vision problems, including vision therapy, neuro-optometric rehabilitation, low vision rehabilitation, and sports vision, as well as a member of the support team for the vulnerable population with conditions including learning disabilities, autism spectrum disorders, intellectual disabilities, and chronic systemic conditions.

OPTOMETRIC VISION THERAPY

Introduction

The American Optometric Association defines optometric vision therapy as a treatment utilizing a sequence of neurosensory and neuromuscular activities individually prescribed and monitored by the doctor to develop, rehabilitate, and enhance visual skills and processing (American Optometric Association, 2009). Treatment with vision therapy can be preventive as part of early detection and treatment of vision problems, rehabilitative to restore a compromised visual system to its original function, or enhancing to improve visual skills for one's activities of daily living (ADL).

Clinical research has demonstrated that optometric vision therapy can be an effective treatment option for both visual input and output problems, such as (College of Optometrists in Vision Development):

- Ocular motility dysfunctions (eye movement disorders)
- Non-strabismic binocular disorders (inefficient eye teaming)
- Strabismus (misalignment of the eyes)
- Amblyopia (poorly developed vision)
- Accommodative disorders (focusing problems)
- Visual information processing (VIP) disorders, including visual-motor integration and integration with other sensory modalities
- Visual sequelae of acquired brain injury
- Learning problems (e.g., dyslexia)

Vision therapy, also called visual rehabilitation, evolved from its origins in orthoptics (the straightening of eyes) into a distinct field of rehabilitative eye care within the discipline of optometry. Vision therapy, as opposed to self-prescribed eye exercises or vision training, emphasizes the interactions between the therapist and patient and is analogous to the doctor-patient relationship found in the allied fields of occupational therapy and physical therapy that requires ongoing professional guidance.

Pediatricians, ophthalmologists, occupational therapists, child psychologist, and physical therapist are the most likely professionals to see and co-manage patients with conditions treated by optometric vision therapy. A constellation of visual deficits treatable by visual rehabilitation can lead to an improvement in patients' quality of life.

What should providers know about optometric vision therapy?

- The visual system is plastic through the lifespan. It is never too late to treat functional visual problems at any age, especially in patients with amblyopia (lazy eye).
- The eyes are an extension of the brain. The eyes are subject to the same stressors that influence development, maintenance, and metabolic equilibrium elsewhere in the body. Chronic, inflammatory conditions weaken the muscle, tendon and collagenous structures of the eye.

- Collaborative patient care includes school learning specialists, eye doctors, medical doctors, and therapists to connect patients who may need care and benefit from vision therapy.

What It Is

Holistic care of the patient's eye and visual function requires professionals to collaborate. Patients of all ages can benefit from receiving vision therapy. It is often after a complete eye and vision examination, taking into consideration patient signs and symptoms and the needs of the patient that a referral is made for a vision therapy consultation. Conditions treated by vision therapy are usually recommended beyond the correction of refractive errors (such as with spectacle lenses or contact lenses), or other surgical treatment. Problems with strabismus, amblyopia, and brain injury are successfully treated with therapeutic interventions for a given individual by the doctor or therapist who can modify lenses, instructional sets, or the choice of sequence of procedures involved, to help the patient perform to optimal levels. Doctors utilize lenses, prisms, filters, specialized clinical equipment, and customized computer-based programs to perform visual activities designed to provide training for days, weeks, and months to improve diagnosed visual dysfunctions. Optometric vision therapy services are usually provided in-office and involves supportive activities performed at home.

There are community resources to locate providers of vision therapy. Once such source is the College of Optometrists in Vision Development (COVD), an international association that provides board certification in vision development, vision therapy and vision rehabilitation .

Vision problems can co-exist with learning problems, sometimes sharing like symptoms such as difficulties with learning to read, and reading to learn (e.g. dyslexia), as well as reversals in writing letters and poor spelling and math skills. In the school setting, students with a suspected learning disability is evaluated by a team (i.e. parent, educator, occupational therapist, speech therapist, teacher, resource teacher, social worker, counselor, principal, psychologist, pediatrician). If a visual dysfunction is suspected, the optometrists may be called to join the evaluation team. IDEA (Individuals with disabilities education act), is a special education law, schools must find and evaluate students thought to have disabilities at no cost to families (U.S. Department of Education). Specific diagnoses qualifies a child under IDEA for special education services, and can include optometric vision therapy (Lee).

It is important to point out that although vision therapy does not treat learning disabilities, it can treat the visual problems that interfere with learning in the classroom (American Academy of Pediatrics Section on Ophthalmology, Council on Children with Disabilities, American Academy of Ophthalmology, American Association for Pediatric Ophthalmology and Strabismus, & American Association of Certified Orthoptists, 2009; American Optometric Association, 1997; Lack, 2010).

In summary, effective therapy requires visual skills to be developed until they are integrated with other systems and become automatic, enabling individuals to achieve their full potential. The goals of a prescribed vision therapy treatment regimen are to achieve desired visual outcomes, alleviate the signs and symptoms, and meet patients' need to improve their quality of life (American Optometric Association, 1999).

How Does One Know When a Patient Can Benefit From Optometric Vision Therapy?

To illustrate, it may be best to share a patient story.

Susan Barry, a neuroscientist was fifty years old when she experienced true depth perception. As a patient she described when she used to see snow falling, it would appear as if the snow were falling in one flat sheet in front of her, or the steering wheel of her car being flat. Since early infancy Dr. Barry had esotropia (a type of strabismus in which one eye turned inward). She received surgery to correct the muscle imbalance, but the brain received conflicting messages from her two eyes. To avoid seeing double, her brain turned off (suppressed) one eye. She documents her amazing journey in discovering brain plasticity in an adult, regaining binocular vision in her book "Fixing My Gaze".

Authors Taub and Schnell have published two volumes of "Vision Therapy Success Stories" (Optometric Extension Program Foundation) consisting of clinical cases collected from practitioners from around the world about actual vision therapy cases in their practices.

NEURO-OPTOMETRIC REHABILITATION

Introduction

Neuro-optometric rehabilitation is an area of optometric practice which involves treating patients with neurological disease caused by trauma, metabolic, or congenital conditions (American Optometric Association). These neurological conditions cause a constellation of issues which are sensory, motor, perceptual, linguistic, cognitive, attentional and/or behavioral in nature. Therefore, it is not surprising that it also adversely impacts the visual system and causes various types of visual deficits such as oculomotor problems, binocular vision problems, visual information processing (VIP) problems, visual motion sensitivity (VMS) problems, visual-field defects, photosensitivity, and visual attentional deficits. These vision related deficits may severely impact one's activities of daily livings (ADL's). These visual deficits could be managed and treated by a neuro-optometrist.

Neuro-optometrists perform various examinations on these patients based on their visual symptoms caused by a specific neurological condition. They usually evaluate these patients by assessing the following visual functions:

1. **Sensory-motor:** This includes assessment of accommodative (i.e., focusing of an ocular lens to see object clearly), vergence (i.e., coordination between two eyes), and oculomotor function in nine cardinal eye positions (i.e., function of six extra-ocular muscles).
2. **Visual information processing:** This includes assessment of the speed of the visual information processing both at the level of primary visuo-cortical area and higher visuo-cortical areas.
3. **Pupillary reflex assessment:** This includes assessment of the pupillary reflex that is constriction and dilation of pupil velocity under different light conditions.
4. **Eye movement recording:** This includes assessment of eye movement recordings (i.e., saccades, fixation etc.) and also comprehension while reading a paragraph.
5. **Electro-diagnostic recoding:** This includes an objective assessment of visual pathway from retina to the primary visual cortex.

These above-mentioned assessments provide the information essential to treat these patients. The treatments include visual rehabilitation/vision therapy (as discussed in the vision therapy section) which treats sensory-motor visual dysfunctions and improves visual information processing in these patients. In addition, these visual symptoms could also be treated by providing a unique treatment technique such as binasal occluders (BNO) to treat patients with abnormal VMS, and to prescribe colored filter lenses to reduce photosensitivity and to improve VIP (Yadav & Ciuffreda, 2014).

As mentioned above, these patients suffer from vision related deficits. Therefore, these patients often need to be referred to the neuro-optometrist. This branch of optometry includes several visual rehabilitation techniques which helps these patients in reducing their visual symptoms. Eventually, this helps these patients in becoming independent in doing their daily vocational and avocational goals. Therefore, it is important that the other healthcare professionals should understand the importance of neuro-optometric services and its impact on the daily life of these patients.

Neuro-optometrists treat patients with a range of neurological conditions. Some of the very common conditions are mentioned below:

- Stroke
- Multiple sclerosis (MS)
- Traumatic brain injury (TBI)/concussion
- Amblyopia (lazy eye)

These patients are referred to the neuro-optometrist by various healthcare professionals, such as neurologists, physiatrists, family medicine physicians, physical therapists, occupational therapists, optometrists/ophthalmologists, and speech therapists. Most of these healthcare professionals work as a team to treat patients with the above neurological conditions. For example, a healthcare team is required to treat patients with TBI/concussion. These TBI/concussion patients suffer from various visual and systemic health problems. Therefore, a team of healthcare professional's is essential to work together to treat these health issues.

This could be better explained by giving an example of Jacob Green a mild TBI patient. Jacob Green is an author of a book entitled "See Change Clearly" (Green, 2019). In this book, he explained in detail his journey about suffering from a mild TBI symptoms to how a team of health professionals worked together to treat him.

These healthcare professionals can only work together if they understand the scope of each other's practices. This could only be possible with the introduction of the interprofessional education (IPE), interprofessional practice (IPP), and interprofessional care (IPC) during their training period. This would prove to be very helpful in treating these patients.

SPORTS VISION

Sports vision is another developing area of optometry. Optometrists with expertise and training in this field are involved in the assessment and improvement of visual skills training for players of different sports teams (American Optometric Association). Sports vision optometrists can recommend prescription eyeglasses or contact lenses which can improve an athlete's contrast sensitivity and vision. Optometrists can also customize a vision therapy treatment plan for players suited for their particular sport. This can translate into improving athlete's performance on the field.

Sports vision optometrists perform examinations that focus on the visual functions of an athlete(International Sports Vision Association), including an evaluation for the following visual skills (Berman, 1993):

1. **Visual Acuity:** This is the most important visual function test for a player (Gao et al., 2015; Zimmerman, Lust, & Bullimore, 2011). If a player has poor visual acuity, their performance may be affected on the field. Therefore, to

improve an athlete's visual acuity, the optometrist can prescribe eyeglasses for athletes engaged in stationary stances such as, archery and shooting, and prescribe contact lenses for players of more dynamic games such as football or soccer.

2. **Contrast Sensitivity Function (CSF):** CSF test is the second important visual function for an athlete (Gao et al., 2015; Zimmerman et al., 2011). CSF is seeing the visual world under different light conditions. Having a good CSF is very important for athletes to play under a range of light conditions. For an athlete with poor CSF, his/her visual activity is negatively affected even if the measured visual acuity is better than 20/20. Better CSF helps players under various lighting conditions to see and track other players or moving targets such as a moving ball. Athletes can experience enhanced CSF by wearing prescription eyeglasses or contact lenses with tints.
3. **Eye Tracking:** Eye tracking is another important visual function for an athlete. Eye tracking helps athletes in tracking other players and balls quickly, clearly, and accurately. There are various eye tracking devices (Piras, Lobietti, & Squatrito, 2010)to evaluate eye tracking skills including fixation, pursuits and saccades. An athlete with abnormal eye movement recordings may experience challenges performing well on the field. To help these athletes, a sports vision optometrist can provide vision therapy to improve their eye tracking (Appelbaum & Erickson, 2018).
4. **Ocular Alignment:** This test evaluates if the two eyes are aligned and how well they work together (normal binocular vision) (Gao et al., 2015). This visual function provides information related to depth judgement. If ocular alignment is disrupted in athletes, it would affect their performance on the field. This could be treated by a sports vision optometrist by providing them vision therapy (Appelbaum & Erickson, 2018).
5. **Ocular Dominance:** Ocular (eye) dominance is eye preference or preference for visual input from one eye to the other. Testing for ocular dominance is important for various sports, such as archery, target shooting, and golf (Gao et al., 2015). Specific training of athletes in using their dominant eye to take aim a target may improve their performance (Mohammadi et al., 2016).
6. **Visual Processing Speed:** Visual processing speed is defined as the brain's ability to receive, analyze, and interpret visual information. On the field, visual processing involves the athlete's ability to visualize and react quickly to moving objects, such as hitting a baseball thrown at different speeds, or catching a football. This can be tested using computerized visual processing speed tests. Optometrists could improve athletes visual processing speed by providing them vision therapy. This can help them develop better hand-eye coordination and faster reaction times (Poltavski & Biberdorf, 2015).

7. **Stereoacuity and Depth Perception:** Testing static and dynamic stereoacuity and depth perception of an athlete provides information about judging the distance of opposing players or the ball with respect to themselves. Sports vision therapists could help the players in improving their stereoacuity and depth perception.

Sport vision optometrists work together with other professionals to improve the visual skills of the sports teams at the high school, college, national, and international levels. They usually work with ophthalmologists, sports physical therapists, athletic trainers, and team coaches.

These healthcare and athletic professionals can only work together if they understand the scope of each other's work. This could only be possible with the introduction of the interprofessional education (IPE) and interprofessional care (IPC) during their training period.

LOW VISION REHABILITATION

Who Are the Patients?

According to the American Optometric Association, there are relatively few people in the United States who are totally without sight (American Optometric Association). A majority of people whom we may categorize as "blind" actually have remaining sight, and are more appropriately thought of as visually impaired. A specialized area of optometric practice, commonly known as "low vision rehabilitation", emphasizes techniques to enhance visual functioning and improve quality of life for people who have uncorrectable vision loss.

On a global level, population-based research estimates 36 million people who are blind, out of 7.33 billion people living in 2015. This compares with 216.6 million people with moderate to severe visual impairment and 188.5 million people with mild visual impairment. From 1990 to 2015, blindness has increased by 17.6%, and moderate and severe visual impairment has increased by 35.5%, with the increase attributable to an overall increase in the population combined with aging of the population (Bourne et al., 2017).

Anyone with reduced vision that cannot be fully restored when using conventional prescription spectacles or contact lenses is considered to be visually impaired (American Optometric Association).

The American Optometric Association's *Optometric Clinical Practice Guideline Care of the Patient with Visual Impairment* further elaborates the description and classification of visual impairment (American Optometric Association, 2007). How we think about visual impairment has changed over time, and varies from different perspectives. Legal blindness is a definition that was adopted by governmental agencies in the United States to determine eligibility for rehabilitation services, vocational training, specialized schooling, disability benefits, and tax exemption programs (Blind; Hoppe, 1992). The U.S. definition of legal blindness is comprised of two parts: a visual acuity of 20/200 or less in the better seeing eye with best conventional correction, or a visual field of 20 degrees or less in the better seeing eye. Definitions of visual impairment have been tied to The International Classification of Diseases for use in medical billing. Previously, Visual impairment was defined as a functional limitation of the eye(s) or visual system (Centers for Disease Control and Prevention, 1996) manifesting as reduced visual acuity or contrast sensitivity, visual field loss, photophobia, diplopia, visual distortion, visual perceptual difficulties, or any combination of the above. ICD-10 codes have expanded the definition and have incorporated perspectives from the definitions recommended by the World Health Organization. Categories were developed to include mild or no visual impairment, moderate impairment, severe impairment, and blindness (Buckholtz, 2017, September 27) as shown in Figure 4.

Figure 4. Categories of Visual Impairment

The International Classification of Diseases 11 (2018) classifies vision impairment into two groups, distance and near presenting vision impairment (World Health Organization, 2018 October 11).

Distance vision impairment:

- Mild – presenting visual acuity worse than 6/12 or 20/50
- Moderate – presenting visual acuity worse than 6/18 or 20/60
- Severe – presenting visual acuity worse than 6/60 or 20/200
- Blindness – presenting visual acuity worse than 3/60 or 20/400

Near vision impairment: Presenting near visual acuity worse than N6 or M0.8 or 20/50 with existing correction.

Visual impairment may result from genetic abnormalities, injuries or trauma, ocular diseases, or ocular manifestations of systemic disease processes. Vision impairment may be from birth, or may occur at any stage of life. However, the majority of patients living with vision impairment experience vision loss later in life (Congdon et al., 2004).

Some of the most common causes of vision impairment from ocular conditions include glaucoma, macular degeneration, and retinitis pigmentosa. Some of the most common causes of vision impairment from systemic conditions are diabetic eye disease, stroke or cerebral vascular accident, or complications from hypertension or hypercholesterolemia. Genetic conditions such as albinism or the effects of premature birth can lead to vision impairment from birth or at a very young age. Vision impairments may affect visual acuity, visual fields or peripheral vision, contrast sensitivity, color vision, visual perception, and cortical visual function. Many people experience more than one type of visual impairment (American Optometric Association, 2007).

Beyond the definitions, classifications, and causes, it is vitally important to understand how visual impairment impacts our patients. A visual impairment may cause a functional disability by significantly reducing a person's ability to perform activities of daily living, to travel safely, and ultimately to function independently. Examples of specific problems have been noted to include loss of the ability to read regular sized print, limitations or loss of ability to drive, difficulty performing work-related tasks, inability to enjoy hobbies, sports, and leisure activities, and social limitations such as the inability to recognize faces or facial expressions. Importantly, when these types of disabilities limit a person's independence or socioeconomic status, then it is noted that a visual handicap is present (West et al., 2002). For people with visual impairments, access to vision rehabilitation is crucial.

The American Optometric Association defines vision rehabilitation as:

Vision rehabilitation is the process of treatment and education that helps individuals who are visually disabled attain maximum function, a sense of well-being, a personally satisfying level of independence, and optimum quality of life. Function is maximized by evaluation, diagnosis and treatment including, but not limited to, the prescription of optical, non-optical, electronic and/or other treatments. The rehabilitation process includes the development of an individual rehabilitation plan specifying clinical therapy and/or instruction in compensatory approaches.

Vision rehabilitation may be necessitated by any condition, disease, or injury that causes a visual impairment which results in functional limitation or disability. In addition to the evaluation, diagnosis and management of visual impairment by an eye care physician (optometrist or ophthalmologist), vision rehabilitation may include, but is not limited to, optometric, medical, allied health, social, educational and psychological services (American Optometric Association, 2007).

Why Is It Important?

Low vision rehabilitation services allow individuals with impaired vision to gain better control of their surroundings which leads to improved independence, lower risk for depression, and better quality of life (Stelmack et al., 2017) (Colenbrander, 2010). The goal of low vision rehabilitation is not to restore sight, but to restore function.

How Do We Integrate Within an IPE Collaboration?

Low vision rehabilitation services involve a team of professions:

- Optometrist/Ophthalmologist
- Occupational therapists, Physical therapists
- Social worker
- Speech-Language Pathologists
- Audiologists
- Orientation and Mobility Specialists
- Vision Rehabilitation Therapists
- Teachers of the Visually Impaired
- Psychological services/ counseling
- Physicians

Health care providers who encounter individuals with visual impairments should be aware of low vision rehabilitation services and should assist patients in seeking appropriate care. Optometrists can work with patients and other members of the health care team to prescribe assistive devices and technology for self-care with a goal maintaining independence. This could involve adaptive technology for medication management such as talking medicine bottles, syringe magnifiers, or even video magnification to be used for inspecting skin and self-care for foot inspection. Doctors of optometry can work with members of the wellness team to prescribe visual devices and specialized filter lenses that improve mobility and allow people with visual impairments to maintain an exercise routine. Optometrists can support other providers by working with their visually impaired patients to ensure that they can accurately read health education materials, instructions for care regimens, and to read labels for good nutrition. Doctors of optometry can also assist in preparing health education materials in alternate formats and can assist in educating other health care providers on how to make their offices and patient care facilities safe and welcoming for people with visual impairments. Because many people with visual impairment also have systemic health conditions and cope with chronic ailments, optometrists also play a role in monitoring overall health and well-being and assist in managing their patients' health with appropriate in-office testing, consultations, and referrals for conditions such as hypertension, diabetes, hypercholesterolemia, cardiovascular disease, and many neurological conditions.

What Should Providers Know?

According to National Eye Institute, 4.2 million Americans are visually impaired with 3 million who have low vision(National Eye Health Education Program). Few people are totally without sight. Most people who are classified as "blind" actually have remaining sight. Progressive vision loss can be congenital or acquired. Visual impairments take many forms and exist in varying degrees. Anyone with noncorrectable, reduced vision is visually impaired. Thanks to developments in low vision rehabilitation services, people with visual impairments can enhance their visual function and improve their quality of life. Visual acuity alone is not a good predictor of a person's vision problems. Someone with relatively good acuity (20/40) can have difficulty functioning, while someone with worse acuity (20/200) might not have any real problems performing daily activities. It is important for health care and social services professionals to identify and encourage those with vision loss to seek care to help them maintain independence and enjoy life.

SUMMARY – DIABETIC CASE

46 year old Hispanic female presented to a community based clinic for a diabetic eye exam with complaints of fluctuating blurred vision at distance and near, left eye worse than the right, for the past 6 months. She was referred to the eye clinic by her primary care physician after being diagnosed with Type 2 Diabetes Mellitus 1 month prior. Her past ocular history is unremarkable. Her past family history was positive for Type 2 Diabetes mellitus in multiple family members. She began taking metformin 1000mg twice a day and atorvastin 20 mg once daily a month ago. She declined alcohol, tobacco or drug use. She was alert and orientated to person, place, and time. Her reported fasting blood sugar was 192. Table 2 provides a summary of the patient's relevant laboratory findings. Table 3 provides a summary of the patient's relevant eye findings.

Table 2. Summary of Laboratory Findings.

Laboratory test	Laboratory Results	Reference range
Endocrine		
Random glucose	209	65/110 mg/dL
Hemoglobin A1C	9.8 %	<5.8%
Lipid Profile		
Cholesterol total	300	<200 mg/dL
Triglycerides	142	<150 mg/dL
HDL	74	>50 mg/ dL
LDL	196	99 mg/ dl

Table 3. Summary of Eye Findings.

Test	Right Eye	Left Eye
Distance Visual acuity	20/40 Pinhole NI	20/50 Pinhole NI
Near visual acuity	20/80	20/160
Pupils	PERRL (-) APD	PERRL (-) APD
Confrontational fields	Full to finger counting	Full to finger counting
Extraocular motility	Full and smooth, no restriction	Full and smooth, no restriction
Cover test	Orthophoria at distance and near	Orthophoria at distance and near
Refraction:	+0.25-0.75x090 BCVA 20/20	+1.75-0.50x085 BCVA 20/40
Slit lamp evaluation	Grade 1 central posterior subcapsular cataract	Trace posterior subcapsular cataract
Dilated fundus examination	Proliferative diabetic retinopathy with clinically significant macular edema	Proliferative diabetic retinopathy with clinically significant macular edema

Figure 5 shows the fundus of patient's right eye, demonstrating findings of neovascularization "everywhere," dot and blot hemorrhages, exudates, and clinically significant macular edema (hazy view from cataract)

Figure 5. Fundus photography right eye.

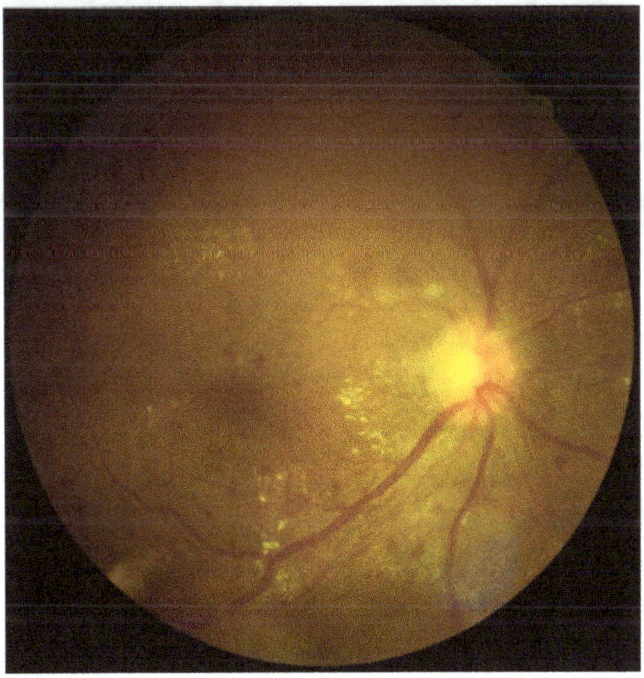

Figure 6 shows the fundus of patient's left eye demonstrating findings of neovascularization "everywhere," dot and blot hemorrhages, pre-retinal hemorrhages, exudates, and clinically significant macular edema.

Figure 6. Fundus photography left eye.

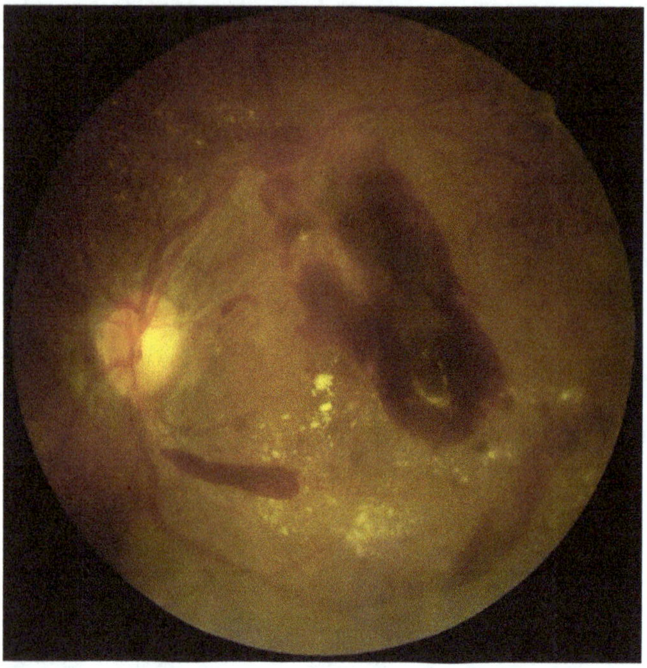

The ocular assessment made for the patient was high risk proliferative diabetic retinopathy with clinically significant macular edema in both eyes. The patient was

Table 4.

CATEGORY	WORSE THAN:	EQUAL TO OR BETTER THAN:
Mild or no visual impairment 0		20/70
Moderate visual impairment 1	20/70	20/200
Severe visual impairment 2	20/200	20/400
Blindness 3	20/400	20/1200
Blindness 4	20/1200	Light Perception
Blindness 5	No light perception	No Light Perception

referred to a retinal ophthalmologist for treatment and management for retinopathy and to a clinical pharmacy to control blood glucose. The patient was asked to return in 6 weeks for a follow up on diabetic retinopathy. The optometrist educated the patient on the importance of tight blood sugar control and adherence of all diabetic medications.

Retinal Ophthalmology

The patient was examined by a retinal ophthalmologist one day later. She was treated with anti-VEGF injections and pan-retinal photocoagulation in both eyes. She continues to see ophthalmology every month until her retinopathy is deemed stable and quiescent

Clinical Pharmacy

The clinical pharmacist assessed the patient's adherence with medication, daily dietary intake, and exercise. The patient notes good compliance with metformin 1000 mg twice a day for blood glucose control. Blood glucose levels taken that morning was 148 and before bed was 214. She stated that she ate 3 meals a day without snacks. A normal meal consisted of bread with ham, salad, rice, chicken and mixed vegetables. The clinical pharmacist educated the patient on restricting carbs, stay adherent to medication and the possible need for additional therapy if no lifestyle changes. The clinical pharmacist's goal for the patient is outlined in Table 5.

Table 5. Clinical pharmacist's patient goals.

Blood pressure	<130/80- patient was currently at goal
Hemoglobin A1c	<7%
Blood glucose	Morning <120 and none >200
Cholesterol therapy	High intensity statin, adjustment of atorvastin from 20mg to 40mg dosage was recommended to primary care.

The patient was asked to follow up with clinical pharmacy in 6 weeks. A referral was placed to podiatry for an assessment of neuropathy.

Primary Care

The patient continues to see primary care every three months until blood sugar and hemoglobin a1C is at goal. A referral was placed to podiatry for an assessment of neuropathy

Optometry Follow Up

The patient continues to be under the care of ophthalmology. Due to the good visual status, no other optometry specialty is needed at this time.

REFERENCES

InfantSEE. (n.d.b)About InfantSEE. Retrieved from https://www.infantsee.org/about-us.xml

American Academy of Pediatrics Section on Ophthalmology. (2009). Joint statement—Learning disabilities, dyslexia, and vision. *Pediatrics*, *124*(2), 837–844. doi:10.1542/peds.2009-1445 PMID:19651597

American Optometric Association. (1997). *Vision, learning and dyslexia*. Retrieved from https://cdn.ymaws.com/www.covd.org/resource/resmgr/position_papers/vision-learning-dyslexia_-_j.pdf

American Optometric Association. (1999). *Vision Therapy Information for Health Care and Other Allied Professionals*. Retrieved from https://cdn.ymaws.com/www.covd.org/resource/resmgr/position_papers/vision-therapy_-_jops_aao_&_.pdf

American Optometric Association. (2007). *Optometric Clinical Practice Guideline Care of the Patient with Visual Impairment (Low Vision Rehabilitation)*. Retrieved from https://www.aoa.org/documents/optometrists/CPG-14.pdf

American Optometric Association. (2009). *Definition of optometric vision therapy*. Retrieved from https://www.aoa.org/Documents/CRG/definition-of-optometric-vision-therapy.pdf

American Optometric Association. (2015). *AOA Optometric Clinical Practice Guidelines- Adult Eye Exam*. Retrieved from https://www.aoa.org/optometrists/tools-and-resources/clinical-care-publications/clinical-practice-guidelines

American Optometric Association. (2017). *Evidence-Based Clinical Practice Guideline: Comprehensive Pediatric Eye and Vision Examination.* Retrieved from http://aoa.uberflip.com/i/807465-cpg-pediatric-eye-and-vision-examination/0?m4=

American Optometric Association. (n.d.a). Retrieved from https://www.aoa.org/optometrists/tools-and-resources/vision-rehabilitation/neuro

American Optometric Association. (n.d.b). *Low Vision. American Optometric Association. Realeyes Program*. Retrieved from https://www.aoa.org/the-realeyes-program

American Optometric Association. (n.d.c). *Sports & Performance Vision*. Retrieved from https://www.aoa.org/optometrists/tools-and-resources/sports-and-performance-vision

American Optometric Association. (n.d.d). *What is a Doctor of Optometry?* Retrieved from https://www.aoa.org/about-the-aoa/what-is-a-doctor-of-optometry

Appelbaum, L. G., & Erickson, G. (2018). Sports vision training: A review of the state-of-the-art in digital training techniques. *International Review of Sport and Exercise Psychology, 11*(1), 160–189. doi:10.1080/1750984X.2016.1266376

Aravamudhan, R., Vitek, M., & Casser, L. (2015). The Implementation and Assessment of an Interprofessional Education Initiative at Salus University. *Optometric Education, 40*(3), 11–15.

Association of Schools and Colleges of Optometry. (n.d.). *Interprofessional Education and Collaborative Practice*. Retrieved from https://optometriceducation.org/interprofessional-education/

Berman, A. M. (1993). Clinical evaluation of the athlete. *Optometry Clinics, 3*(1), 1–26. PMID:8324319

Blind, A. F. t. (n.d.). *Blindness and Low Vision.* Retrieved from https://www.afb.org/blindness-and-low-vision

Borsting, E., Mitchell, G. L., Kulp, M. T., Scheiman, M., Amster, D. M., Cotter, S., ... Group, C. S. (2012). Improvement in academic behaviors after successful treatment of convergence insufficiency. *Optometry and Vision Science, 89*(1), 12–18. doi:10.1097/OPX.0b013e318238ffc3 PMID:22080400

Bourne, R. R. A., Flaxman, S. R., Braithwaite, T., Cicinelli, M. V., Das, A., Jonas, J. B., ... Vision Loss Expert, G. (2017). Magnitude, temporal trends, and projections of the global prevalence of blindness and distance and near vision impairment: A systematic review and meta-analysis. *The Lancet. Global Health*, *5*(9), e888–e897. doi:10.1016/S2214-109X(17)30293-0 PMID:28779882

Buckholtz, R. (2017, September 27). *Looking at new ICD-10-CM Codes for Blindness*. Retrieved from https://www.icd10monitor.com/looking-at-new-icd-10-cm-codes-for-blindness

Centers for Disease Control and Prevention. (1996). *International Classification of Diseases, Ninth Revision, Clinical Modification (ICD-9-CM)*. Retrieved from https://www.cdc.gov/nchs/icd/icd9cm.htm

Centers for Disease Control and Prevention. (n.d.). *Keep an Eye on Your Vision Health*. Retrieved from https://www.cdc.gov/features/healthyvision/index.html

Christian, L. W., MacIver, S., & Alfieri, M. (2015). Evaluation of Interprofessional Education and Collaboration in Optometry. *Optometric Education*, *40*(3), 16–22.

Colenbrander, A. (2010). Assessment of functional vision and its rehabilitation. *Acta Ophthalmologica*, *88*(2), 163–173. doi:10.1111/j.1755-3768.2009.01670.x PMID:20039847

College of Optometrists in Vision Development. (n.d.a). *Locate a Doctor*. Retrieved from https://www.covd.org

College of Optometrists in Vision Development. (n.d.b). *Research on Vision Therapy*. Retrieved from https://www.covd.org/page/research

Congdon, N., O'Colmain, B., Klaver, C. C., Klein, R., Munoz, B., & Friedman, D. S. (2004). Causes and prevalence of visual impairment among adults in the United States. *Archives of Ophthalmology*, *122*(4), 477–485. doi:10.1001/archopht.122.4.477 PMID:15078664

Donahue, S. P., & Nixon, C. N., Section on Opthamology, A. A. o. P., Committee on, P., Ambulatory Medicine, A. A. o. P., American Academy of, O., . . . American Association of Certified, O. (2016). Visual System Assessment in Infants, Children, and Young Adults by Pediatricians. *Pediatrics*, *137*(1), 28–30. doi:10.1542/peds.2015-3596 PMID:29756730

Dowd, L., & Smith, J. P. (2015). Incorporating Interprofessional Education into a VA Optometric Residency. *Optometric Education*, *40*(3), 38–41.

Fishman Hellerstein, L. B. I. F. (1999). Collaboration Between Occupational Therapists and Optometrists. *Journal of Behavioral Optometry*, *10*, 147–152.

Francis, J., & Abraham, S. (2014). Clinical pharmacists: Bridging the gap between patients and physicians. *Saudi Pharmaceutical Journal*, *22*(6), 600–602. doi:10.1016/j.jsps.2014.02.011 PMID:25561874

Gao, Y., Chen, L., Yang, S. N., Wang, H., Yao, J., Dai, Q., & Chang, S. (2015). Contributions of Visuo-oculomotor Abilities to Interceptive Skills in Sports. *Optometry and Vision Science*, *92*(6), 679–689. doi:10.1097/OPX.0000000000000599 PMID:25930979

Granet, D. B., Gomi, C. F., Ventura, R., & Miller-Scholte, A. (2005). The relationship between convergence insufficiency and ADHD. *Strabismus*, *13*(4), 163–168. doi:10.1080/09273970500455436 PMID:16361187

Green, J. (2019). *See Change Clearly: Leveraging Adversity to Sharpen Your Vision and Build Resilient Teams*. Lioncrest Publishing.

Hartmann, E. E., Block, S. S., & Wallace, D. K. (2015). Vision and eye health in children 36 to <72 months: Proposed data system. *Optometry and Vision Science*, *92*(1), 24–30. doi:10.1097/OPX.0000000000000445 PMID:25562478

Hendrick, A. M., & Maria, V. (2015). Diabetic Retinopathy. *Primary Care Clinical Office Practice*, *42*(3), 451–464. doi:10.1016/j.pop.2015.05.005 PMID:26319349

Hodge, C., Chan, C., Zantos, S., Kokkinakis, J., Stapleton, F., & Sutton, G. (2015). Therapeutic treatment of keratoconus: A survey of local optometric practice criteria. *Clinical & Experimental Optometry*, *98*(4), 312–318. doi:10.1111/cxo.12233 PMID:26104590

Hoppe, E. (1992). Evaluating the laws defining blindness. *Journal of the American Optometric Association*, *63*(6), 390–394. PMID:1634739

International Sports Vision Association. (n.d.). *Dynamic Visual Skills for Sports*. Retrieved from https://www.sportsvision.pro

Jaiswal, S., Asper, L., Long, J., Lee, A., Harrison, K., & Golebiowski, B. (2019). Ocular and visual discomfort associated with smartphones, tablets and computers: What we do and do not know. *Clinical & Experimental Optometry*, *102*(5), 463–477. doi:10.1111/cxo.12851 PMID:30663136

Krumholtz, I. (2004). Educating the educators: Increasing grade-school teachers' ability to detect vision problems. *Optometry (St. Louis, Mo.)*, *75*(7), 445–451. doi:10.1016/S1529-1839(04)70159-1 PMID:15296377

Lack, D. (2010). Another joint statement regarding learning disabilities, dyslexia, and vision—A rebuttal. *Optometry (St. Louis, Mo.)*, *81*(10), 533–543. doi:10.1016/j.optm.2009.11.007 PMID:20728412

Lasher, S. K. (2015). *IDOC: Interpreting Data from the Oyler Clinic Thesis*. Academic Press.

Lawrenson, J. G., Hull, C. C., & Downie, L. E. (2017). The effect of blue-light blocking spectacle lenses on visual performance, macular health and the sleep-wake cycle: A systematic review of the literature. *Ophthalmic & Physiological Optics*, *37*(6), 644–654. doi:10.1111/opo.12406 PMID:29044670

Lee, A. M. I. (n.d.). *Individuals With Disabilities Education Act (IDEA): What You Need to Know*. Retrieved from https://www.understood.org/en/school-learning/your-childs-rights/basics-about-childs-rights/individuals-with-disabilities-education-act-idea-what-you-need-to-know

Long, D. D., & Rosen, I. (2017). Social Work and Optometry: Interprofessional Practice Revisited. *Health & Social Work*, *42*(2), 117–120. doi:10.1093/hsw/hlx002 PMID:28339798

Long, J., & Helland, M. (2012). A multidisciplinary approach to solving computer related vision problems. *Ophthalmic & Physiological Optics*, *32*(5), 429–435. doi:10.1111/j.1475-1313.2012.00911.x PMID:22540950

Marsh-Tootle, W. L., Russ, S. A., & Repka, M. X. (2015). Vision and eye health in children 36 to <72 months: Proposed data definitions. *Optometry and Vision Science*, *92*(1), 17–23. doi:10.1097/OPX.0000000000000444 PMID:25562477

Maternal and Child Health Bureau. (n.d.). Retrieved from https://mchb.hrsa.gov/

McLeod, A., & Bush, S. (2015). Pilot Assessment of Teaching Anterior Segment Evaluation to Develop Interprofessional Education Programs. *Optometric Education*, *40*(3), 42–47.

Mohammadi, S. F., Aghazade Amiri, M., Naderifar, H., Rakhshi, E., Vakilian, B., Ashrafi, E., & Behesht-Nejad, A. H. (2016). Vision Examination Protocol for Archery Athletes Along With an Introduction to Sports Vision. *Asian Journal of Sports Medicine*, *7*(1), e26591. doi:10.5812/asjsm.26591 PMID:27217923

Murphy, J. (2013 November 15). *Current Trends in Comanagement*. Retrieved from https://www.reviewofoptometry.com/article/current-trends-in-comanagement-44930

National, P. T. A. (2005). *Position Statement - Elements of Comprehensive Health Programs*. Retrieved from https://www.pta.org/home/advocacy/ptas-positions/Individual-Position-Statements/Position-Statement-Elements-of-Comprehensive-Health-Programs

National Academies of Practice. (n.d.). *14 Health Professions Joining Together*. Retrieved from https://napractice.org/About-NAP/Academies/Optometry%20accessed%20on%208/16/19

National Association of School Nurses. (2017). *Vision and eye health*. Retrieved from https://www.nasn.org/nasn-resources/practice-topics/vision-health

National Eye Health Education Program. (n.d.). *Vision Rehabilitation: Helping People with Low Vision*. Retrieved from https://nei.nih.gov/sites/default/files/nehep-pdfs/Low_Vision_Fact_Sheet_v3.pdf

InfantSEE. (n.d.a). Retrieved from https://www.infantsee.org/

Nehmad, L., Reynolds, S. A., & Anderson-Worts, P. (2015). Interprofessional Education on a Mission. *Optometric Education*, *40*(3), 51–54.

OneSight. (n.d.). *Vision Center at Oyler School*. Retrieved from https://www.cincinnati-oh.gov/health/assets/File/Oyler%20Vision%20Center.pdf

Optometric Extension Program Foundation. (n.d.). *Shop OEPF*. Retrieved from https://www.oepf.org/

Piras, A., Lobietti, R., & Squatrito, S. (2010). A study of saccadic eye movement dynamics in volleyball: Comparison between athletes and non-athletes. *The Journal of Sports Medicine and Physical Fitness*, *50*(1), 99–108. PMID:20308980

Poltavski, D., & Biberdorf, D. (2015). The role of visual perception measures used in sports vision programmes in predicting actual game performance in Division I collegiate hockey players. *Journal of Sports Sciences*, *33*(6), 597–608. doi:10.1080/02640414.2014.951952 PMID:25142869

Remick, K. (2018). *Eyes On Track; Ages 4-Adult: A manual to improve vision processing*. Academic Press.

Roch-Levecq, A. C., Brody, B. L., Thomas, R. G., & Brown, S. I. (2008). Ametropia, preschoolers' cognitive abilities, and effects of spectacle correction. *Archives of Ophthalmology*, *126*(2), 252–258. doi:10.1001/archophthalmol.2007.36 PMID:18268218

Rodriguez, E., Srivastava, A., & Landau, M. (2018). Increasing Screening Follow-Up for Vulnerable Children: A Partnership with School Nurses. *International Journal of Environmental Research and Public Health*, *15*(8), 1572. Advance online publication. doi:10.3390/ijerph15081572 PMID:30044383

Sanchez-Diaz, P. C., Ann Parker, R. A., Valdes, M. S., Ramirez, M. N., Narayanan, S., Dominguez, D. G., & Jones, M. E. (2015). Shaping Student Attitudes Toward Healthcare Teams Through a Hybrid and an Online Interprofessional Education Course: Results from a Pilot Study. *Optometric Education*, *40*(3), 23–30.

Stelmack, J. A., Tang, X. C., Wei, Y., Wilcox, D. T., Morand, T., Brahm, K., ... Group, L. I. S. (2017). Outcomes of the Veterans Affairs Low Vision Intervention Trial II (LOVIT II): A Randomized Clinical Trial. *JAMA Ophthalmology*, *135*(2), 96–104. doi:10.1001/jamaophthalmol.2016.4742 PMID:27978569

U.S. Department of Education. (n.d.). *IDEA Individuals with Disabilities Education Act*. Retrieved from https://sites.ed.gov/idea/

U.S. Preventive Services Task Force. (2011). U.*S. Preventive Services Task Force Issues Final Recommendation Statement for Vision Screening in Children Ages 1 to 5*. Retrieved from https://www.uspreventiveservicestaskforce.org/Announcements/News/Item/us-preventive-services-task-force-issues-final-recommendation-statement-for-vision-screening-in-children-ages-1-to-5

InfantSEE. (n.d.c). *InfantSEE. Ways to help infant vision development.* Retrieved from https://www.infantsee.org/parents-center/ways-to-help-infant-vision-development.xml

West, S. K., Rubin, G. S., Broman, A. T., Munoz, B., Bandeen-Roche, K., & Turano, K. (2002). How does visual impairment affect performance on tasks of everyday life? The SEE Project. Salisbury Eye Evaluation. *Archives of Ophthalmology*, *120*(6), 774–780. doi:10.1001/archopht.120.6.774 PMID:12049583

World Health Organization. (2015). *The impact of myopia and high myopia*. Retrieved from https://www.who.int/blindness/causes/MyopiaReportforWeb.pdf

World Health Organization. (2018 October 11). *Blindness and vision impairment*. Retrieved from https://www.who.int/news-room/fact-sheets/detail/blindness-and-visual-impairment

Yadav, N. K., & Ciuffreda, K. J. (2014). Effect of binasal occlusion (BNO) and base-in prisms on the visual-evoked potential (VEP) in mild traumatic brain injury (mTBI). *Brain Injury: [BI]*, *28*(12), 1568–1580. doi:10.3109/02699052.2014.939718 PMID:25058498

Yeu, E., Donnenfeld, E., & Chang, D. H. (2018 February 21). *Five secrets to success with co-management*. Retrieved from https://www.ophthalmologytimes.com/article/five-secrets-success-co-management

Yumori, J. W., Dickter, D. N., Napier-Dovorany, K., Wren, V. Q., Tegzes, J. H., & Stielstra, S. (2015). Optometry Students' Knowledge-Based Performance within Interprofessional Education Courses. *Optometric Education*, *40*(3), 31–36.

Zimmerman, A. B., Lust, K. L., & Bullimore, M. A. (2011). Visual acuity and contrast sensitivity testing for sports vision. *Eye & Contact Lens*, *37*(3), 153–159. doi:10.1097/ICL.0b013e31820d12f4 PMID:21378574

Chapter 12
Development of a Well-Being Mentorship Program for Clinical Clerkships

Raúl René Cantú-Hernández
https://orcid.org/0000-0001-6653-3799
Escuela de Medicina y Ciencias de la Salud, Tecnologico de Monterrey, Mexico

Manuel Emiliano Quiroga Garza
https://orcid.org/0000-0002-5237-240X
Escuela de Medicina y Ciencias de la Salud, Tecnologico de Monterrey, Mexico

David Leonardo Flores-Marín
https://orcid.org/0000-0001-5310-9649
Escuela de Medicina y Ciencias de la Salud, Tecnologico de Monterrey, Mexico

Irma Elisa Erana-Rojas
https://orcid.org/0000-0002-9022-3739
Escuela de Medicina y Ciencias de la Salud, Tecnologico de Monterrey, Mexico

Mildred Vanessa López Cabrera
https://orcid.org/0000-0002-6965-6636
Escuela de Medicina y Ciencias de la Salud, Tecnologico de Monterrey, Mexico

ABSTRACT

Clinical clerkships allow students to transition from exclusively academic to real professional settings. This stressful transition can lead to burnout. Recent awareness has led to the creation of mentorship programs focused on improving students' well-being. A mentorship program was developed for students in the clinical clerkships to monitor and foster habits for well-being based on a six-pillar model: mental,

DOI: 10.4018/978-1-7998-3066-5.ch012

social, emotional, academic, nutritional, and physical health. The purpose of the chapter is to present the model and preliminary results of a study that assessed the program's effects through the mentor's perception. A qualitative approach with semi-structured interviews was used. Results indicate impact on mental (85%) and emotional health (85%), as evidenced by the identification of multiple red-flag cases. The implementation of programs must effectively foster students' self-assessment and allows them to develop better coping mechanisms.

INTRODUCTION

Medical education has been in constant evolution throughout history. Since the Flexner report (1910) in the early twentieth century, a study of more than 150 medical schools in the United States and Canada, several transition phases in the teaching and learning processes have been identified which require teachers to assume new roles and skills as medical educators (Olivares and Valdez, 2017). Olivares and Valdez recognized four historical stages in medical education: Science Based Learning, Problem Based Learning, Competency Based Learning, and Perspective Based Learning. The major transitions had a focus on developing a student reasoning profile and a corresponding faculty profile. It is presented in table 1.

Table 1. Historical stages in medical education of Olivares and Valdez (2017)

Historical Stage	Student Reasoning Profile	Required Faculty Profile
Science Based Learning	Students work to develop deductive reasoning.	Faculty know as a lecturer.
Problem Based Learning	Students gather information, infer, and use inductive reasoning to find a solution.	Faculty that works as a facilitator, work as tutors during the sessions were students work.
Competency Based Learning	Students practice a skill until they are able to demonstrate mastery of it.	Faculty participate as an assessor for students competency.
Perspective Based Learning	Students develop transformative reasoning to question traditions and paradigms, to make co-built solutions with the community that is sustainable for the environment.	Faculty act as a mentor for students to solve challenges.

Medical education is designed for students to gain skills and independence until, gradually, they can be responsible for the patient's health and well-being. Although ideally, training should provide sufficient practice opportunities for all students, this is time and resource constricted (López and Valdez-García, 2019). Learning in the clinical setting is highly iñuenced by several trends on care, such as the decrease of patients, the impact of cost optimization, and a tendency on reducing the number of in-hospital hours by the implementation of patient-safety procedures. Programs, faculty, and universities should adapt and reorient their efforts to continue preparing physicians that would revolutionize patient care.

The context in which these learning experiences take place is a determinant of behavior; the experiences integrate five focal terms: curriculum, environment, climate, quality, and change (Genn, 2001). The curriculum describes the desired educational impact to guarantee an alumni profile. The environment must be patient centered where the objective is to provide the best care possible while trying to honor patient requests. The climate refers to a culture that promotes the construction of a learning community, where everybody involved has a voice and should be heard. The quality elements translate to the level of care that is delivered for the patient and their families. There are several factors that influence or drive change, such as the improvement of educational practice and innovation, the incorporation of technology, the transition in healthcare models, and some others attributed to epidemiological factors (Valdez-García, 2004).

The clinical clerkship experience is considered the base or standing point for acquiring most of the clinical competencies declared; though, there is no consensus on the volume or nature of the patient encounters that a student must be involved in to achieve the learning outcomes that are targeted in any undergraduate program (Wimmers, Schmidt and Splinter, 2006). A clinical clerkship refers to the last stage in training before becoming a primary care practitioner. During this period, students rotate through different specialties and hospital settings, having the opportunity to be active participants in patient care under the supervision of specialized medical faculty. However, medical schools cannot rely merely on the clerkship stage to train students in essential clinical skills, these should be incorporated through the curriculum, using other experiences like standardized patients, clinical simulation or computer simulations to build on them(Remmen, Derese, Scherpbier, Denekens, Hermann, Van der Vleuten, Royen and Bossaert, 2002).

Evidence shows that the level of involvement and participation medical students get during their clinical years not only correlates with their satisfaction, but also with the ability to attain the adequate skills for further training (Kandiah, 2017). According to Byrne and Cohen (1973), the focus has been on balancing educational and service activities. However, the students' responsibilities on a program vary widely across departments, it can depend on the scope of training each program has declared and the operation it runs, the faculty's perception of the students' responsibility or the area of growth they observe is necessary for the fulfillment of requirements. As well as, the students' willingness to seek for further responsibilities, as it may give them a sense of growth, confidence, competitivity, and probably the opportunity to shine in the stakeholders ' eyes.

Based on the same principle and the necessity of standardizing learning experiences in different medical schools, the Association of American Medical Colleges (AAMC) (1999) issued a declaration of the required learning objectives for the medical curriculum However, there is no consensus among educational institutions on how to do an implementation of those objectives in a homogeneous program. Therefore, the focus and activities during the clinical years vary on domains of learning.

In medical school, students complete a 1-year internship in which they experience different clerkships in both public and private hospitals. The goal of this stage of the undergraduate program is to consolidate the theoretical and practical knowledge that trainees acquire throughout their years of preparation, keeping the patients' best interests at the center of care (Tapia, 2007). They have the responsibility of reviewing and updating medical chart data, going on medical rounds, carrying out minor procedures, and assisting in major ones, while simultaneously fulfilling their academic responsibilities.

In this demanding setting, medical students experience mistreatment at some point, whether it is by a faculty member or a fellow resident (Cook, 2015). Unfortunately, these practices have become enrooted in the learning environment to the extent that many consider them part of a hidden curriculum that builds resilience. But, in fact, what has been proven is that students who experience physical or psychological mistreatment, present higher rates of stress, depression, and even suicidal ideation (Haglund, 2009). Medical professionals are at the highest risk of suicide compared to the general population (Schernhammer, 2005). Dyrbye (2008) suggests that this problem is a consequence of burnout, high workload, lack of sleep, and competitiveness.

The objective of this chapter is:

- Describe the effects of burnout and well-being on medical students.
- Analyze the contribution of mentorship programs based on the six-pillar model for the development of well-being.
- Present the preliminary results of a study that assessed the effects of a mentorship program through the six-pillar model.

EFFECTS OF BURNOUT AND WELL-BEING

Burnout can be defined as a syndrome in the aftermath of severe stress and holding oneself to high ideals, leading to emotional exhaustion, depersonalization, and a decreased sense of personal accomplishment (McCray, 2008). The exhaustion influences negatively academic and professional accomplishments through the lack of warm, trust, tolerance, and dutifulness (Hojat, Vergare, Isenberg, Cohen, and Spandorfer, 2015). For Muñoz, Medina, Carrasco, Pérez, and Ortiz (2016) burnout could affect every professional in three dimensions: emotional exhaustion, depersonalization, and lack of personal fulfillment. It has been identified in undergraduate students derived from the academic and social demands that they face during this intense period of training (Pérez, Parra, Fasce, Ortiz, Bastías and Bustamante, 2012).

Physicians, and particularly those still in training such as residents and medical students, are susceptible to burnout due to the traditionally long hours spent at work, the vast amount of knowledge to master in a short time frame, and the challenges of achieving work-life balance. Emotional factors include the burden of caring for the sick, delivering bad news, and dealing with death. Other stress factors are of a more logistical nature and include working odd-schedules, managing an ever-increasing bureaucratic workload, and not receiving proper work recognition due to their low position on the medical hierarchy. An estimation has been made that about 25-60% of physicians show burnout, varying across different medical specialties (Gazelle, Liebschutz, and Riess, 2014). This is especially true in countries with vulnerable working conditions such as Mexico, where burnout is barely recognized as a distinct phenomenon even though it is estimated that about 75% of the working population suffer from it (Forbes, 2017).

Universities have the responsibility and compromise to respond to this rising problem that is having a worldwide negative impact on students affecting their psychological, social, and physical well-being. For Kemp, Hu, Bishop, Forrest, Hudson, Wilson, Teodorczuk, Rogers, Roberts, and Wearn (2019) the key aspects are designing curricula that progressively increases complexity, foster spaces to develop coping strategies among students, promote physical activity, and provide mental health promotion, and suicide prevention initiatives.

The conversation must be shifted from burnout to the importance of well-being on medical education. Well-being is the experience of health, happiness, and prosperity resulting in achieving a sense of meaning or purpose. It is composed of emotional, physical, social, and workplace elements (Davis, 2019). Other authors integrate the family, school and cultural setting to describe emotional and social health (Muñoz, Medina, Carrasco, Pérez and Ortiz, 2016). For Pérez, Parra, Fasce, Ortiz, Bastías, and Bustamante (2012) there is a direct relationship between the academic setting and the mental health of students and faculty members, as performance shapes attitude and self-esteem of participants. Gazelle, Liebschutz, and Riess (2014) describe that life-wellness is made of domains in which an individual must work to achieve fulfillment: physical, career, money, health, friends and family, romance, personal grown, and recreation.

The well-being of medical students can be described as an integration model of six-pillars that monitor and foster habits: mental, social, emotional, academic, nutritional, and physical health (figure 1).

Figure 1. Six-pillar model for well-being

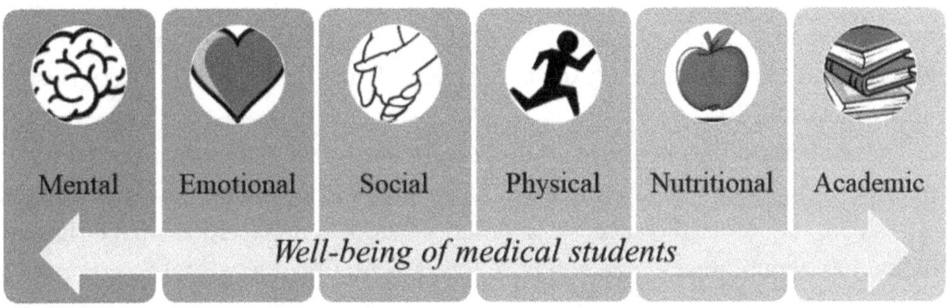

The mental pillar refers to the inner balance in which an individual is at peace with himself (Bughra, Till, and Sartorius, 2013). Consequently, the student is able to look after his basic and higher function needs. A student without the mental health pillar would feel frustrated, finished or with lack of motivation to pursue new challenges. Gazelle, Liebschutz, and Riess (2014) describe this as the personal growth domain. If it has not been achieved, students would present higher rates of stress, depression, and even suicidal ideation (Haglund, 2009). Suicide is a growing public health issue. According to the World Health Organization (2014), it is committed by more than 1 million people yearly, and in the past 45 years, this rate has skyrocketed by a staggering 60% (WHO, 2014). Medical professionals are one of the populations at highest risk of suicide and reports among medical students indicate that it is higher than age-matched population (Schernhammer, 2005). This problem could be traced back to medical school years, as a consequence of the burnout of high workload, lack of sleep, and competition to be the best (Dyrbye, 2008).

Although commonly included within mental health and sometimes even used interchangeably, the emotional pillar refers to understanding and respecting your own feelings, as well as acknowledging and respecting the feelings of others (Smith, 2014). By contrast, the lack of emotional health could produce burnout in students by being emotionally drained due to studying-related activities and by doing an extenuating effort to incorporate to early-morning activities after the exhaustion lived during an academic day (Pérez, Parra, Fasce, Ortiz, Bastías and Bustamante, 2012). According to Friederike (2017), there is a positive association between emotional well-being and academic achievement, and that is what learning communities try to nurture.

The social pillar consists of nourishing healthy relationships with the people around you and at the same time contributing to the growth of the community. It refers to the longitudinal relationships among students and between students and faculty, in a way that the students develop a deeper sense of learning and belonging (Tackket, 2018). Students should work on incorporating friends, family, and romance through a significant-other relationship (Gazelle, Liebschutz and Riess, 2014). A student without the social health pillar would not be able to understand how other people feel and would have a hard time dealing with problems, as well as laking the ability to work in teams in a relaxed atmosphere (Pérez, Parra, Fasce, Ortiz, Bastías and Bustamante, 2012).

The academic pillar encompasses the performance of the student in his educational endeavors. Academic achievement has been found to influence self-concept and self-esteem, therefore the success or failure in studies impacts the image that the student has about himself, and can have lower aspirational levels when comparing to other students (Muñoz, Medina, Carrasco, Pérez and Ortiz, 2016). The sense of being able to plan a career and achieve learning goals can contribute to improving the level of satisfaction (Gazelle, Liebschutz and Riess, 2014). Clinical and research activity, as well as other educational demands, need to be monitored to ensure optimal performance in this period.

The nutritional pillar refers to maintaining a balanced diet in order to bind every other pillar together by providing one's body with adequate-quality nutrition. Although it has been assumed that medical students have a greater knowledge about healthy lifestyle and dietary habits, there is no evidence that indicates this knowledge translates to maintaining good health (Rao, Darshan, Das, Rajan, Bhogun and Gupta, 2012). For instance, the emerging field of nutritional psychiatry has evidenced the fact that the quality of the diet is related to the risk of some mental disorders, such as depression (Jacka, 2017).

This, in turn, influences the physical pillar, which refers to caring for one's body to stay healthy. Physical activity is consistently related to higher levels of self-esteem and self-concept and lower levels of anxiety and stress. Physicians who are physically active are more likely to counsel patients about exercise and thus promote the well-being of the community (Dacey, 2014).

MENTORSHIP FOR THE DEVELOPMENT OF WELL-BEING

Support systems are being established to reach out to struggling students, but the efforts are scarce as there are no regulations or requirements from the government or educational regulation association to respond to these issues. An alternative that has been widely adopted is the implementation of a mentoring program (Jordon, 2005).

Mentoring originates from an ancient Greek word that could be translated as "enduring"; it refers to a myth that before entering a long voyage Odysseus trusted an old friend called Mentor, the training and guidance of his son Telemachus (Taherian and Shekarchian, 2009). This story exemplifies the heart of the definition of a mentor, the guidance of a counseling partner. Several definitions are widely on use, like the one on the Oxford dictionary that describes a mentor as an experienced person who advices and helps somebody less experienced over a period of time (Oxford Dictionaries, 2019). Sambunjak, Straus, and Marusic (2006) performed a systematic review of mentoring in medicine and identified more than 3,640 citations describing mentorship. There is an agreement that it is a catalyst of career success, advancement, and productivity because it influences personal development, career guidance, career choice, and research productivity (Straus, Chatur and Taylor, 2009).

Mentoring is defined as a reciprocal trust relationship between an experienced individual with a mentee, fostering adequate personal and professional development in which the young colleague gains experience through the professional life of the mentor. The target, facilitated by active listening, is to foster growth via self-questioning and examination of ideas and principles citation. Mentoring provides a protected space to work in the metacognitive elements of learning while facilitating productivity, career, and personal satisfaction for both mentees and mentors (Bhatia, 2013). Selection of mentors with adequate personality traits is vital for a program design that promotes space for reflection and introspection (McLaughlin, 2013).

Entering a medical career involves the assimilation of a vast amount of scientific content, by students who at a very young age decided to enter a high-performance program. This makes them particularly vulnerable to feel the stress or fatigue of integrating into such a demanding environment so that various coping or support mechanisms have been informally implemented to help them assimilate the transition. However, these efforts have been limited because they are individual, and due to the volume of work required, they can only provide care and support to a limited group of students (Aveiro, Castro, Martins, Costa, Castro, Veronese and Almedia, 2009).

These types of programs are based on learning theories as social participation in which the adoption of practices and the construction of identity in relation to the community to which they belong is described (Wenger, 2002). For Wenger, participation in these communities defines the ways in which individuals act, who they are, and how they interpret the meanings of events. He classifies this interaction into four components: meaning, practice, community, and identity, which are described in Figure 2. Meaning has to do with the interpretation they give to the experience of the world. The practice describes the historical background that provides a shared perspective of the daily exercise of his profession. The community describes the vision that the participation of its group is perceived as valuable within its social order. Identity is the past stories that define the group and personal learning that describes who are the members of the specific community.

Figure 2. Components of Wenger's (2002) social participation theory.

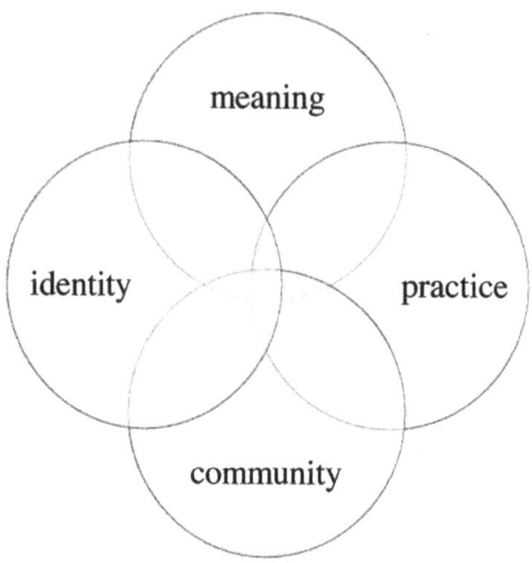

Mentoring started in the United States in the 1970s, where companies encouraged these programs to develop and support young staff entering a career in business. Since then, it has been widely used in different areas of business or militia, in which distinctions of terms are made between tutor, advisor, role model, and mentor, making the differentiation of these terms in relation to the economic remuneration received, the objective of the relationship and the context where it unfolds. A tutor has an academic character and develops in the academic context in order to achieve an educational objective. A counselor can support at a specific time to give recommendations that support the decision, even without knowing the particular context or case. A role model is just an example of how to conduct yourself positively in your discipline. A mentor includes an active role in personal and professional development while solving the balance between work and personal life (Frei, Stamm and Buddeberg-Fischer, 2010).

Informally, a mentor is described as a reliable and experienced counselor who has an interest in the development and education of another individual (Garmel, 2004). Mentoring is described more as a process than an end, in which two individuals intentionally relate the mentor and the apprentice for the promotion of growth and development. Being based on a relationship between people, with the passage of time and as the roles change between participants, the mentoring relationship evolves, is suspended or even terminated.

This relationship of power, in which the mentor has a higher level of knowledge or experience, seeks care and attention toward the apprentice, having a paternalistic and condescending approach, does not become one of professional competition. But, as the trainee acquires experience and approaches his mentor with similar job opportunities and access to research funds and prestige, they become colleagues and begin to compete for the same resources, possibly harming the relationship. It is in that sense that it is healthy for the apprentice to have multiple mentors in a given time, without this being interpreted as a mentor's failure (Garmel, 2004), each of them simply has a personal or academic quality that generates a bond specific with the apprentice. An apprentice can choose a mentor because of a specific quality, or he can observe his mentors and determine which qualities to model and absorb in from each one to start building their own professional and personal identity.

Program design varies amongst institutions, with some opting for student-selected mentors, whereas others have them pre-assigned. The format can also vary from approaches that consider one-on-one mentor relationship, to others that consider a group-based strategy (Fornari, 2014). The results have benefited organizations as they nurture healthier working environments that help physicians and students to thrive and feel more valued (Taherian & Shekarchian, 2008). Some of the benefits are the direct impact on reducing barriers for seeking help, they promote safe cultures, and implement and monitor policies to promote well-being (Kemp, Hu, Bishop, Forrest, Hudson, Wilson, Teodorczuk, Rogers, Roberts and Wearn, 2019).

Regarding the daily operation of the program, the logistics considered that every mentor, according to the clinical clerkship they were participating in, should provide support for eight students. Mentors received formal training to perform these duties. There were six mentors for each clerkship: pediatrics, internal medicine, obstetrics/gynecology, and surgery. The meetings occurred every two weeks throughout the students' clinical clerkships to discuss their academic progress and potential drawbacks. Initially, the students were followed longitudinally, with one assigned mentor that would guide them across different clerkships. However, when students changed department, the mentor had issues regarding matching schedules and did not felt confident enough to counsel and give academic advice on a different specialty department. Students perceived that a mentor with a stronger knowledge of the operations and management of the clinical rotation they were at the moment was more enriching for their learning experience and for their appreciation of the mentor-apprentice meetings, so they made a plea to return to the old model. The observations were analyzed and the previous model was re-established, providing again students with a mentor within their clerkship rotation.

The setting varied according to the mentor and participants, some approaches considered informal gatherings for lunch or dinner and others were more structured, booking regular meetings during office hours. A study was performed to understand the effects of the program through the perspective of the mentors that participated in the sessions. The described six-pillar model was used as a reference framework. A qualitative approach was used to explore and understand the effects of the mentorship program in a complex and holistic way (Maxwel, 2013).

The method used was a framework analysis because of its systematic and flexible approach to analyze data, as it identifies commonalities and differences focusing on relationships between different parts of the data (Gale et al., 2013). An analytical framework was developed based on the model of well-being. Semi-structured interviews were conducted with the mentors participating in the program.

This data was transcribed and contrasted with field notes from participant observation to enrich the understanding of social situations. Categories and codes were extracted through iteration between the members of the research team, obtaining 13 categories that associate to the well-being pillars, as presented in table 1. The sample consisted of seven mentors, two females and five males' physicians with a mean of 12 years of clinical experience and 8 years as medical educators. According to their medical specialties, there were three pediatricians, two gynecologists, one general surgeon, and one plastic surgeon.

Incidence on the impact of the program, as described by the interviewed mentors, was in the mental (85%), emotional (85%), social (100%) and academic (85%) pillars (table 2). Results indicate a direct impact on mental health, the extracts of the interviews evidence the identification of burnout and suicidal ideation cases.

The mentors explained that regarding the emotional pillars, students confessed severe stress and depression for not being able to fulfill the expectations of their supervisor and of the program. All of the professors reported that the mentorship program helped students in the social pillar. Mentions were about the strength in the learning community, fostered by faculty and students' interactions. Making evident the emphasis of the program on interpersonal interaction through scheduled meetings.

According to mentors, the academic pillar was developed through the interactions of students and professors. Finding an academic guide through clinical clerkships has proven to be an advantage to accompany them on gaining disciplinary skills.

Finally, the nutritional and physical health pillars were the least influenced by the program, mentors described that students often forgo a balanced diet and frequent exercise in favor of more study time or rest from their long working hours.

Table 2. Extracts of mentor interviews

Well-being Pillars	Categories	Extract From the Interview Transcription
Mental 85%	Red-flag cases	"There is a strong impact on the mental sphere, we have detected several red flags on 5th year students and risky situations that could lead to a problem within a group of students.
	Detect and refer	"If it had not been for the mentorship program, we (the faculty) would not have noticed these cases. We would not be able to intervene and refer them to the appropriate services"
	Systematic detection	"A lot of students were on, or above average mental health risk. Implementing mentorship through a system helped to detect particular suicidal ideation cases and reach out to them in time."
Emotional 85%	Stress	"We have had cases in which the students have confessed that they are very stressed out regarding the clinical clerkship year and that they are depressed because of it"
	Coping strategies	"Students do not feel they are able to deal with their clinical clerkships"
Social 100%	Community	"A social network between students and professors has been created"
	Identity	"…there is a strong bond between the different participants of the mentorship program"
Physical 28%	Self-care	"... the framework we have created allows students to focus not only on the academic aspects of education but also allows them to be more cautious and self-conscious about their physical well-being."
	Physical activity	"The implementation of active sessions such as the Challenge allows integration of professors and students through physical activity"
Nutritional 0%		*It was not mentioned directly in any of the interviews.
Academic 85%	Guidance	"As tutors, we stand by their side through the whole process so that they can reach their full academic potential"
	Tutor	"Students are becoming closer with professors and finding within them academic tutors, especially when it comes to their clinical clerkships"

This implementation contributes to designing an effective program that fosters the student's self-assessment and allows them to develop coping strategies. A systematic follow-up tool is needed to document the effects of the program, gathering real-time information to act accordingly. Although initially developed for medical students, this program can also be beneficial for residents' mentorship. It is also a valuable program that contributes to identifying red-flag cases regarding mental health issues and low academic performances. A limitation of this study was that the implementation included student engagement and adherence to the program and meeting schedule. Its success is based on the quality time shared between participants.

CONCLUSION

To work in an environment where the patient is the center implies high demands for professional performance. Students need to gain experience in a safe environment that fosters formal and academic training. It is in this sense that the role of teachers and training institutions dedicated to medical education needs to produce spaces for mentoring that support the teaching-learning process, as well as the holistic development as individuals and professionals integrated into a health system.

In these reflection processes all actors, students or teachers, benefit. Mentors have the possibility of visualizing their work in a different dimension that includes increasing their professional satisfaction by being of service for someone else, increasing their participation in the organization, and by their involvement in the educational process (Jordon, 2005).

Documenting the mentorship program contributes to the student process of self-assessment and helps the medical school to identify critical points of struggle during each specific clerkship, allowing them to respond accordingly. An important question to answer is the extent of responsibility the universities and mentors have on the detection and follow-up of these situations. However, this proximity between faculty and students reduces considerable barriers to seeking help.

Focusing on physician and student well-being is a responsibility that must be taken seriously, as the quality of care depends on it. There is a wide variety of approaches that can be implemented to monitor and improve it. Any organization would benefit from applying programs based on this six-pillar model, however a personalized approach would target specific short-comings in any setting. Special interest must be granted to self-reflection and supportive safe-environments for personal improvement.

Interprofessional settings prepare medicine and health practitioners that would provide patient care in a collaborative environment; however, little has been studied about how these settings can favor a culture of self-care and health spread within a community. Professionals, and particularly those still in training are susceptible to burnout due to the traditionally long hours spent at work. This has proven to be a red flag, as those professionals are the ones responsible for the well-being of others. By embracing wellness habits and healthy lifestyles, as well as recognizing the lack of it, could have a positive impact on health professionals that could also be translated to better patient care.

ACKNOWLEDGMENT

We would like to recognize the hard work of all the community involved in implementing the Mentorship program of Sociedades Académicas in the school, the deans, the coordinators, and leaders that have made this program have a positive impact on the life of students. Particularly the work of the mentors that have helped build the learning communities by voluntarily dedicating their time to foster a safer environment for students, residents, and staff to interact, and grow.

REFERENCES

AAMC. (1999). Learning objectives for medical student education–guidelines for medical schools. *Academic Medicine*, *74*(1), 13–18. doi:10.1097/00001888-199901000-00010 PMID:9934288

Aveiro, M. F., Castro, M., Martins, C., Costa, A. D., Castro, J. F., Veronese, M. L., & Almedia, L. E. (2009). Group mentoring for junior Medical students: Perceptions of mentees and mentors. *Revista Brasileira de Educação Médica*, *33*(4), 670–675. doi:10.1590/S0100-55022009000400019

Bhatia, A., Singh, N., & Dhaliwal, U. (2013). Mentoring for first year medical students: Humanising medical education. *Indian Journal of Medical Ethics*, (2). Advance online publication. doi:10.20529/IJME.2013.030 PMID:23697488

Bhugra, D., Till, A., & Sartorius, N. (2013). What is mental health? *The International Journal of Social Psychiatry*, *59*(1), 3–4. doi:10.1177/0020764012463315 PMID:23349505

Byrne, N., & Cohen, R. (1973). Observational study of clinical clerkship activities. *Academic Medicine*, *48*(10), 919–927. doi:10.1097/00001888-197310000-00005 PMID:4728311

Cook, A. F., Arora, V. M., Rasinski, K. A., Curlin, F. A., & Yoon, J. D. (2014). The Prevalence of Medical Student Mistreatment and Its Association with Burnout. *Academic Medicine*, *89*(5), 749–754. doi:10.1097/ACM.0000000000000204 PMID:24667503

Dacey, M., Kennedy, M., Polak, R., & Phillips, E. (2014). Physical activity counseling in medical school education: A systematic review. *Medical Education Online*, *19*(1), 24325. doi:10.3402/meo.v19.24325 PMID:25062944

Dyrbye, L. N., Thomas, M. R., Massie, F. S., Power, D. V., Eacker, A., Harper, W., Durning, S., Moutier, C., Szydlo, D. W., Novotny, P. J., Sloan, J. A., & Shanafelt, T. D. (2008). Burnout and Suicidal Ideation among U.S. Medical Students. *Annals of Internal Medicine, 149*(5), 334. doi:10.7326/0003-4819-149-5-200809020-00008 PMID:18765703

Forbes. (2017). Mexicanos, los más estresados del mundo por su trabajo. *Forbes México*. Retrieved from https://www.forbes.com.mx/mexicanos-los-mas-estresados-del-mundo-por-su-trabajo/

Fornari, A., Murray, T., Menzin, A., Woo, V., Clifton, M., Lombardi, M., & Shelov, S. (2014). Mentoring program design and implementation in new medical schools. *Medical Education Online, 19*(1), 24570. doi:10.3402/meo.v19.24570 PMID:24962112

Frei, E., Stamm, M., & Buddeberg-Fischer, B. (2010). Mentoring programs for medical students – a review of the PubMed literature 2000 – 2008. *BMC Medical Education, 10*(32), 1–14. PMID:20433727

Friederike-Grabel, B. (2017). *The relationship between wellbeing and academic achievement A systematic review* (Master's thesis).

Gale, N. K., Heath, G., Cameron, E., Rashid, S., & Redwood, S. (2013). Using the framework method for the analysis of qualitative data in multi-disciplinary health research. *BMC Medical Research Methodology, 13*(1), 117. Advance online publication. doi:10.1186/1471-2288-13-117 PMID:24047204

Garmel, G. M. (2004). Mentoring Medical Students in Academic Emergency Medicine. *Academic Emergency Medicine, 11*(12), 1351–1357. doi:10.1197/j.aem.2004.06.013 PMID:15576528

Gazelle, G., Liebschutz, J., & Riess, H. (2014). Physician Burnout. Coaching a Way Out. *Journal of General Internal Medicine, 30*(4), 508–513. doi:10.100711606-014-3144-y PMID:25527340

Genn, J. M. (2001). AMEE Medical Education Guide No. 23 (Part 2): Curriculum, environment, climate, quality and change in medical education – a unifying perspective. *Medical Teacher, 23*(5), 445–454. PMID:12098364

Haglund, M. E. M., aan het Rot, M., Cooper, N. S., Nestadt, P. S., Muller, D., Southwick, S. M., & Charney, D. S. (2009). Resilience in the Third Year of Medical School: A Prospective Study of the Associations Between Stressful Events Occurring During Clinical Rotations and Student Well-Being. *Academic Medicine, 84*(2), 258–268. doi:10.1097/ACM.0b013e31819381b1 PMID:19174682

Hojat, M., Vergare, M., Isenberg, G., Cohen, M., & Spandorfer, J. (2015). Underlying construct of empathy, optimism, and burnout in medical students. *International Journal of Medical Education*, *6*, 12–16. doi:10.5116/ijme.54c3.60cd PMID:25633650

Jacka, F. (2017). Nutritional Psychiatry: Where to Next? *EBioMedicine*, *17*, 24–29. doi:10.1016/j.ebiom.2017.02.020 PMID:28242200

Jordon, J. (2005). *Mentorship and Preceptorship. Teaching Learners in Clinical Practice*. School of Health Studies.

Kandiah, D. (2017). Perception of educational value in clinical rotations by medical students. *Advances in Medical Education and Practice*, *8*, 149–162. doi:10.2147/AMEP.S129183 PMID:28223855

Kemp, S., Hu, W., Bishop, J., Forrest, K., Hudson, J. N., Wilson, I., Teodorczuk, A., Rogers, G. D., & Wearn, A. (2019). Medical student wellbeing – a consensus statement from Australia and New Zealand. *BMC Medical Education*, *69*(19). Advance online publication. doi:10.118612909-019-1505-2 PMID:30832630

López, M.V., & Valdez-García, J.E. (2019). Virtual reality in residents training. *Annals of Eye Science*. doi:10.21037/aes.2019.08.01

Maxwell, J. (2013). *Qualitative research design*. SAGE Publications.

McCray. (2008). Resident physician burnout: Is there hope? *Family Medicine*, *40*(9), 626–632. https://www.ncbi.nlm.nih.gov/pubmed/18830837 PMID:18830837

McLaughlin, K., Veale, P., McIlwrick, J., de Groot, J., & Wright, B. (2013). A practical approach to mentoring students with repeated performance deficiencies. *BMC Medical Education*, *13*(1), 56. Advance online publication. doi:10.1186/1472-6920-13-56 PMID:23597111

Muñoz, F., Medina, A., Carrasco, D., Pérez, C., & Ortiz, L. (2016). Burnout en estudiantes de Odontología y su relación con sus características sociodemográficas y antecedentes académicos. *Educación Médica Superior*, *30*(2). http://www.ems.sld.cu/index.php/ems/article/view/762/375

Olivares, S. L., & Valdez, J. E. (2017). *Aprendizaje Centrado en el Paciente*. Editorial Médica Panamericana.

Oxford Dictionary. (2019). *Definition of mentor noun*. Retrieved from: https://www.oxfordlearnersdictionaries.com/us/definition/english/mentor?q=mentor

Pérez, C., Parra, P., Fasce, E., Ortiz, L., Bastías, N., & Bustamante, C. (2012). Estructura factorial y confiabilidad del inventario de burnout de Maslach en universitarios chilenos. *Revista Argentina de Clínica Psicológica*, *21*(3), 255–263.

Rao, C., Darshan, B., Das, N., Rajan, V., Bhogun, M., & Gupta, A. (2012). Practice of Physical Activity among Future Doctors: A Cross Sectional Analysis. *International Journal of Preventive Medicine*, *3*(5), 365–369. PMID:22708033

Remmen, R., Derese, A., Scherpbier, A., Denekens, J., Hermann, I., Van der Vleuten, C., Royen, P. V., & Bossaert, L. (2002). Can medical schools rely on clerkships to train students in basic clinical skills? *Medical Education*, *33*(8), 600–605. Advance online publication. doi:10.1046/j.1365-2923.1999.00467.x PMID:10447847

Sambunjak, D., Straus, S. E., & Marusic, A. (2006). Mentoring in Academic Medicine A Systematic Review. *Journal of the American Medical Association*, *296*(9), 1103–1115. doi:10.1001/jama.296.9.1103 PMID:16954490

Schernhammer, E. (2005). Taking Their Own Lives — The High Rate of Physician Suicide. *The New England Journal of Medicine*, *352*(24), 2473–2476. doi:10.1056/NEJMp058014 PMID:15958803

Smith, S., Shochet, R., Keeley, M., Fleming, A., & Moynahan, K. (2014). The Growth of Learning Communities in Undergraduate Medical Education. *Academic Medicine*, *89*(6), 928–933. doi:10.1097/ACM.0000000000000239 PMID:24871245

Straus, S., Chatur, F., & Taylor, M. (2009). Issures in the Mentor-Mentee relationship in academic medicine: A qualitative study. *Academic Medicine*, *84*(1), 135–139. doi:10.1097/ACM.0b013e31819301ab PMID:19116493

Tackett, S., Wright, S., Colbert-Getz, J., & Shochet, R. (2018). Associations between learning community engagement and burnout, quality of life, and empathy among medical students. *International Journal of Medical Education*, *9*(1), 316–322. doi:10.5116/ijme.5bef.e834 PMID:30504524

Taherian, K., & Shekarchian, M. (2008). Mentoring for doctors. Do its benefits outweigh its disadvantages? *Medical Teacher*, *30*(4), e95–e99. doi:10.1080/01421590801929968 PMID:18569651

Valdez-García, J. E. (2004). Brevísima Historia de la Educación Médica. *Avances*, *1*(3), 37–38.

Valdez-García, J. E., & Uscanga, V. M. (2006). Nuevos campos clínicos en la educación médica: Análisis comparativo campos clínicos hospitalario y ambulatorio. *Avances*, *9*, 33–40.

Villanueva, T., Núñez Tapia, R. M, Syr Salas Perea, R., & Rodríguez-Orozco, A. R. (2007). The undergraduate medical internship and the clinical competences: Mexico in the Latin American context. *Educación Médica Superior, 21*(4). Retrieved from http://scielo.sld.cu/scielo.php?script=sci_arttext&pid=S0864-21412007000400005&lng=es&tlng=en

Wenger, E. (2002). *Comunidades de práctica.* Paidós.

Wimmers, P., Schmidt, H., & Splinter, T. A. (2006). Influence of clerkship experiences on clinical competence. *Medical Education, 40*(5), 450–458. Advance online publication. doi:10.1111/j.1365-2929.2006.02447.x PMID:16635125

World Health Organization. (2019). *Preventing suicide: A global perspective.* Retrieved from https://apps.who.int/iris/bitstream/handle/10665/131056/9789241564878_eng.pdf;jsessionid=0E95072A30E5F3DF4DB15AE4CEA79C33?sequence=8

ADDITIONAL READING

Cordero Díaz, M. A., Félix Arce, C., & Dávila Rivas, J. A. (2016). Promoting an Optimal Clinical Learning Environment for Residency Education and Patient Care (presented at ICRE 2016 Niagara Falls). *Investigación en Educación Médica, 6*(22), 135–136. doi:10.1016/j.riem.2017.01.136

Gómez, P., Pérez, C., Parra, P., Ortiz, L., Matus, O., McColl, P., Torres, G., & Meyer, A. (2015). Relación entre el bienestar y el rendimiento académico en alumnos de primer año de medicina. *Revista Medica de Chile, 143*(7), 930–937. doi:10.4067/S0034-98872015000700015 PMID:26361031

Hammick, M., Olckers, L., & Campion-Smith, C. (2009). Learning in interprofessional teams: AMEE Guide no 38. *Medical Teacher, 31*(1), 1–12. doi:10.1080/01421590802585561 PMID:19253148

Harden, R. M. (2009). Stress, pressure and burnout in teachers: Is the swan exhausted? *Medical Teacher, 21*(3), 245–247. doi:10.1080/01421599979482

Sandars, J. (2009). The use of reflection in medical students: AMEE Guide No. 44. *Medical Teacher, 31*(8), 685–695. doi:10.1080/01421590903050374 PMID:19811204

Sandars, J., Patel, R., Steele, H., & McAreavey, M. (2014). Developmental student support in undergraduate medical education: AMEE Guide No. 92. *Medical Teacher, 36*(12), 1015–1026. doi:10.3109/0142159X.2014.917166 PMID:25072412

Taherian, K., & Shekarchian, M. (2008). Mentoring for doctors. Do its benefits outweigh its disadvantages? *Medical Teacher*, *30*(4), 1015–1026. doi:10.1080/01421590801929968 PMID:18569651

KEY TERMS AND DEFINITIONS

Academic Pillar: It encompasses the performance of the student in his or her educational endeavors. It could also integrate the long-career goal planning.

Clinical Clerkship: Is the last stage in training that a medical student has to become a primary care practitioner. During this period, students rotate through different specialty and hospital settings, allowing them to be active participants in patient care, under the supervision of medical specialists.

Emotional Health: Is understanding and embracing the individual emotions and feelings, acknowledging and validating the feelings of others, and regulating them in a respectful understanding.

Mental Health: Is the state of peace where an individual finds inner balance between the problematical situations that challenge daily life, and the coping mechanisms to overcome them.

Mentorship: Is a reciprocal trust relationship between an experienced individual with a mentee, fostering adequate personal and professional development in which the young colleague gains experience through the professional life of the mentor.

Nutritional Health: It refers to maintaining a balanced diet in order to bind every other pillar together by providing one's body with adequate-quality nutrition.

Physical Health: It refers to caring for one's body to stay healthy. Physical activity is consistently related to higher levels of self-esteem and self-concept and lower levels of anxiety and stress.

Social Health: Refers to nourishing healthy and harmonious relationships with the people around an individual and contributing to the growth of the community to which he belongs.

Well-Being: Is the state of being that integrates healthy lifestyle, self-awareness and fullness of living in an individual.

Chapter 13
Interprofessional Education: A Perspective From India

Izhar Faisal
https://orcid.org/0000-0003-3761-6303
Medeor Hospital, India

Saima Salam
https://orcid.org/0000-0003-3139-8771
Lal Ded Hospital-Government Medical College, Srinagar, India

Manisha Arora
Delhi Pain Management Centre, India

ABSTRACT

With an ever worsening shortage of healthcare workers, there has been a global shift towards strengthening of interprofessional education (IPE). IPE has existed as a powerful tool in developed countries, but in developing countries like India, it is still in its infancy. Several models of interprofessional education exist, yet India lags behind in implementing these models in academic curricula. Rudimentary curriculum, inefficient healthcare system, and maldistribution of health professionals are some of the potential barriers. A complete overhaul of the healthcare system along with progressive strategies of incorporation of IPE needs to be debated, and associated limitations need to be addressed. Adequate institutional support, well-constructed protocols, infrastructural revamp, and change of workplace culture are vital for IPE to succeed and be sustainable. This chapter provides an overview of IPE and collaborative practice in Indian settings and presents an account of an Indian institution utilizing IPP approach and highlights potential challenges in incorporating IPE in the academic curriculum.

DOI: 10.4018/978-1-7998-3066-5.ch013

"Interprofessional education is a necessary step in preparing a collaborative practice-ready health workforce that is better prepared to respond to local health needs" (WHO, 2010)

INTRODUCTION

Interprofessional Education (IPE) is not a recent concept; it has existed as a powerful tool in developed countries for past several years. Early initiative dates back to 1940s in USA, 1960s in Canada, 1970s in Sweden and Australia (Nisbet, Lee, Kumar, Thistlethwaite, & Dunston, 2011) and 1980s in United Kingdom (Barr, 2014) . The World Health Organization (WHO) reports, "Continuing Education for Physicians" (World Health Organization [WHO], 1973) and "Learning together to work together for health" (WHO, 1988) in late 1980s were the main driving force for popularity of IPE. The 59th World Health Assembly (WHA) recognized that shortages of the health workers are interfering with efforts to achieve the internationally agreed health related development goals (WHO, 2006). It urges member states to use innovative approaches to teaching with state of the art teaching materials and continuing education through the innovative use of information and technology (WHO, 2006).

With the ever-worsening shortage of health care workers globally, a constant rise of ageing population and increasing incidence of chronic and complex conditions as well as professional silos, wherein health professions are educated and practice separately, the change of vision and strategy for education of health care professionals has become imperative. A thorough understanding of roles and responsibilities of each health profession and collaborative practice is need of the hour.

According to Centre for the Advancement of Interprofessional Education (CAIPE), the aim of interprofessional education is to improve patient care through an interactive learning process wherein two or more professionals learn with, from and about each other to improve collaboration and the quality of care (Centre for the Advancement of Interprofessional Education [CAIPE], 2002).

WHO has been a supporter of Interprofessional Education for Collaborative Practice (IPECP) and to facilitate implementation; it came up with recommendations and framework for Action (WHO, 2010) for interprofessional education. With regards to IPE, it states that 'Health professional's education and training institutions should consider implementing interprofessional education in both undergraduate and postgraduate programmes' while recognizing that the quality of the evidence supporting this recommendation is low, and the strength of the recommendation is conditional (WHO, 2013).

The past decade or so has seen global shift towards strengthening of IPE, however in developing countries like India it's still in nascent stages. At present, India lags behind developed countries in implementation of IPE, therefore, there is a dire need to support interprofessional education within the Indian academic curriculum. Academic programmes must be tailored to train students, both academically and experientially, in concepts and practices of IPE so that a workforce is created that can educate and train other educators, practicing professionals and future practitioners in this field.

Interprofessional Education

Evidences suggested that fragmentation, compartmentalization and poor interprofessional communication resulted in underutilization of talent of healthcare professionals as well as wastage of human resources. Therefore, education within healthcare system began to undergo a major transformation with main focus on implementation of interprofessional education. WHO envisioned worldwide improvement in quality and effectiveness of healthcare by an educational system that promotes Interprofessional Learning (IPL) with those outside their disciplines.

As per WHO, the main aim of interprofessional education is to "prepare all health profession students for deliberately working together with the common goal of building a safer and better health care system" (Interprofessional Education Collaborative Expert Panel, 2011).

Interprofessional education occurs when participants from two or more professions in health care and social care (such as medical, dental, nursing, physiotherapy, psychology, psychotherapy or allied health sciences) learn about, from and with each other during entire or part of their professional training with the intent of cultivating collaborative practice for providing better patient-centered healthcare (CAIPE, 1997; Barr, Koppel, Reeves, Hammick, & Freeth, 2005; Craddock, O'Halloran, Borthwick, & McPherson, 2006).

IPE act as a platform of coordinated care thereby reinforcing a team based approach towards collaborative practice.

Why Interprofessional Education

With the establishment of corporate-health culture, team-based and collaborative approach to health care is becoming a norm. Although healthcare team is supposed to work as a single unit, blame game for patient's problems and unfavorable health outcomes is not an uncommon site. Modern health care delivery system requires ability to work in a team, yet we never sensitize healthcare providers about the essence of team work.

The evidences suggest that failure to learn and work as healthcare team is resulting in poor patient-related outcomes. Also, reports attributed 70% of avoidable patient-related adverse events to 'compartmentalized and fragmented' approach of patient care (Kohn, Corrigan, & Donaldson, 2000), thus emphasizing that coherent and collaborative approach to learn and work is essential in present scenario. Further, it is assumed that interprofessional learning facilitates professional progress and improved patient services thereby improving clinical outcome and quality of patient care (Reeves et al., 2016).

Health care is not only limited at focusing disease alone, rather it encompasses to deal with aspects like mental, social, behavioral and psychological health too. Apart from dealing with disease alone one has to deal with stresses of daily life. Trend is to provide overall quality care to patient. Collaborative practice can decrease patient complications, errors in patient management, duration of hospital stay and overall morbidity and mortality. In the long run these practices of collaborative learning will benefit individuals as they would be under care of a rehabilitation team rather than one health professional so as to provide comprehensive care.

Comprehensively planned and meticulously introduced and conducted Interprofessional Program (IPP) can not only augment flexible, compatible, patient centered and cost-effective synergism in interprofessional teams but also acknowledges prerequisite of each profession in the team and safeguarding profession-specific identity (Barr, Gray, Helme, Low, & Reeves, 2016). The resultant collaborative practice and interprofessional care is expected to be a symbolic intervention to provide efficient, cost-effective and quality healthcare (Frenk et al., 2010; Baker, Gustafson, Beaubien, Salas, & Barach, 2003; Nelson et al., 2014).

Key Considerations for IPE

Since its inception, IPE has been a topic of debate. To some, it was a tool to resolve interprofessional misunderstanding and tensions (Hall, 2005). To others, it was a method of improving teamwork or reforming professional education (Interprofessional Education Collaborative Expert Panel, 2011). While some opined that occasional IPE presentation were sufficient to produce and sustain a collaborative workforce, yet others insisted that IPE could be productive only if its thoroughly imbedded in the healthcare profession curriculum (Blue, Mitcham, Smith, Raymond, & Greenberg, 2010; Cook, 2005; Solomon, 2011). Some argued that IPE must be introduced before pre-licensure studies, while others vouched for a more delayed exposure (Charles, Bainbridge, & Gilbert, 2010; Ho et al., 2008; Langton, 2009).

Although there is consensus regarding effectiveness of IPE but the means to achieve are not very clear within the professionals. One should realize that interprofessional education and collaborative learning are not a goal but a means to achieve better healthcare for individuals and community. Therefore, no one model can fit in all the clinical situations and needs individualization according to local needs.

Figure 1. Key considerations for interprofessional education
(Adapted from the WHO Framework for Action on Interprofessional Education and Collaborative Practice)

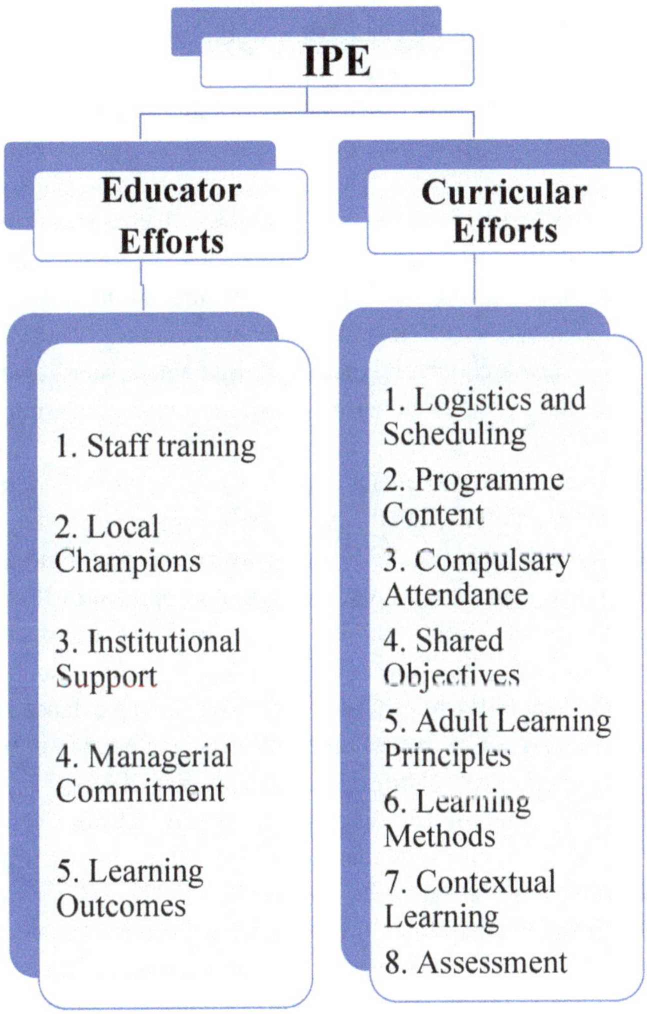
IPE
Educator Efforts
Curricular Efforts
1. Staff training
2. Local Champions
3. Institutional Support
4. Managerial Commitment
5. Learning Outcomes
1. Logistics and Scheduling
2. Programme Content
3. Compulsary Attendance
4. Shared Objectives
5. Adult Learning Principles
6. Learning Methods
7. Contextual Learning
8. Assessment

The successful implementations of IPE require educator as well as curricular efforts. Educators consist of the team involved in developing, teaching and managing IPE. All staff involved in teaching, developing and managing IPE requires a shared vision and good understanding of the benefits of IPL (WHO, 2010). A major change in workplace culture is required with implementation of shared communication, decision making and conflict resolution. Local champions with ability to undertake cross-disciplinary collaboration activities, identifying barriers to progress and capacity to effectively guide the institutional directions towards IPE need to come forth (WHO, 2010). The effectiveness of any program depends on team leader who may not necessarily be a doctor and should be dictated by context in which team operates. The leader should promote communication and cooperation between groups. The objectives should include team work, understanding one's role and responsibilities in team dynamics and concept of ethical practice.

One of the important aspects for encouraging future interest and development of IPE is that the initial experiences of staff as well as students remain positive (WHO, 2010).

The primary aim of IPE is to create a workforce that can work in synergy to meet heath needs of population effectively. To achieve this goal a definite change in workplace culture and institutional support structure is imperative. The institute should provide adequate space, infrastructure and funding. The institute might need to incorporate few architectural (activity-based workspaces) changes and few facilities like simulation clinics or virtual spaces to enhance learning experience (WHO, 2010).

Curricular efforts towards IPE include developing a flexible schedule and making attendance mandatory (WHO, 2010). Although a logistical challenge towards a shared curriculum is a major concern, well-constructed problem-based learning aided with real-world experiences are a must for development of IPE.

The interprofessional fellowship programme should be introduced in various academic institutes having multiple specialties to empower nation's health. The content of the course should be relevant and attractive. Having balanced membership in the team is essential for its success providing avenue for acquiring maximum knowledge and skills (Dargahi, Shirazi, & Yazdanparast, 2012).

Various methodologies of IPE like patient-driven didactic lectures, journal clubs, clinical case simulations, telemedicine, and community/family visit based experiential learning exist and are becoming popular in US undergraduate medical education (UME) (Interprofessional Education Collaborative Expert Panel, 2011; Coggeshall, 1966).

The IPE approach will help in assimilation of knowledge, attitude and skills of healthcare providers as well as development of teams of future healthcare workers who will work together in a respectful manner and with a positive attitude to provide better healthcare services to the patients and the community.

Benefits of Interprofessional Learning

Table 1. Benefits of Interprofessional Learning

Educational Benefits	Health Policy Benefits
1. Students will work in practical and realistic conditions and will encounter real world experiences. 2. Faculty from distinct professions will contribute to development and implementation of the program thereby bringing in diverse range of experience. 3. Will reinforce mutual respect and trust among professionals involved. 4. Will provide opportunities to develop competent skills to work as a team and acquire leadership qualities. 5. Will provide better insight about professional roles. 6. Enhanced communication and negotiation skills and professionalism. 7. Students will have better understanding of skills and modalities of other professional streams.	1. Better utilization of the resources. 2. Improved workplace based practices. 3. Improved patient/client-centered care and quality enhancement. 4. Improved clinical and patient outcomes. 5. Improved morale, self confidence and self-esteem. 6. Collaborative and team based work culture leading to enhanced patient safety. 7. Cost-effective health care. 8. Better access to health-care facilities. 9. Improved emergency patient care and disaster management.

Interprofessional Education in Indian Context

With changing healthcare trends globally, there is a dire need of interprofessional education especially in developing countries like India. Although models and tools for IPE exist, they have not been implemented widely.

India has a huge medical education system with broad network of institutions that produces a large number of doctors, nurses, pharmacist and allied health professionals every year. The concept of IPE is highly relevant in current context of healthcare situation in India to work for patient centered care. Interprofessional practice (IPP) is increasingly being implemented in several specialties in India such as dentistry, pediatrics and primary health care settings. There is growing need of such programmes as developing countries lack in providing basic health needs and there is shift of paradigm of increasing prevalence of number of chronic illnesses and multifactorial diseases. There exist various inefficiencies in health system (largely privatized health care, inadequate public service and differences in payment mechanism) and geographic maldistribution of health care providers make healthcare inaccessible to a large proportion of rural and disadvantaged communities (Balasubramanian, Short, & Gallagher, 2018).

Developmental-Behavioral Pediatrics (DBP)

Developmental-behavioral pediatrics (DBP), an emerging subspecialty in India has utilized and implemented the concept of IPE to provide services to children suffering from neurodevelopmental disorders.

DBP emerged as a subspecialty in well-established department of pediatric neurology of Lokmanya Tilak Municipal General Hospital (LTMGH), Mumbai, India more than 2 decades ago. The service driven, clinical care model was started with the aim to diagnose and treat children with neurological diseases and developmental disorders. Initial model was based on the concept of single physician provider with referrals to other specialties (psychology, social work, etc.) as and when required, however fragmented care, non-adherence to follow-up and intercommunication failure between various specialties resulted in falling through of this model and an indispensable need of a trained interprofessional team was realized. In 1995, recognition and approval by the state government for assessment and certification of children with specific learning disabilities led to integration of independent practice model into the dedicated "Learning Disability" centre. Concurrently, the awareness about need to support children with developmental disorders in the educational setting became popular among policy makers, law-makers and in public domain as well.

With recognition of DBP as a subspecialty, need for the expansion of armamentarium beyond assessments of learning disorders to other neurodevelopmental disorders like autism, spectrum disorders, attention issues, language disorders, intellectual disabilities and other behavioral issues was realized. As most of these disorders require multidisciplinary approach, the essence of IPE was further recognized.

Over the years centre evolved from diagnostic-only center to multimodal center with facilities like career planning, remediation, and behavioral and counselling strategies. As of today, the centre serves as a regional model of IPE and includes developmental pediatricians, psychiatrists, clinical psychologists, special educators, speech-language pathologists, and occupational therapists who work cordially to provide comprehensive patient care.

With the success of DBP model of Lokmanya Tilak Municipal Medical College (LTMMC), need to train young pediatricians in this emerging specialty was felt and moving forward in the direction, an approval for a state-university affiliated fellowship programme in developmental pediatrics was obtained in year 2013. The curriculum was based on US post-graduate fellowships model in DBP. The model emphasized on components of IPE, viz. defined responsibility and shared decision-making. It also marked a change of practice from traditional patient-physician archetype to a more holistic approach. However, the lack of trained educators was realized soon and the process led to the international collaboration and DBP education via videoconferencing was started (Soares, Gajre, & Manglani, 2016). This internationally collaborated educational videoconferencing model included biweekly sessions over the period of two years, with focus on case-based training of team members by their international counterparts, mentoring trainees on research projects and refined development of the fellowship programme. Successful outcomes of the videoconferencing modality included contentment of Indian participants in interacting with subject specialists, greater reliance in their ability to diagnose and manage neurodevelopmental disorders, access to regular updates and new guidelines, presentations at international conferences and publications in reputed journals. Also, their counterparts attained a better understanding of international IPE and cultural aspects of DBP care in India.

At the Pediatric Neurodevelopmental (PND) Center, LTMMC, apart from case-based discussions and video-conferencing, exposure of subspecialty fellows and pediatric residents to collaborative case discussions and immersive learning as well as working with different professionals help trainees acquire IPE skills and learn a systematic collaborative approach (Kelly, 2013) .

Developmental Paediatrics Clinic, LMTGH

The Developmental Paediatrics Clinic at Lokmanya Tilak Municipal General Hospital (LMTGH), Mumbai, India caters to children with chronic neurological problems such as neurodegenerative, neurometabolic, neuromuscular and neurodevelopmental disorders. A multidisciplinary team comprising of a pediatric neurologist, developmental pediatrician, pediatric occupational and physiotherapist, pediatric orthopedician, social worker and rehabilitation consultant work together for comprehensive evaluation including genetic diagnosis, prenatal diagnosis, counseling and therapeutic interventions. The centre acts as a referral hospital for expert opinion and thorough evaluation of these patients. Apart from evaluation and interventions, parent education programme is conducted every year wherein parents and children are educated regarding normal developmental milestones with an aim to detect developmental delay at the earliest.

Autism Intervention Centre

Autism Intervention Centre was started in urban health centre, Dharavi, in collaboration with Hi media laboratories in the year 2016.

The centre was started in joint collaboration with the Department of Occupational Therapy and Psychiatry, Lokmanya Tilak Municipal Medical College (LTMMC) and Lokmanya Tilak Municipal General Hospital (LTMGH). This centre has dedicated, experienced and professionals inter-disciplinary team to provide comprehensive care to children with autism. This centre offers comprehensive care to these children i.e. diagnosis, evaluation, therapy and certification. The services include Developmental paediatrician evaluation, Psychiatric evaluation, Occupational therapy (Sensory Integration), Speech and language therapy, Behavioural therapy, Special education, Parental counselling and support groups and workshops for parents and professionals.

Interprofessional Education and Its Implications for Dentistry in India

Indian dental education system is the largest dental education system in the world with over 300 institutions producing approx 25,000 dental graduates per year. India also has an exceptionally competent medical education system which actively produces a large number of physicians, nurses, pharmacists, and allied health professionals. Yet educational silos leading to practice silos are evident when these young graduates enter the real world.

Although oral health models, focused at improving cooperation amongst various members of dental team viz. dentists, dental hygienists, dental therapists, dental technicians, and dental assistants as well as other healthcare professionals such as medical, nursing, pharmacy, and allied health exist in developed nations, it's a distant dream for dental education system of India.

Various inefficiencies in Indian dental health system like inadequate provision of public health care, privatized healthcare sector, and geographic maldistribution of healthcare providers make dental healthcare inadequate and inaccessible to vast majority of rural population.

Transformation in dental education system in the direction which expands horizons of oral health providers towards promotion and prevention as well as brings Indian dentistry closer to general healthcare is need of the hour. Dental schools need to work in synergy with other health schools and develop curriculums based on interprofessional education and collaborative practice. As there is not a single accepted model of IPE in India, experimentation with various models in compliance with local needs of the population and institutional interests can be done but care should be taken to ensure a positive early experience for staff and students involved.

Recently, the La Cascada Declaration proposed an overhaul of the dental education system as a means of reformation of dentistry so that dental profession is in sync with the needs of the population (Cohen, et al., 2017a; Cohen, et al., 2017b). Pattern of dental care must address the needs of lower income groups and underprivileged communities and should shift focus from restorative/surgical services to diagnostic and preventive care as evidences suggest that shift toward minimum intervention dentistry will steer novel approaches in interprofessional education and collaborative practice (Brennan, Balasubramanian, & Spencer, 2015). Educational leaders, health planners and policy-makers must realize that interprofessional education is an important measure to improve access to healthcare and health outcomes of the population and they should facilitate an effective cultural change, guide favorable governance mechanisms, and encourage dedicated staff to establish integrated, people-centric health workforce that is in line with the needs of the population in India.

Maxillofacial Rehabilitation and Indian Module of Interprofessional Education

Rehabilitation of maxillofacial deformities is a challenging task as it not only requires expertise and great skills but also integration between various specialties (like prosthodontist, head and neck oncology, ear, nose & throat (ENT), plastic surgery, radiology, speech therapist, and other related disciplines) for favorable outcome.

Successful rehabilitation of the patients largely depends on the treatment plan involving all specialties. However by and large prosthodontist is not a part of the team formulating treatment plan and is consulted only after surgery which adversely affects the prognosis and improvement in quality of life. A dire need of creating awareness among referring surgeons and physicians was perceived and implementing an interprofessional education module to improve interprofessional communication was deemed necessary. Therefore, moving forward in this direction, Department of Prosthodontics and Implantology, VSPM (Vidya Shikshan Prasarak Mandals) Dental College and Research centre, Nagpur, Maharashtra, India, conducted a study to evaluate the impact of IPE module on attitudes of health-care providers involved in rehabilitation of maxillofacial defects.

Figure 2. Study Methodology

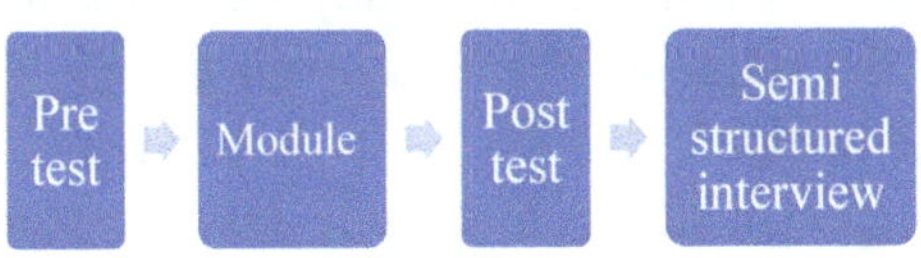

An IPE module to facilitate better understanding of limitations, expectations and individual roles of team members involved in maxillofacial prosthetic rehabilitation was designed and peer validated.

Module involving residents and faculty from three disciplines (Department of ENT, Department of Oral Surgery and Department of Prosthodontics) of three different institutes (two dental colleges and one medical college) was conducted as day long activity and involved presentations and discussion on basic and advanced techniques in management and rehabilitation of jaw malignancies (Fig. 3).

Figure 3. IPE Module

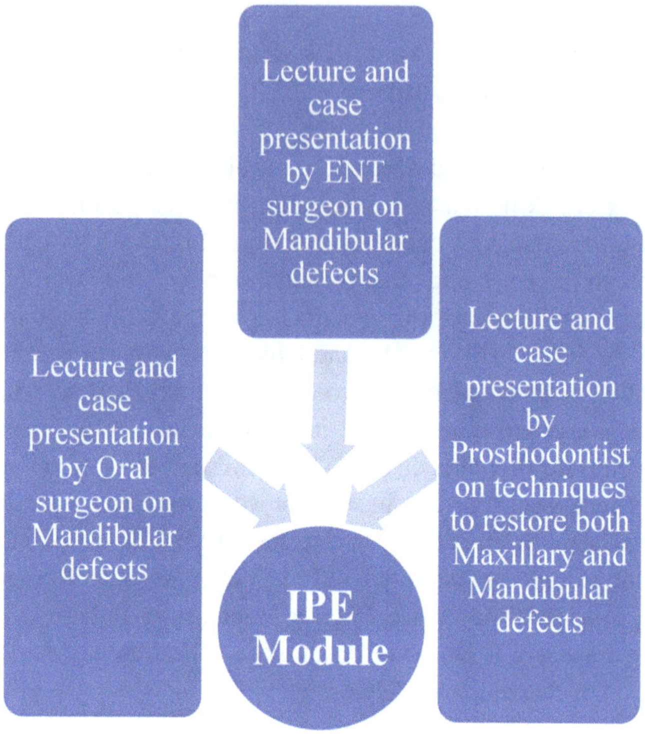

The primary research question of the study was "whether participation in an IPE module changes the attitude/perception of health-care professionals involved in maxillofacial rehabilitation"

Quantitative evaluation of change of attitude was done using standard Attitudes toward Health Care Teams (ATHCTS) questionnaire (Curran, Sharpe, & Forristall, 2007; Robben et al., 2012) both before and after the module. Semi- structured interview with selected participants provided the qualitative feedback. Participants opined that the module provided a common platform that helped them in better understanding of role and responsibility of other profession. They also expressed their view that they understood the scope of maxillofacial prosthetic rehabilitation in better manner after this module.

The module was well received and constructive as it enhanced the knowledge and skills of the participants and improved their outlook regarding collaborative practices thereby mandating that such initiatives can be pivotal in development of interprofessional education and improvement of health-care services.

Primary Health Care (PHC) Settings and Collaborative Practice in India

The World Health Organization (WHO) defined primary health care (PHC) as an "essential health care based on practical, scientifically sound and socially acceptable models and technology made universally accessible to individuals and families in the community through their full participation and at the cost that the community can afford to maintain at every stage of their development in the spirit of self-reliance and self-determination" (WHO, 2016).

The growing body of literature suggesting that effective interprofessional education enables effective collaborative practice and an increasing emphasis on the ability of healthcare professionals to work as a team, and in understanding how interprofessional education may contribute to primary health care has been main driving force to identify and establish methods for collaborative practices in primary health care.

In India, the programme was started by Catholic Health Association of India (CHAI), the largest non-governmental heath care network with 3537 member institutions which includes hospitals, health centers, nursing schools and social service societies. Apart from health care institutions and social service societies, CHAI has 780 care and support centers for People Living with HIV, children and youth with disabilities, the terminally ill, and so on.

The Catholic Health Association of India envisioned 'health for all' and upholding its commitment to deliver health-care services at the grass-roots level, CHAI has been effectually delivering much needed critical services to poor and marginalized people in India for 75 years.

In order to realize the vision of 'health for all', CHAI endeavors to

1. Promote COMMUNITY HEALTH, understood as a process of enabling the people, especially the poor and the marginalized, to be collectively responsible to attain and maintain their health and demand health as a right, and ensure availability of quality health care at reasonable cost.
2. Prevent and control communicable and non-communicable diseases as they cause a huge public health burden as well as take a heavy toll of human life in the country.
3. Ensure relief and rehabilitation to persons with disabilities.
4. Provide relief to disaster victims in the country and bring the affected to normal level of functioning.

5. Sustain advocacy for the cause of poor and needy.

Thrust areas of CHAI

1. Achieving universal access to health through national and international networking, and through the process of capacity building and advocacy.
2. Addressing communicable diseases and related issues through specific interventions of awareness, capacity building, advocacy and networking.
3. Assisting in promoting indigenous systems of medicine for enabling and empowering people to manage health problems as well as working towards becoming an accrediting institution in Integrated Systems of Medicine.

Key projects of CHAI in Community Health

1. With assistance from Misereor, Germany, CHAI has been executing project "Provision of Community Health Services and Scale-up of Interventions on Communicable Diseases" in 6 regional units in India, with an aim to ensure that "Access to health and developmental services is improved through decreased coverage gaps in provision of health services".

The project is committed to facilitate collaboration between Catholic Health Care Facilities (CHFs) and various national disease-control programmes such as, National Vector-borne Diseases Control Programme, Leprosy Programme, Blindness Programme, Revised National Tuberculosis Control Program (RNTCP), and HIV/AIDS Programme [particularly for provision of PPTCT (prevention of parent to child transmission) or ICTC (integrated counseling and testing centre) services through public-private partnership mode] as well implementing health and developmental interventions in villages.

2. CHAI, with support from Kindermissionswerk, Germany, pioneered a pilot project "Promoting Mother and Child Health through Mother's Clubs." The project covers seven states providing comprehensive maternal health care to 1000 pregnant women, identified through CHAI's Member Hospitals in rural areas, over a period of 1000 days up to the child's 2nd birthday. Also, Action Research is undertaken scaling up the model at sustainable level.
3. Supported by UNICEF (United Nations International Children's Emergency Fund), a project "Social Behavior Change Communication (SBCC)'' is being implemented by CHAI in 100 villages of India. The main objective of the project is to contribute towards the creation of a protective environment for children in which they can be protected against various diseases by newborn

care & immunization, and adolescents against getting married before the legal age, and to ensure that families and communities have safe and hygiene surroundings through systematically coordinated intensive SBCC.

4. Decentralization of HIV/AIDS services to PHC level in India has been pivotal especially for rural and remote population as it paved the way to counselling and testing services, which in turn provide access to entire range of HIV/AIDS services. Initially the services were available only at sub-district and district levels; however, the Center for Disease Control and Prevention (CDC) in collaboration with its partners decentralized those services to PHC level by piloting this PHC enhancement project. CHAI facilitated this PHC programme in Andhra Pradesh, fifth largest state in India, with 73% of total population living in rural areas and with 0.97% estimated prevalence of HIV/AIDS among adults (among 6 Indian states with highest prevalence). The programme was distinct as for the first time HIV/AIDS-related services were freely available and easily accessible to rural population at PHC level. The model of programme was unique as it involved service delivery through a novel "task shifting model" whereby nurses were trained for extended roles as counsellor, lab technician and outreach worker. Stringent monitoring and evaluation, supervision of nurses by the PHC Medical Officer and nurse supervisors and qualitative human recourse (HR) assessment of PHC nurses was implemented. Positive results (especially with respect to role of nurses) of the programme were indicated on subsequent evaluations.

Indian Interprofessional Education and Practice Network IndIPEN

Following the principles enunciated in the Framework for Action on Interprofessional Education and Collabrative Practice which is a product of WHO Study Group, IndIPEN (Indian Interprofessional Education and Practice Network) has been started in India. IndIPEN is a collaborative initiative of Manipal-FAIMER (Foundation for Advancement of International Medical Education and Research) institute for leadership in Interprofessional Education (M-FILIPE) with academy of Health Professions Educators (AHPE). The intent of this initiative is to develop a group of like-minded health professionals who have keen interest in development and advancement of health professions education in India. It has a mission to provide national leadership in moving all health providers, teams and organizations towards improved interprofessional collaboration in health professional education and healthcare practice with vision to improve health of all Indians.

Objectives

1. To create awareness and significance about interprofessional education and practice in the Indian context.
2. To stimulate networking of interprofessional education and practice across academic institutions, healthcare delivery systems, professional, academic and patient organizations in India.
3. To share promising practices in interprofessional education, collaboration and practice within the region.
4. To advance interprofessional collaboration across the healthcare system.
5. To advance research in all aspects of interprofessional education of person centered collaborative practice.

The Manipal University-FAIMER International Institute for leadership in Interprofessional Education (MUFILIPE) is a first of its kind two-year fellowship program in India that emphasizes development of leadership competencies for Interprofessional Practice (IPP). It provides opportunities for interaction with recognized leaders in IPP, collaboration with peers, and implementation of interprofessional projects. The fellowship includes two annual one-week residential session at Manipal University, Karnataka, India and two 11-month online learning sessions following the residential sessions. Participants of this program also receive mentoring and support from experts, faculty, and fellows who will be connected throughout the program and beyond.

Plans for Next 2 Years

1. Organize a national survey to collate and document health professions' faculty perceptions on IPE and IPP.
2. To develop and promote strategic partnerships with organizations that can introduce and integrate interprofessional collaboration.
3. To develop certificate courses in IPE.
4. Develop grant applications.
5. Promote academic scholarship in IPE by encouraging faculty to conduct research and publish in the field of IPE.

This program elucidates major conceptual and philosophical aspects of IPE pedagogy. The program includes faculty exchanges, interprofessional simulation, debriefing and team based learning.

Future Research in India

A recent study conducted among 250 dental undergraduate students in India have shown positive view towards interprofessional learning. They agreed that it can improve their knowledge and skills after interaction with students of other profession which is requisite for benefits of the patient or the community as a whole (Sibyl, Bennadi, kshetrimayum, & Reddy, 2018). The limitation of study is small number of sample size and all the students were from a single dental college from India. Further such studies should be undertaken taking view of multiple institutions and multiple specialities.

Another study conducted at Dr. D. Y. Patil College of Physiotherapy, Pimpri, Pune, India to find out the perception of faculty from different health sciences faculties regarding IPE have demonstrated positive outcomes. A modified version of the Readiness for Interprofessional Learning Scale (RIPLS) was used to find out the faculty perception regarding IPE. 118 teachers from medical, physiotherapy and nursing responded to the survey. Majority of them did not have any experience of IPE. Study concluded that IPE will prepare students for collaboration in healthcare teams, and felt that teaching as well as learning in interprofessional groups is possible in Indian context. Shared learning will help students to think positively about health professionals from professions other than their own. Faculty training in IPE is required (Baxi & Palekar, 2015). The feedback from such studies can gather the momentum to convince policy makers in incorporation of formal IPE training at undergraduate level.

Teaching and Learning Approaches in Interprofessional Education

Till date, not a single comprehensive interprofessional education module that fits all situations has been validated due to the differences in the structure, organizational culture, physical environment and country specific needs, however some of the proposed methods for teaching and learning in an interprofessional education setting include (Nelson, White, Hodges, & Tassone, 2017; Kusnoor & Stelljes, 2016; Hosny, Kamel, El-Wazir, & Gilbert, 2013; Kesten, 2011; Aebersold, Tschannen, & Sculli, 2013, Garbee et al., 2013; “Progressive education,” n.d.; Shumer, 1994).

1. Physician shadowing
2. Team-based learning
3. Community-based learning

Table 2. Methods for teaching and learning in an interprofessional education setting

Physician Shadowing	Team-based Learning	Community-based Learning
Students acquire knowledge and skills by observing a health care professional in the real-life setting.	Sensitizing the learner about the importance and attitudes of working as and for interprofessional team by means of interactivity, roleplays and problem based learning.	Experiential learning in the community. Real-life scenario within the community equips students with enhanced adjustment in an interprofessional practice.

Keeping students focused and involved using varied sources and methods of learning form an integral part of delivering interprofessional education. Irrespective of the module of interprofessional education used, it should be interactive, reflective, and experiential and patient oriented as well as should lead to the effective synergism amongst professionals involved.

Assessment of IPE (Barr et al., 2016)

Sustenance of any programme depends on its proper evaluation and documentation. The concept of IPE is relatively new and tools for its assessment are also limited. It can be either summative or formative assessment.

Questionnaires, Learning logs, Objective Structured Clinical Examinations (OSCEs) and Reflective diaries are most commonly used for evaluation.

I. Questionnaire

Readiness for Interprofessional Learning Scale (RIPLS) is a well-established form of questionnaire used for assessment of IPE.

The questionnaire consists of 27 items, grouped under five categories

1. Collaboration in healthcare teams
2. Professional boundaries
3. Teaching identity
4. Teaching practices and
5. Person centeredness

There are various other questionnaire based tools but they are not good indicator of learning as they can only evaluate attitudes and perceptions of learners (Parsell & Bligh, 1999).

II. Learning logs

Learning logs is keeping record of one's own learning in response to challenges set by teacher. It also gives the opportunity to provide the feedback. Thus, it is simple but revolutionary.

III. Objective Structured Clinical Examinations (OSCE)

The Objective Structured Clinical Examinations can assess collaborative knowledge, skills, behaviors and attitude by structured observation (Simmons et al. 2011).

A modified version ITOSCE (Interprofessional Team Objective Structured Clinical Examination) has been suggested by Symonds et al. (2003)

IV. Reflective Diaries

Reflective diaries are the most common and handy tool used for assessment of IPE. It is a reflective report by learners which should include reflection before action, reflection in action and reflection on action. Since it's a self-assessment tool, one can always underestimate or overestimate their learning which is an inherent drawback.

Challenges in Adopting IPE in Indian Scenario

Although changing demands and needs of the patients and the health care services focuses on the need for reframing the existing curriculum and incorporation of

Figure 4. Assessment tools of IPE

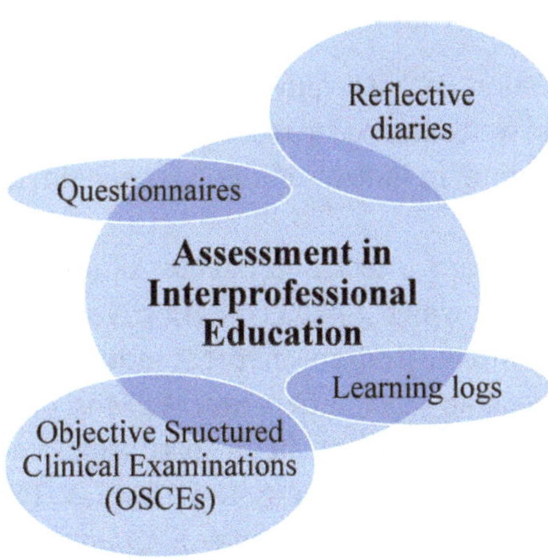

Figure 5. Challenges in adopting IPE

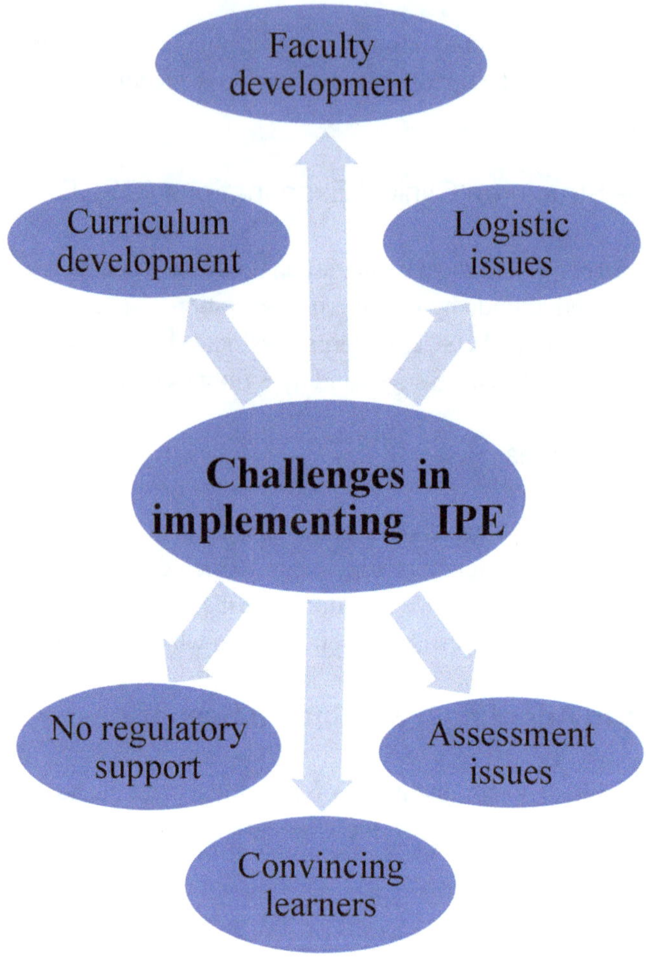
Faculty development
Curriculum development
Logistic issues
Challenges in implementing IPE
No regulatory support
Assessment issues
Convincing learners

interprofessional education, so that health care professionals understand their global responsibilities and are well equipped to meet these changes but introduction of IPE into the medical curriculum in Indian settings has been difficult due to

1. Lack of awareness: there is lack of awareness of role of other disciplines and multimodal approach which will be cost effective too.
2. Professional identity: Indian medical education system is highly compartmentalized into separate departments. Most of the training in medical education system is in isolation. Interdepartmental cooperation and IPE is lacking in our medical education system (Baxi & Palekar, 2015). Losing one's own professional identity and interdisciplinary identity is also one of

the biggest fears putting obstacle in propagating idea of IPE. Breaking barrier of fixed ideology is a must.

3. Time constraint: IPE is time consuming as it requires interaction of students from different fields over weeks or months.
4. Faculty development concerns: the content and tools for training in IPE is quite different from usual medical teaching. Most of the faculty teach in an enclosed environment and do not have skills required to teach in interdisciplinary manner and joint efforts. Lack of leadership or trained faculty to facilitate interaction within students from different fields is a big challenge in implementing IPE in various health institutes in India.
5. Curriculum development: development of common academic curriculum involving different departments, attitudes and different level of understanding with consensus among all is one of the difficult tasks. The curriculum needs to be reformed, incorporating knowledge and skills to promote collaborative practices through interprofessional teaching and learning (Sibyl, Bennadi, kshetrimayum, & Reddy, 2018).
6. Logistic issues: constructing a common timetable, standardization of timings to bring learners, faculty and professionals together at a commonplace, accommodating large number of students and undertaking a common activity at same time and setting is logistically challenging. It is recommended to develop a flexible schedule with compulsory attendance as necessary steps toward success of programme (WHO, 2010). Apart from these issues, every health institute may not have learners from multiple disciplines and implementing the concept of IPE may not be feasible in such scenario. In such scenario, it may be required to bring in more than one institute in collaboration to make IPL possible.
7. Assessment issues: Interprofessional education in India is still in infancy so are the assessment tools. Serious steps towards development of assessment modules are a must so as to boost the concept of interprofessional education.
8. Convincing learners: learners are the major contributors and backbone of interprofessional education programme and convincing them about application and utilization of such modules remains area of concern. Learners needs to be motivated and encouraged to enrol in such programmes for training by highlighting applicability and benefits of IPE to community.
9. Lack of regulatory support: lack of dedicated interprofessional facilitators/ administrators and no regulations per se about implementation of interprofessional education is the biggest challenge. Bringing the regulatory authorities and policy makers on a common platform forms an integral part of changing the perspectives of interprofessional education in India. Policy making at national level can solve few of these challenges. Involvement of policy

makers can help sustain the programme efficiently. Educational leaders should facilitate favorable government policies and ensure supportive dedicated staff to set the pace for smooth functioning of system that works for integrated health workforce that is people-centric and in line with needs of Indian population (Langton, 2009).

10. In India, health care system is a mix of public and private set-up and public health care system is far lacking behind in many aspects of health care system delivery.

CONCLUSION

Healthcare outcomes has definitely improved in India due better education, immunization, sanitation, health related schemes, infrastructure (Hedge, Gajre, Shah, & Soares, 2016) but health professional education system is still fragmented and outdated with static curriculum that fails to facilitate graduates to meet challenges of healthcare sector in real world. Interprofessional education is a viable tool to transform this obsolete educational module, but unfortunately in resource constrained countries like India; interprofessional education is still in emerging phase. Accordingly, there remain clear and compelling opportunities for improvement. Bridging interprofessional education between academic settings and real world practice, encouraging new models of interprofessional education and collaborative practice across dental, medical, and allied health care setups, implementation of creative approach, progressive strategies and interactive methods of interprofessional education into existing health policy, as well as nurture administrative interest to overcome barriers in implementation of interprofessional education and collaborative practices are some of the important measures to improve healthcare outcomes in India.

REFERENCES

Aebersold, M., Tschannen, D., & Sculli, G. (2013). Improving nursing student's communication skills using crew resource management strategies. *The Journal of Nursing Education*, *52*(3), 125–130. doi:10.3928/01484834-20130205-01 PMID:23380022

Baker, D. P., Gustafson, S., Beaubien, J., Salas, E., & Barach, P. (2003, October 20). *Medical Teamwork and Patient Safety: The Evidence-Based Relation*. Rockville, MD: Agency for Healthcare Research and Quality. Available from: https://archive.ahrq.gov/research/findings/final-reports/medteam/medteamwork.pdf

Balasubramanian, M., Short, S. D., & Gallagher, J. E. (2018). Dental professionals for a new century: Transforming dentistry through interprofessional education and collaborative practice. *Indian Journal of Dental Research*, *29*(4), 401–403. doi:10.4103/ijdr.IJDR_495_18 PMID:30127184

Barr, H. (2014). *Leading the way: Leadership Development for Interprofessional Education and Practice* (D. Forman, M. Jones, & J. E. Thistlethwaite, Eds.). Palgrave.

Barr, H., Gray, R., Helme, M., Low, H., & Reeves, S. (2016). *CAIPE- Interprofessional Education Guidelines: Centre for Advancement of Interprofessional Education.* Available from: https://www.caipe.org/resources/publications/barr-h-grayr-helmem-low-h-reeves-2016-interprofessional-education-guidelines

Barr, H., Koppel, I., Reeves, S., Hammick, M., & Freeth, D. (2005). *Effective interprofessional education: argument, assumption and evidence*. Blackwell. doi:10.1002/9780470776445

Baxi, G., & Palekar, T. (2015). Health science teacher's attitude towards interprofessional education. *National Journal of Integrated Research in Medicine*, *6*(3), 84–87.

Blue, A. V., Mitcham, M., Smith, T., Raymond, J., & Greenberg, R. (2010). Changing the future of health professions: Embedding interprofessional education within an academic health center. *Academic Medicine*, *85*(8), 1290–1295. doi:10.1097/ACM.0b013e3181e53e07 PMID:20671454

Brennan, D. S., Balasubramanian, M., & Spencer, A. J. (2015). Trends in dental service provision in Australia: 1983-1984 to 2009-2010. *International Dental Journal*, *65*(1), 39–44. doi:10.1111/idj.12141 PMID:25371293

CAIPE. (2002). *Defining IPE*. Available at: http://caipe.org.uk/about-us/defining-ipe

Centre for the Advancement of Interprofessional Education (CAIPE). (1997). Interprofessional education - a definition. *CAIPE Bulletin, 13*, 19. Retrieved from www.caipe.org/resources/publications/archived

Charles, G., Bainbridge, L., & Gilbert, J. (2010). The University of British Columbia model of interprofessional education. *Journal of Interprofessional Care*, *24*(1), 9–18. doi:10.3109/13561820903294549 PMID:20001544

Coggeshall, L. T. (1966). Planning for medical progress through education. *Journal of the American Medical Association*, *197*(11), 909–912. doi:10.1001/jama.1966.03110110133032 PMID:5952783

Cohen, L. C., Dahlen, G., Escobar, A., Fejerskov, O., Johnson, N. W., & Manji, F. (2017). Dentistry in crisis: Time to change. La cascada declaration. *Australian Dental Journal, 62*(3), 258–260. doi:10.1111/adj.12546 PMID:28793371

Cohen, L. C., Dahlen, G., Escobar, A., Fejerskov, O., Johnson, N. W., & Manji, F. (2017). Why a radical overhaul of dentistry is needed. *Indian Journal of Dental Research, 28*(5), 471–474. doi:10.4103/ijdr.IJDR_449_17 PMID:29072204

Cook, D. A. (2005). Models of interprofessional learning in Canada. *Journal of Interprofessional Care, 19*(supl), 107–115. doi:10.1080/13561820500082354 PMID:16096149

Craddock, D., O'Halloran, C., Borthwick, A., & McPherson, K. (2006). Interprofessional education in health and social care: Fashion or informed practice. *Learning in Health and Social Care, 5*(4), 220–242. doi:10.1111/j.1473-6861.2006.00135.x

Curran, V. R., Sharpe, D., & Forristall, J. (2007). Attitudes of health sciences students towards interprofessional teamwork and education. *Medical Education, 41*(9), 892–896. doi:10.1111/j.1365-2923.2007.02823.x PMID:17696982

Dargahi, H., Shirazi, M., & Yazdanparast, S. A. (2012). Interprofessional learning: The attitudes of medical, nursing and pharmacy students to shared learning at Tehran University of Medical Sciences. *Thrita J Med Sci, 1*(2), 44–48. doi:10.5812/thrita.5203

Frenk, J., Chen, L., Bhutta, Z.A., Cohen, J., Crisp, N., Evans, T., . . . Zurayk, H. (2010). Health professionals for a new century: Transforming education to strengthen health systems in an interdependent world. *Lancet, 376*(9756), 1923-58. DOI:(10)61854-5 doi:10.1016/S0140-6736

Garbee, D. D., Paige, J. T., Bonanno, L. S., Rusnak, V. V., Barrier, K. M., Kozmenko, L. S., ... Nelson, T. K. (2013). Effectiveness of teamwork and communication education using an interprofessional high-fidelity human patient simulation critical care code. *Journal of Nursing Education and Practice, 3*(3), 1–12. doi:10.5430/jnep.v3n3p1

Hall, P. (2005). Interprofessional teamwork: Professional cultures as barriers. *Journal of Interprofessional Care, 19*(supl), 188–196. doi:10.1080/13561820500081745 PMID:16096155

Hedge, S., Gajre, M. P., Shah, H., & Soares, N. S. (2016). Interprofessional Education and practice in an Indian setting. *J Taibah Univ Med Sci, 12*(3), 265–267. doi:10.1016/j.jtumed.2016.08.005 PMID:31435249

Ho, K., Jarvis-Selinger, S., Borduas, F., Frank, B., Hall, P., Handfield-Jones, R., Hardwick, D. F., Lockyer, J., Sinclair, D., Lauscher, H. N., Ferdinands, L., MacLeod, A., Robitaille, M.-A., & Rouleau, M. (2008). Making interprofessional education work: The strategic roles of the academy. *Academic Medicine*, *83*(10), 934–940. doi:10.1097/ACM.0b013e3181850a75 PMID:18820523

Hosny, S., Kamel, M. H., El-Wazir, Y., & Gilbert, J. (2013). Integrating interprofessional education in community-based learning activities: Case study. *Medical Teacher*, *35*(sup1), S68–S73. doi:10.3109/0142159X.2013.765550 PMID:23581899

Interprofessional Education Collaborative Expert Panel. (2011). *Core competencies for interprofessional collaborative practice: report of an expert panel.* Retrieved from www.umassmed.edu/.../collaborativepractice

Kelly, D. P. (2013). Interdisciplinary collaborative future for developmental-behavioral pediatrics: Barriers and opportunities. *Journal of Developmental and Behavioral Pediatrics*, *34*(7), 523–528. doi:10.1097/DBP.0b013e31829d1f44 PMID:24042083

Kesten, K. S. (2011). Role-play using SBAR technique to improve observed communication skills in senior nursing students. *The Journal of Nursing Education*, *50*(2), 79–87. doi:10.3928/01484834-20101230-02 PMID:21210611

Kohn, L. T., Corrigan, J. M., & Donaldson, M. S. (2000). *To Err is Human: Building a Safer Health System*. National Academy Press. Available at http://www.nap.edu/books/0309068371/html

Kusnoor, A. V., & Stelljes, L. A. (2016). Interprofessional learning through shadowing: Insights and lessons learned. *Medical Teacher*, *38*(12), 1278–1284. doi:10.1080/0142159X.2016.1230186 PMID:27647042

Langton, H. (2009). *Interprofessional education in higher education institutions: Models, pedagogies and realities*. Palgrave Macmillan. Retrieved from www.worldcat.org/title/interprofessional

Nelson, S., Turnbull, J., Bainbridge, L., Caufield, T., Hudon, G., Kendel, D., & Sketris, I. (2014). *Optimizing Scopes of Practice: New Models for a New Health Care System: Report of the Expert Panel Appointed by the Canadian Academy of Health Sciences*. Canadian Academy of Health Sciences. Retrieved from www.cahs-acss.ca/completed-projects

Nelson, S., White, C. F., Hodges, B. D., & Tassone, M. (2017). Interprofessional team training at the prelicensure level: A review of the literature. *Academic Medicine*, *92*(5), 709–716. doi:10.1097/ACM.0000000000001435 PMID:27782914

Nisbet, G., Lee, A., Kumar, K., Thistlethwaite, J., & Dunston, R. (2011). *Interprofessional Health Education: A Literature Review. Overview of international and Australian developments in interprofessional health education (IPE).* Retrieved from www.health.wa.gov.au/wactn/docs/IPEAUSlitreview2011

Parsell, G., & Bligh, J. (1999). The development of a questionnaire to assess the readiness for health care students for interprofessional learning (RIPLS). *Medical Education, 33*(2), 95–100. doi:10.1046/j.1365-2923.1999.00298.x PMID:10211258

Progressive Education. (n.d.). In *Wikipedia*. Available from: https://en.wikipedia.org/wiki/Progressive_education.

Reeves, S., Fletcher, S., Barr, H., Birch, I., Boet, S., Davies, N., McFadyen, A., Rivera, J., & Kitto, S. (2016). A BEME systematic review of the effects of interprofessional education: BEME Guide No. 39. *Medical Teacher, 38*(7), 656–668. doi:10.3109/0142159X.2016.1173663 PMID:27146438

Robben, S., Perry, M., van Nieuwenhuijzen, L., van Achterberg, T., Rikkert, M. O., Schers, H., Heinen, M., & Melis, R. (2012). Impact of interprofessional education on collaboration attitudes, skills, and behavior among primary care professionals. *The Journal of Continuing Education in the Health Professions, 32*(3), 196–204. doi:10.1002/chp.21145 PMID:23008082

Shumer, R. (1994). Community-based learning: Humanizing education. *Journal of Adolescence, 17*(4), 357–367. doi:10.1006/jado.1994.1032

Sibyl, S., Bennadi, D., Kshetrimayum, N., & Reddy, C.V.K. (2018). Readiness for interprofessional learning among dental undergraduate students: An institutional study. *J Indian Assoc Public Health Dent, 16*(4), 328-32. Doi:10.4103/jiaphd.jiaphd_59_18

Simmons, B., Egan-Lee, E., Wagner, S. J., Esdaile, M., Baker, L., & Reeves, S. (2011). Assessment of interprofessional learning: The design of an interprofessional objective structured clinical examination (iOSCE) approach. *Journal of Interprofessional Care, 25*(1), 73–74. doi:10.3109/13561820.2010.483746 PMID:20645683

Soares, N. S., Gajre, M. P., & Manglani, M. V. (2016). Building developmental-behavioral pediatrics in low-middle income countries through international collaboration. *Journal of Developmental and Behavioral Pediatrics, 37*(6), 508–510. doi:10.1097/DBP.0000000000000306 PMID:27366958

Solomon, P. (2011). Student perspectives on patient educators as facilitators of interprofessional education. *Medical Teacher, 33*(10), 851–853. doi:10.3109/0142159X.2010.530703 PMID:21942483

Symonds, I., Cullen, L., & Fraser, D. (2003). Evaluation of a formative interprofessional team objective structured clinical examination (ITOSCE): A method of shared learning in maternity education. *Medical Teacher*, *25*(1), 38–41. doi:10.1080/0142159021000061404 PMID:14741857

World Health Organization. (1973). Continuing education for physicians. Report of a WHO expert committee. *World Health Organization Technical Report Series*, *534*, 1–32. eric.ed.gov/?id=ED102917 PMID:4204010

World Health Organization. (1988). Learning together to work together for health. Report of a WHO study group on multiprofessional education of health personnel: The team approach. *World Health Organization Technical Report Series*, *769*, 1–72. https://apps.who.int/iris/handle/10665/37411 PMID:3140499

World Health Organization. (2006). *Rapid Scaling Up of Health Workforce Production. World Health Assembly. WHA59.23*. Retrieved from https://www.who.int/workforcealliance/knowledge/resources/wha_scalingup/en

World Health Organization. (2010). *Framework for Action on Interprofessional Education and Collaborative Practice*. Retrieved from www.who.int/hrh/resources/framework_action

World Health Organization. (2013). *Transforming and scaling up health professional's education and training: World health organization guidelines*. Retrieved from www.who.int/hrh/resources/transf_scaling_hpet/en

World Health Organization. (2016). *Declaration of Alma-Ata: Adopted at the International Conference on Primary Health Care, Alma-Ata, USSR*. Retrieved from www.who.int/publications/almaata_declaration_en.pdf

Chapter 14
A History of Interprofessional Education and Assessment at WesternU

David N. Dickter
https://orcid.org/0000-0001-9567-3918
Western University of Health Sciences, USA

Daniel C. Robinson
https://orcid.org/0000-0002-5538-2910
Western University of Health Sciences, USA

ABSTRACT

This chapter traces the early history and progress of a pioneering interprofessional practice and education (IPE) program at Western University of Health Sciences (WesternU), whose growth and development can be viewed in the context of the broader IPE field, that of a nascent movement within the United States to recognize and facilitate collaborative, patient-centered healthcare. This chapter provides some of the background and details from the early design years at WesternU. The IPE movement in the U.S. worked with general principles and broad conceptual outcomes such as safety and quality but it took time to delineate more specific guidelines and practices. Over the years, frameworks and standards for education, practice, and outcomes assessment have developed that have helped to guide the program. Similarly, WesternU has developed and refined its education and assessment methods over time.

DOI: 10.4018/978-1-7998-3066-5.ch014

"The whole is greater than the sum of its parts" – Aristotle

INTRODUCTION

This chapter traces the early history and progress of a pioneering interprofessional practice and education (IPE) program at Western University of Health Sciences (WesternU), whose growth and development can be viewed in the context of the broader IPE field, that of a nascent movement within the United States to recognize and facilitate collaborative, patient-centered healthcare. This chapter provides some of the background and details from the early design years at WesternU. The IPE movement in the U.S. worked with general principles and broad conceptual outcomes such as safety and quality but it took time to delineate more specific guidelines and practices. Over the years, frameworks and standards for education, practice, and outcomes assessment have developed that have helped to guide the program. Similarly, WesternU has developed and refined its education and assessment methods over time.

Healthcare and High-Functioning Teams

It would be hard to argue that well-functioning teams are capable of producing better outcomes than individuals working in isolation, particularly when dealing with complex tasks. This could be said for many industries, but it has special importance in health care.

Society has every right to expect that the delivery of health care should be a well-choreographed process in which all members of the health care enterprise work in concert to ensure the best possible results for the patients and populations they serve. But where does the concept of teamwork in health care come from? As students celebrate their transition to practicing professionals, they often take a pledge or oath signifying their commitment to the highest ethical and moral values and the wellbeing of their patients. Yet, there are no references to teamwork, collaboration or working with others to improve patient care or outcomes in the Hippocratic Oath, The Oath of a Pharmacist, Florence Nightingale Pledge (derived from the Hippocratic Oath and often modified for contemporary use), or the Dentist's Pledge.

Where do we see evidence of effective interprofessional teams? Pandemics and epidemics place sudden and intense demands on health systems. Teams often respond. Natural disasters and humanitarian crises bring health professionals together in relief efforts. The key elements that make teams work in these settings is a workforce shortage, adding to the value of each contributing member; a shared situation awareness such as a hurricane, earthquake, or flood; and a common goal. Everyone knows why they are there and they know what has to be done. There will also be a less formal delineation of roles as everyone is needed to the full extent of their abilities.

The healthcare literature offers numerous examples of high functioning health care teams, particularly in interdependent care situations such as emergency rooms, trauma settings and surgical teams (Courtenay, Nancarrow & Dawson, 2019; Wilson et.al, 2005). In these settings it is of paramount importance to have a common team mental model: a shared understanding about roles, responsibilities and tasks, and the ability to anticipate teammates' responses and adapt to situations (Mathieu, Heffner, Goodwin, Salas, & Cannon-Bowers, 2000). With these teams there is a shared situation awareness, a free flow of information and a common goal. If those are the components of high functioning teams, however, should there not be numerous examples in the literature for all practice settings? As Mitchell et al. (2012) state (p. 3):

Teams in health care take many forms, for example, there are disaster response teams; teams that perform emergency operations; hospital teams caring for acutely ill patients; teams that care for people at home; office-based care teams; geographically disparate teams that care for ambulatory patients; teams limited to one clinician and patient; and teams that include the patient and loved ones, as well as a number of supporting health professionals. Teams in health care can therefore be large or small, centralized or dispersed, virtual or face-to-face—while their tasks can be focused and brief or broad and lengthy.

Other examples of team-based health care include the field of Geriatrics (as is discussed in another chapter in this volume by Meyer and Hoffman) and the treatment of chronic illnesses and conditions requiring coordination of care and interprofessional collaboration (van Dongen et al., 2016).

The Origins of Interprofessional Education

The origins of interprofessional care teams have been largely borne out of concerns for patient safety in the health care setting (Kohn, Corrigan & Donaldson, 2000) and not through any coordinated effort at team-based education across the health care professions. In October 1972, the Institute of Medicine (IOM) sponsored a conference on the Interrelationships of Educational Programs for Health Professionals. A steering committee was composed of luminaries in their respective fields, bringing together 120 leaders from five health professions including Medicine (4), Nursing (3), Pharmacy (2), Dentistry (1), and Allied Health (1).[1]

This two-day conference is significant for two important reasons. First, it was considered a pioneering event and its findings created the first published IOM Report, based on 2,400 pages of tape recorded transcripts. And second, the interrelationship of health professions educational programs was the spark that launched a nearly 50 year history of IOM reports. (The name was changed to National Academy of Medicine in 2015.) In his opening remarks at the 1972 conference, committee chairman Edmund Pellegrino stated:

Few subjects are more appropriate for consideration by the Institute of Medicine than the one of interprofessional education. It reflects the breadth of membership of the Institute and its concern for issues that transcend particular professions. More important, however, it bespeaks the dedication of the Institute to emergent issues of national importance in health. (IOM, 1972, p.4)

Recommendations of the report that followed included the following (IOM, 1972, see preamble Highlights of Recommendations):

- Academic health centers must recognize an obligation to engage in interdisciplinary education and patient care, and regional consortia of health professional schools not otherwise associated with academic health centers should be formed to foster educational teamwork;
- Methods must be developed within institutions to relate interdisciplinary education to the practical requirements of health care;
- Clinical care, and particularly ambulatory care, offers a setting with the most immediate promise for successful interdisciplinary education, while classroom instruction appears to initially be more feasible in the humanities and the social and behavioral sciences associated with health care;
- Interdisciplinary instruction will require that faculties develop new skills, present new role models, and work to understand the impediments that have accumulated to hamper cooperation among health professions;
- A clearinghouse should be established to collect and distribute information on programs of interdisciplinary education and models of health care teams;
- Government agencies should support innovative interdisciplinary health education, new health care models associated with educational programs, and research on the obstacles to interprofessional cooperation;
- The Institute of Medicine should further the lines of investigation opened by this conference and advance the concepts of interdisciplinary education in the health professions.

Unfortunately, decades passed before interprofessional education began to take hold. The 2001 Institute of Medicine Report, Crossing the Quality Chasm, provides a partial explanation as to why it has taken so long to embrace interprofessional team-based care:

Existing team interactions often fall short of expectations because medical education emphasizes hierarchy and the importance of assuming individual responsibility for decision making. An emphasis on personal accountability comes at the price of losing valuable contributions from other qualified providers. (IOM, 2001, p. 132)

The IOM revisited the subject in 2003 as part of its *Quality Chasm Series* with Health Professions Education: A Bridge to Quality. The opening sentence in the Executive Summary reads: "*Education for the health professions is in need of major overhaul.*" Their major premise was that clinical education has not kept pace with rapid transformations in health care delivery, the explosion of knowledge, advances in technology, and a focus on improving quality. As a result, the report authors created a *New Vision for Health Professions Education* (p. 3):

All health professions should be educated to deliver patient-centered care as members of an interdisciplinary team, emphasizing evidence-based practice, quality improvement approaches, and informatics.

In identifying challenges facing the health care system, the report questions whether it is a system at all. Rather, it is a dizzying array of highly decentralized sectors that do not talk to each other. According to Mary Naylor, School of Nursing, University of Pennsylvania, (paraphrased) "We have a culture and organization that separate care into distinct systems – hospitals, home care, skilled nursing facilities – with little formal communication … and providers who don't see that they're responsible for what happens as patients move from one level of care to another" (IOM 2003, p. 30). This provided further clarity to the need for better communications, team-based care, and attention to transitions of care.

The 2003 report also pointed to the need for health professions education accrediting organizations to include the following five competencies in their educational standards: 1) Quality improvement; 2) patient-centered care; 3) informatics; 4) interdisciplinary teams; and 5) evidence-based practice. Based on their review at the time, the five competencies were part of the standards for only medical residencies (ACGME, AOA-Grad), pharmacy residencies (ASHP), pharmacy (ACPE), and occupational therapy (ACOTE). Furthermore, none of the licensing exams assessed for competency in informatics and only nursing (NCLEX-RN) had content on interdisciplinary teams.

INTERPROFESSIONAL EDUCATION AT WesternU

Program Goals and Early Planning; Collaboration across the University

The vision of interprofessional education is that collaborative practice is essential to ensuring safe, high quality, accessible, patient-centered care. Therefore, the stated mission of the IPE program at WesternU is "to produce humanistic healthcare professionals who practice and promote collaborative patient-centered care."

In November 2006, Provost Ben Cohen convened the Interprofessional Education Program "Kick-Off Meeting" in the Saul Bernat Boardroom at WesternU. Participants were sent preparatory questions to solicit opinions, goals and objectives relative to interprofessional education. The leading question asked "When you hear the term Interprofessional Education (IE), what does that conjure in your mind for the University? How would you (begin to) accomplish that process?" With the additional background that we would be using a case/problem-based learning format, the following questions were included: "A) Who will write the case/problem studies? B) Who will assess the students? C) What will be the learning objectives? D) What are the goals of such a program? E) How will (academic) credit be given for the course? F) Can we delete any curricular overlaps? G) How will this program be administered?"

While participants offered a large variety of responses regarding curriculum and logistics, there was general consensus that a successful IPE program would require the University's full support including financial and personnel resources and a "top-down" approach that empowers faculty and engages students in extra-curricular activities (i.e., clubs, special events, etc.). This initial meeting and accompanying working sessions was facilitated by LuAnn Wilkerson, EdD, Professor of Medicine and Senior Associate Dean for Medical Education at the University of California – Los Angeles David Geffen School of Medicine. All participants were involved in two exercises; first, define IPE and list its associated competencies, and second, identify items (actions) that would be necessary to initiate an IPE program. At the conclusion of the session the Next Steps action items were identified: 1) Recruit a Director; 2) Provide ongoing faculty development to ensure effective facilitation expertise; 3) Assign a dedicated team for case writing; 4) Initiate IPE program for all 1st and 2nd year students in the 2009-2010 academic year. The development and implementation of IPE at WesternU was possible because a group of dedicated and passionate educators got together and embraced a common goal.[2]

The timing of the 2006 WesternU meeting was particularly relevant and fortuitous. The University consisted of five colleges (Osteopathic Medicine, Allied Health, Pharmacy, Graduate Nursing, and Veterinary Medicine) at this time and plans were underway to add three additional professional programs, Dental Medicine, Podiatric Medicine and Optometry. WesternU had the benefit of having representatives from the three new programs as we began planning for the launch of interprofessional education simultaneously with the opening of the new colleges.

Committee activities continued into 2007 with the IPE Committee being subdivided into work streams. The Communications Work Stream was charged with communicating our progress to both internal and external stakeholders through website development, updated postings, town hall meetings, and print media. The Clinical Work Stream would identify examples of interprofessional clinical experiences that existed for WesternU students, whether through clinical rotations, health fairs or other community outreach activities. They also examined the possibility of having a truly interprofessional onsite clinic. The Pilot Project Work Stream was asked to address some key structural issues such as whether to use a face to face or distance format. If distant, would it be synchronous or asynchronous? Would limited participation be a challenge for certain disciplines because of scheduling conflicts? Would there be sufficient faculty available as facilitators? With all of these questions it was decided to develop two pilot cases (Obesity and West Nile Virus) first and deal with logistics once we were assured that we had sufficient administrative support to move forward with other decisions. The Program Evaluation Work Stream would create a framework for assessment to determine how well the program and its various activities met their objectives. The Environmental Scan Work Stream would gather information on interprofessional education activities in existence at WesternU and other health sciences universities in the United States and Canada. This work was done through a literature search, navigating university websites and/or calling universities directly. Overall, the findings indicated that Interprofessional Education was not widespread with the exceptions of a few model programs, particularly in Canada.

On September 13, 2007, the IPE Committee met to report its findings from the Work Stream groups, in addition to proposing an acceptable definition of Interprofessional Education that would guide our work moving forward. We adopted the definition proposed by Freeth, et al. (2005, p. 11): interprofessional education "occasions when (students) from two or more professions learn with, from and about each other to improve collaboration and the quality of care."

Further, to demonstrate interprofessional competence, the committee determined that the student should:

1. Share a common language that facilitates communication among health care professionals.
2. Demonstrate an understanding of the health professions – understanding the value that each profession adds to the delivery of health care.

3. Work effectively as a team that utilizes the unique and complementary talents of each member through interprofessional courses, seminars, activities, clinical experiences and research projects.
4. Be able to promote interprofessional delivery of health care in all practice settings.

The IPE program launched in January 2010. As reported by Aston, Mackintosh and Orzoff (2010), the launch included 850 first-year students in a case-based course and 151 participating faculty. Ninety-four groups, consisting of approximately 9 students each, met with a faculty facilitator in breakout rooms on campus.

WesternU IPE Model

As described above, the initial model for the program was developed by a team of faculty from nine WesternU programs in conjunction with the IPE Strategic Planning Oversight Committee. Over 50 WesternU faculty and staff had provided oversight to the development of the IPE program. Aston et al. (2012) have described the educational model and phases of the IPE program at WesternU. The program was designed with three phases: a didactic, case-based small group course (1st year); an online phase to include principles of teamwork in healthcare (2nd year); and a clinical phase to include clinical experiences on campus and at off-campus rotations (3rd and 4th years). The didactic phase was developed to provide an opportunity for newly matriculated students to discuss realistic cases while developing non-technical competencies such as communication, teamwork principles, and professional roles (Aston et al., 2012). As described earlier, specific diseases were selected for emphasis in the cases based on their prevalence and applicability across the broad range of programs at WesternU. The IPE course would illustrate how collaborative care is essential.

During the development of WesternU's IPE program, there was little guidance in terms of nationally recognized educational competencies. This changed with the formation of the Interprofessional Education Collaborative (IPEC) and the expert panel that was charged with developing Core Competencies for Interprofessional Collaborative Practice (IPEC, 2011)[3], described in the next section. WesternU's didactic phase grew to include the IPEC competencies as well as skills from the TeamSTEPPS curriculum. TeamSTEPPS (Team Strategies and Tools to Enhance Performance and Patient Safety; King et al., 2008) is a framework developed by Department of Defense and the Agency for Healthcare Research and Quality for practicing effective team performance. The framework provides information about teamwork principles in healthcare and includes techniques, communication scripts, and assessment tools (e.g., American Institutes for Research, 2010).

Crafted over a two-year period, the first year of WesternU's program was informed by pilot research on the course design, including on-line versus face-to-face delivery modality. Pilot study results revealed that students and faculty preferred face-to-face rather than online small group meetings, as well as the three-week versus the six-week version of the case delivery. To address the preference for face-to-face group meetings, a dedicated IPE class time was created, Wednesdays from 3-5 pm. (This dedicated time still stands today for the first year of IPE.) Bringing the professions together in a conceptual sense also required unification in a tangible sense: alignment of calendars across all colleges and programs to provide sufficient meeting time (for example, one common spring break period). Such challenges involving time, staffing and space[4] are important considerations for IPE as they likely await any new program (Abu-Rish et al., 2012). Fortunately, practical guides and other resources now exist for meeting these challenges (e.g., Evans et al., 2019; Hall & Zierler, 2015; Kahaleh et al., 2015).

The second phase (2nd year) included online education and asynchronous student collaboration, as it was not possible to align the schedules for meeting on Wednesdays (or any other day). Students in some professions also departed campus for rotations during this year. Students participated in team projects and obtained further practice with TeamSTEPPS and other teamwork concepts. WesternU experimented with different types of team activities, from general team exercises in which anyone could contribute and practice teamwork skills, to more healthcare-specific cases and exercises. Student surveys and focus groups pointed to stronger acceptance of IPE activities that were based on realistic cases and exercises that allowed students to problem-solve and practice their skills. The third phase (3rd year) was designated for interprofessional case conferences, simulations, rotations and other experiences involving patients. WesternU had an on-campus clinic but was not an academic health center, and students left campus for hundreds of geographically dispersed locations. Therefore, creating and coordinating WesternU interprofessional experiences for all students posed a challenge. Some students participated in an optional case conference, and others took part in an interprofessional activity with simulated patients. (Piloting and development of new cases continues to this day.)

GOALS IN DEVELOPING THE PROGRAM

Educational Philosophy, Case-Based Approach, Early/Didactic Years

The IPE program was developed keeping in mind the range of health care settings in which WesternU's graduates will work. While some may ultimately work in acute care, others will work in in-patient, chronic care facilities and still others in ambulatory (outpatient) settings. Thus, the care team may be synchronous or asynchronous; teams may meet in-person, virtually, or may not meet at all, collaborating only through their shared work on medical health care records systems. As stated in the 1972 IOM report, ambulatory care could immediately benefit from IPE. WesternU was graduating students into ambulatory care environments who would navigate these various team situations.

In its opening years, WesternU's IPE program had an educational philosophy, but limited examples to build upon from other IPE initiatives in the United States. While numerous educational and organizational theories were relevant to this new field, theoretical perspectives were underutilized in IPE, with most initiatives having been established without a theoretical foundation to build upon (Barr et al., 2005). However, Reeves et al. (2007) had provided a scoping review of education and organizational theories that are relevant to IPE, including theories from the domains of adult learning, social psychology, sociology, and industrial/organizational psychology, and identified over 30 potentially useful theories. Sargeant (2009) had noted that IPE at the time was built on theories of social and experiential learning (see Chorazy & Klinedinst, 2019), requiring, among other elements, student interaction with those in other professions, challenging assumptions about how they and others would work as members of a team, and self-reflection about what they were learning. At WesternU, self-regulated learning theory was employed as a guiding theoretical framework for the continued development of the IPE curriculum. According to this theory, students are actively engaged to take responsibility for their own learning and skills development (see Lopez & Tegzes chapter in this volume). This included Problem-Based Learning (PBL; Barrows & Tamblyn, 1980; Azer, 2008), in which student teams take upon themselves the responsibility for following up on topics that are addressed during case meetings. Students revisited these topics during the three-case meetings and also reflected individually on what they had learned.

Due to the novel nature of IPE programs in the U.S., in the early years of WesternU's IPE program there was little national guidance from accrediting bodies or educational institutions about learning objectives. When the program was implemented in January 2010, the Accreditation Council for Pharmacy Education and a few others had issued accreditation standards or guidelines. However, there were no national IPE outcomes identified across the professions. Therefore, WesternU had to recognize the limitations within the field of IPE and break new ground.

Descriptions of interprofessional competencies and educational frameworks is a relatively new development in the United States, with the first report of the Interprofessional Education Collaborative (IPEC) appearing in 2011 and undergoing revisions five years later (IPEC, 2016). IPEC included representatives from osteopathic medicine, allopathic medicine, pharmacy, nursing, dentistry, and public health, who published the often-cited framework listing four interprofessional core competencies: values/ethics for interprofessional practice; knowledge of one's own and other professions' roles and responsibilities; interprofessional communication; and teamwork. In 2010, the Canadian Interprofessional Health Collaborative had described six competency areas: role clarification, team functioning, interprofessional communication, patient/client/family/community-centered care, collaborative leadership, and interprofessional conflict resolution (Canadian Interprofessional Health Collaborative, 2010). Such competencies are now an integral part of IPE and are included in the accreditation standards of most healthcare professions. These standards require that core curricula prepare students to provide coordinated and collaborative care with members of other health professions. Reviewing accreditation documentation for a range of professions, Zorek and Raehl (2013) found over 60 statements in which education programs are held accountable for IPE learning outcomes, including medicine, pharmacy, nursing, physical therapy, physician assistant studies, occupational therapy, and public health.

Competencies/Educational Objectives

Model educational outcomes, originally described by Kirkpatrick (1967), were later adapted by Freeth, et.al. (2002) to include interprofessional competencies, as a hierarchy of outcomes as measured by the following (see Figure 1):

1. Learner reactions (e.g., course evaluations/surveys, opinions rendered during focus groups);
2. Attitudes about other professions and IPE itself (2nd tier);
3. Knowledge and functional skills, such as about IPEC competencies and TeamSTEPPS;
4. More complex outcomes including the behavior of interprofessional health care teams; and on up to
5. Quality of care delivery and specific benefits to patients (Reeves, Boet, Zierler,& Kitto, 2015)

The top three levels of the pyramid remain elusive for IPE due not only to their complexity but also the distal relationship between the education of students and their subsequent professional practice. In that sense the problem of measurement is not unlike outcomes measurement for the rest of higher education.

The early literature on reactions to the delivery of IPE indicated an appreciation by students of its importance in light of the IOM publications on quality of care. In the early 2000s, IPE outcomes research was predicated on the assumption that a change (improvement) in attitudes is a prerequisite for successful interprofessional

Figure 1. An IPE Outcomes Evaluation Model

Note: Adapted from Kirkpatrick's (1967) model of educational outcomes, as modified by Freeth et al. (2002) and others.

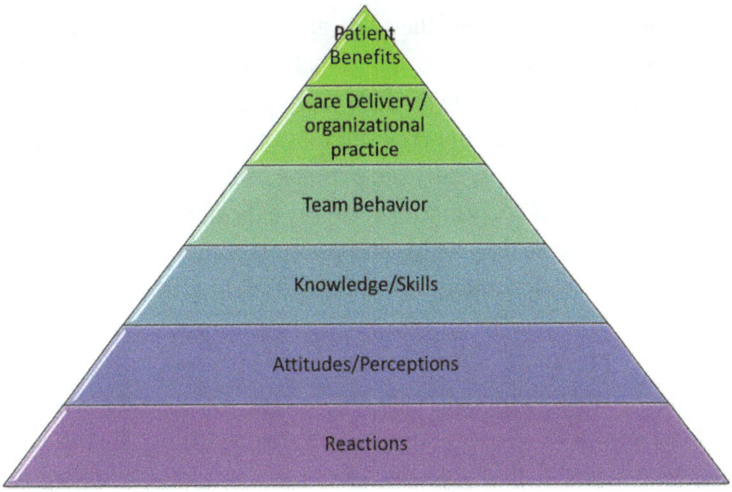

collaboration (i.e., the second level of the pyramid in Figure 1). The published IPE assessment tools available at the time prioritized measuring student attitudes toward interprofessional learning such as the Readiness for Interprofessional Learning Scale (RIPLS; Reid, Bruce, Allstaff, & McLernon, 2006). Abu-Rish et al.'s review of the literature (2012) found that 77% of IPE outcomes studies investigated attitudes and only 30% investigated skills. The research on attitudes extended from the theoretical emphasis at the time, that of contact between the professions as a necessary step to breaking down professional silos and fostering an understanding of the roles and contributions of a range of health professions. This work extended from Allport's Intergroup Contact Theory (Allport, 1954), known more widely as the Contact Hypothesis. This theory, that contact between groups reduces prejudice, has been applied to perceptions and stereotypes about professions different from one's own (Hoffman & Redman-Bentley, 2012). In IPE, the line of thinking was that by breaking down silos and permitting interprofessional learning early on, unproductive stereotypes about different professions (some of which may have formed by learning apart from them, and others from misconceptions about these professions and those who practice them) would be less likely to form. Students would more readily accept interprofessional collaboration as a necessary aspect of health care. Numerous studies have indeed found pre-post improvements on attitudes scales such as the RIPLS, particularly before and after short-term interprofessional training events (e.g., see Freeth, Hammick, Koppel, Reeves, & Barr, 2007). There is also ample evidence of the existence of stereotypes about the health professions, though the effects of IPE program on stereotyping has been mixed (Thurston et al., 2017). However, at professional conferences, IPE researchers began to discuss a curious finding, that RIPLS scores for IPE programs (including WesternU's) may begin at the higher ranges of the scale and then decline over time. Hammick et al.'s (2007) literature review had found that outcomes studies of attitudes and perceptions were more mixed than those of knowledge and skills, and they did note reports of declines in attitudes in some samples over time. At WesternU, students were already proponents of IPE early on, perhaps from the successful efforts by the University to market this concept and the resulting exposure and self-selection among applicants. While breaking down silos and counteracting or preventing stereotypes makes sense intuitively, this outcome is an insufficient criterion for the successful IPE program. Much of the field has moved away from attitudes and perceptions assessments as the primary evaluation criteria and instead focused on higher levels of the outcomes evaluation model, including interprofessional knowledge, practice skills, and behaviors.

The literature offers a variety of outcomes measures based on knowledge, such as assessments of acquisition of IPEC competencies (Brandt, Lutfiyya, King, & Chioreso, 2014) and knowledge about TeamSTEPPS techniques (Chen, Yau, Revere, & Swails, 2019). WesternU has included knowledge assessments (e.g., a final exam on interprofessional competencies and skills) in its IPE program. Skills training and pre-post assessments for practicing healthcare professionals are prevalent in the research literature (Brand et al., 2014), but there is much work needed to advance these assessments for educational settings. In didactic education there are limited opportunities to assess practicing skills in clinical environments, among other reasons due to, for example:

- the educational stage of the learner
- the resources of the educational institution (which may comprise an academic health center or as at WesternU, may not); and
- the assessor/preceptor's opportunity or commitment to observe and evaluate interprofessional skills (especially when the preceptor works at another institution where the student is on rotation)

Self-ratings of skills may be used for pre-post evaluations, but have often been found to be subject to inflation or distortion about one's skills (Alicke & Govorun, 2005; this has been WesternU's experience in IPE as well).

Present State

IPE and WesternU have made progress in outcomes assessment: both have traveled partway up the Kirkpatrick pyramid, from reactions and attitudes to knowledge and skills and team behavior (described further below). Still, measurement of IPE outcomes at the levels of Team Behavior and higher are at an early stage. Research on teams and team training is robust and demonstrates it to be effective for team outcomes. For example, in a meta-analysis by Salas et al., team training can be explained, conservatively, at least 12-19% of improvement in outcomes, including cognitive, affective, teamwork processes and team performance outcomes (Salas, DiazGranados, Klein, Buke, Stagl, Goodwin et al., 2008). Numerous individual studies exist on team training programs for health care in particular (e.g., Hughes, et al., 2016). However, establishing a link (perhaps tenuous) between IPE and the behavior of teams whose members received IPE is challenging. Even more challenging is the effort to gather evidence about care delivery and benefits to patients, families and communities. The National Center for Interprofessional Practice and Education at the University of Minnesota has engaged a network of institutions (including WesternU) to begin to gather evidence for these outcomes (Brandt et al., 2014).

IPE researchers have the benefit of hundreds of team- and healthcare-related assessments, including IPE and teamwork tools measuring team attitudes, knowledge of collaboration and teamwork principles and skills (Canadian Interprofessional Collaborative, 2012). In reviewing the literature, it may seem a standard practice to point out that reliability and data on the published tools are limited; however, this is a conclusion that continues to apply (Wooding, Gayle, & Maynard, 2019; Peltonen et al., 2019). In particular, few tools exist to measure team-related skills, such as through behavior observation rubrics or checklists (Wooding et al., 2019). Peltonen et al.'s review (2019) finds that many interprofessional collaboration instruments tend to focus on only two professions, medicine and nursing. Researchers have not yet agreed upon a set of measures of interprofessional collaboration that could be used broadly for systematic studies (IOM, 2015) and aggregated into scoping reviews and meta-analyses.

Some educators have assembled a "consensus statement" from an international panel of IPE scholars about what and how to assess IPE competencies (Rogers et al., 2016). Included in the statement are that outcomes assessment should include the familiar IPEC competencies of (communication, teamwork, roles/responsibilities, values) as well as coordination, collaborative decision-making, self-reflection. The statement includes the importance of focusing on minimal competencies or standards for summative assessment. Measures of attitudes or perceived confidence are not recommended for conclusion in summative outcome assessments (Rogers et al., 2016).

WesternU includes interprofessional competencies as rated by observers, in the form of preceptor evaluations, and is participating in research on a multi-site study of an interprofessional rating scale (Frost et al., 2019) for individual students training on interprofessional teams under a preceptor, as well as researching interprofessional learning based on a program at an on-site clinic. And given the challenges in assessing interprofessional performance in academic settings, including WesternU's, simulating interprofessional care environments makes sense. Such simulations are already included in many professions' educational standards or licensing, for example in pharmacy (Accreditation Council for Pharmacy Education (ACPE), 2016), medicine (e.g., simulation on the COMLEX-USA Level 2 examination to assess skills including professionalism and interpersonal skills; National Board of Medical Examiners, 2019) and nursing (e.g., Hayden, Smiley, & Gross, 2014). Objective structured clinical examinations (OSCEs) have long been included in healthcare education in medicine, pharmacy, nursing and other professions, and OSCEs represent a burgeoning aspect of assessment for IPE (Palaganas, Brunette, & Winslow, 2016). Students participate in a variety of team care scenarios such as simulated disasters, emergent care situations, case meetings and ambulatory care situations (Palaganas et al., 2016). These simulations advance evidence-based educational experiences and provide outcomes assessment for knowledge and skills/behaviors essential in IPE. WesternU has developed interprofessional simulations to assess student skills using reliable, validated assessments of performance of individual students participating with standardized patients and clinicians (e.g., see Dickter et al., 2013); Dickter, Stielstra, & Lineberry, 2015). WesternU students have participated either solo, with all other patients and healthcare practitioners simulated by actors, or together with other student teams (for example in a case conference and interprofessional patient consultation). Students have found these experiences provided realistic practice opportunities and deepened their knowledge about other healthcare professions.

In the Freeth et al. (2002) diagram, WesternU's emphasis on the knowledge/skills level is evident in other ways as well. Early on, the curriculum consisted of five cases in the first year with attempts to provide subject matter that was relevant to most if not all nine health professions. In each case, students learned to address patient-centered care as a team, with a focus on communication, teamwork, and collaboration between the professions (Hoffman et al., 2014). While the curriculum changes frequently and will be different by the time this chapter is published, the current state includes a range of new activities designed for active, experiential learning. In the first year, students work together on a realistic problem-based learning case, the Johnson Family, which includes patients for students in all nine of WesternU's professions to consider (dental medicine, optometry, osteopathic medicine, nursing, pharmacy, physical therapy, physician assistant studies, podiatric medicine and veterinary medicine). Students collaborate to uncover problems in the case and make recommendations, which can be scored to assess the team's performance. The first year also includes large- and small-group facilitation and a range of multi-media learning materials about errors in healthcare and the consequences of interprofessional collaboration, and the final exam tests students' knowledge of interprofessional concepts, competencies and skills, notably the TeamSTEPPS skills that are now included many other IPE programs (Chen et al., 2019). The second year involves blended learning: online and a face-to-face capstone, as well as the students' choice of team projects or a standardized patient simulation. At the end of the second year, students also earn certifications through online modules from the Institute for Healthcare Improvement. Some students participate in the second and/or third years in the interprofessional simulations (OSCEs) mentioned earlier. The use of simulations has enabled WesternU to apply formative assessment of interprofessional skills, primarily communication, collaboration, and understanding roles and responsibilities of different professions.

FUTURE OF IPE AT WesternU AND AS A FIELD

The IPE curriculum at WesternU changes every year. WesternU plans to increase the use of learning activities allowing for skills practice. In addition to simulations involving patient consultations and interprofessional case conferences, the University is developing team-based, gamified learning. Educational technology is being employed for delivery of virtual-based team experiences and the collection and analysis of collaborative behaviors. Students in some of the programs also participate in interprofessional community-based education experiences (Friedrichsen, Martinez, Hostetler, & Tang, 2014) that in the future may be woven into IPE more formally.

Much is still unknown about the nature and frequency of interprofessional collaboration in healthcare. Schot, Tummers, and Noordegraaf (2019) reviewed over 21,000 studies to describe how practicing healthcare professionals collaborate. The authors described three categories of collaboration: "bridging gaps," "negotiating overlaps," and "creating spaces" (Schot et al, 2019). Bridging gaps includes overcoming differences in professional opinions about treating patients, managing emotions and communications effectively while working together, relaying or translating information and jargon between the professions, and helping others by conducting tasks that are not part of their formal role. Negotiating overlaps involves working through ambiguity of roles where more than one profession may have responsibility, as well as ambiguity about who should carry out which tasks when different professions are on the same care team. Creating spaces involves organizing how the team will work together, which, beyond physical space, refers more to organizing the work processes and dealing with organizational barriers such as bureaucracy (Schot et al., 2019).

Changing healthcare requires broader thinking about how students who enter the workforce will employ their learning in healthcare organizations. Part of this process necessarily involves building more of a theoretical foundation to underpin IPE programs. For example, Suter et al. (2013) described eight organizational and system theories that could be applied to IPE, such as socio-technical theory (Trist & Bamforth, 1951). This theory was originally developed to explain how people and technology work together for organizational effectiveness, and has been since applied to a variety of technological and social subsystems that must be considered collectively in order to optimize performance (Hummels, 2000). Suter et al. (2013) argue that the theory can "provide insights into the interplay between the nature of interprofessional collaboration and organizational reward systems and management structures" (p.60). One way to do this might be to better prepare students to work within these structures and hierarchies in organizations, and to develop their leadership skills to that they may become change agents.

Ultimately, IPE should show a macro-level benefit for healthcare, expressed often as the Triple Aim (Berwick et al., 2008) of quality of healthcare (safety, and patient outcomes), experience (patients' and providers') and costs. Brandt et al. (2014) conducted an extensive review of the literature, finding that most studies focused on assessments and outcomes related to IPE program participants or interprofessional practices, few on patient health outcomes, and none on reducing the cost of healthcare. A recent review of interprofessional collaborative healthcare and patient health outcomes (Lutfiyya, Chang, McGrath, Dana, & Lipsky, 2019) identified 20 studies between 2010-2018, the majority of which identified health benefits, including improvements in blood glucose, hypertension, and pain management, and no study reported negative outcomes.

With its inclusion of ambulatory care in IPE, WesternU is well-positioned to continue to contribute to the IPE field. Schot et al. (2019) found that most studies focus on team settings within hospitals; research in ambulatory care environments – the focus of many WesternU graduates – is lacking, thus providing opportunities for the University to contribute to education and research.

REFERENCES

Abu-Rish, E., Kim, S., Choe, L., Varpio, L., Malik, E., White, A. A., Craddick, K., Blondon, K., Robins, L., Nagasawa, P., Thigpen, A., Chen, L., Rich, J., & Zierler, B. (2012). Current trends in interprofessional education of health sciences students: A literature review. *Journal of Interprofessional Care*, *2*(6), 444–445. doi:10.3109/13561820.2012.715604 PMID:22924872

Accreditation Council for Pharmacy Education (ACPE). (2016). *Accreditation standards and key elements for the professional program in Pharmacy leading to the Doctor of Pharmacy degree*. Retrieved from https://www.acpe-accredit.org/pdf/Standards2016FINAL.pdf

Alicke, M. D., & Govorun, O. (2005). The Better-Than-Average Effect. In M. D. Alicke, D. A. Dunning, & J. I. Krueger (Eds.), *Studies in self and identity. The Self in Social Judgment* (pp. 85–106). Psychology Press.

Allport, G. W. (1954). *The nature of prejudice*. AddisonWesley.

American Institutes for Research. (2010). *TeamSTEPPS Teamwork Perceptions Questionnaire (TPQ)*. Manual.

Association of American Medical Colleges. (2017). *Core entrustable professional activities for entering residency*. https://www.aamc.org/download/484778/data/epa13toolkit.pdf

Aston, S., Mackintosh, S., & Orzoff, J. (2010). Interprofessional Education program, Western University of Health Sciences. *Journal of Allied Health*, *39*(Suppl1), e137–e138. PMID:21174033

Aston, S. J., Rheault, W., Arenson, C. F., Tappert, S., Stoeker, J., Orzoff, J., Galitski, H., & Mackintosh, S. (2012). Interprofessional education: A review and analysis of programs from three academic health centers. *Academic Medicine*, *87*(7), 949–955. doi:10.1097/ACM.0b013e3182583374 PMID:22622216

Azer, S. (2008). *Navigating problem-based learning*. Elsevier.

Barr, H., Koppel, L., Reeves, S., Hammick, M., & Freeth, D. (2005). *Effective interprofessional education: Assumption, argument and evidence*. Blackwell. doi:10.1002/9780470776445

Barrows, H., & Tamblin, R. (1980). *Problem based Learning*. Springer Publications.

Berwick, D. M., Nolan, T. W., & Whittington, J. (2008). The triple aim: Care, health, and cost. *Health Affairs*, *27*(3), 759–769. doi:10.1377/hlthaff.27.3.759 PMID:18474969

Brandt, B., Lutfiyya, M. N., King, J. A., & Chioreso, C. (2014). A scoping review of interprofessional collaborative practice and education using the lens of the Triple Aim. *Journal of Interprofessional Care*, *28*(5), 393–399. doi:10.3109/13561820.2014.906391 PMID:24702046

Canadian Interprofessional Health Collaborative. (2010). *A National Interprofessional Competency Framework*. University of British Columbia. Retrieved from http://www.cihc.ca/files/CIHC_IPCompetencies_Feb1210.pdf

Canadian Interprofessional Health Collaborative. (2012). *An inventory of quantitative tools measuring interprofessional education and collaborative practice outcomes*. Retrieved from http://cihc.ca

Chen, A. S., Yau, B., Revere, L., & Swails, J. (2019). Implementation, evaluation, and outcome of TeamSTEPPS in interprofessional education: a scoping review. *Journal of Interprofessional Care*. Advanced online publication. https://doi:10.1080/13561820.2019.1594729

Chorazy, M. L., & Klinedinst, K. S. (2019). Learn by doing: A model for incorporating high-impact experiential learning into an undergraduate public health curriculum. *Frontiers in Public Health*, *7*, 31. doi:10.3389/fpubh.2019.00031 PMID:30863743

Courtenay, M., Nancarrow, S., & Dawson, D. (2013). Interprofessional teamwork in the trauma setting: A scoping review. *Human Resources for Health*, *11*(1), 57. doi:10.1186/1478-4491-11-57 PMID:24188523

Dickter, D. N., Stielstra, S., & Lineberry, M. (2015). Interrater reliability of standardized actors versus nonactors in a simulation based assessment of interprofessional collaboration. *Simulation in Healthcare*, *10*(4), 249–255. doi:10.1097/SIH.0000000000000094 PMID:26098494

Dickter, D. N., Stielstra, S., Mackintosh, S., Garner, S., Finocchio, V. A., & Aston, S. J. (2013). Development of the Ambulatory Team Observed Structured Clinical Evaluation (ATOSCE). *Medical Science Educator*, *23*(3S), 554–558.

Evans, S., Ward, C., Shaw, N., Walker, A., Knight, T., & Sutherland-Smith, W. (n.d.). Interprofessional education and practice guide No. 10: Developing, supporting and sustaining a team of facilitators in online interprofessional education. *Journal of Interprofessional Care, 31*, 1-7. Advanced online publication. https://doi:10.1080/13561820.2019.1632817

Freeth, D., Hammick, M., Reeves, S., Koppel, I., & Barr, H. (2005). *Effective interprofessional education: Development, delivery & evaluation*. Blackwell Publishing. doi:10.1002/9780470776438

Freeth, D., Hammick, M., Reeves, S., Koppel, I., & Barr, H. (2007). A critical review of evaluations of interprofessional education. King's College, London: Higher Education Academy.

Friedrichsen, S., Martinez, T. S., Hostetler, J., & Tang, J. M. W. (2014). Innovations in interprofessional education: Collaborative practice skills. *California Dental Association Journal*, *42*(9), 629–635. PMID:25265729

Frost, J. S., Hammer, D. P., Nunez, L. M., Adams, J. L., Chesluk, B., Grus, C., Harvison, N., McGuinn, K., Mortensen, L., Nishimoto, J. H., Palatta, A., Richmond, M., Ross, E. J., Tegzes, J., Ruffin, A. L., & Bentley, J. P. (2019, January 2). The intersection of professionalism and interprofessional care: Development and initial testing of the interprofessional professionalism assessment (IPA). *Journal of Interprofessional Care*, *33*(1), 102–115. doi:10.1080/13561820.2018.1515733 PMID:30247940

Greiner, A., & Knebel, E. (2003). Health professions education: A bridge to quality. Washington, DC: National Academies Press.

Hall, L. W., & Zierler, B. (2015). Interprofessional education and practice guide No. 1: Developing faculty to effectively facilitate interprofessional education. *Journal of Interprofessional Care*, *29*(1), 3–7. doi:10.3109/13561820.2014.937483 PMID:25019466

Hammick, M., Freeth, D., Koppel, I., Reeves, S., & Barr, H. (2007). A best evidence systematic review of interprofessional education: BEME guide no. 9. *Medical Teacher*, *29*(8), 735–751. doi:10.1080/01421590701682576 PMID:18236271

Hayden, J. K., Smiley, R. A., & Gross, L. (2014). Simulation in Nursing Education: Current Regulations and Practices. *Journal of Nursing Regulation*, *5*(2), 25–30. doi:10.1016/S2155-8256(15)30084-3

Hean, S., Craddock, D., Hammick, M., & Hammick, M. (2012). Theoretical insights into interprofessional education: AMEE Guide No. 62. *Medical Teacher*, *34*(2), e78–e101. doi:10.3109/0142159X.2012.650740 PMID:22289015

Hoffman, J., Pham, D.Q., & Robinson, D. (2014). Interprofessional education: The road to interprofessional practice. *California Pharmacist*, 42-44.

Hoffman, J., & Redman-Bentley, D. (2012). Comparison of faculty and student attitudes toward teamwork and collaboration in interprofessional education. *Journal of Interprofessional Care, 26*(1), 66–68. doi:10.3109/13561820.2011.602441 PMID:22233371

Hughes, A. M., Gregory, M. E., Joseph, D. L., Sonesh, S. C., Marlow, S. L., Lacerenza, C. N., Benishek, L. E., King, H. B., & Salas, E. (2016). Saving lives: A meta-analysis of team training in healthcare. *The Journal of Applied Psychology, 101*(9), 1266–1304. doi:10.1037/apl0000120 PMID:27599089

Hummels, J., & de Leede, J. (2000). Teamwork and morality: Comparing lean production and socio-technology. *Journal of Business Ethics, 26*(1), 75–88. doi:10.1023/A:1006242516664

Institute of Medicine. (1972). *Educating for the health team: Report of the conference on the interrelationships of educational programs for health professional*. Washington, DC: National Academy of Sciences. Available through http://books.google.com

Institute of Medicine. (2001). *Crossing the quality chasm: A new health system for the 21st Century*. National Academy Press.

Institute of Medicine. (2015). *Measuring the Impact of Interprofessional Education on Collaborative Practice and Patient Outcomes*. The National Academies Press., doi:10.17226/21726

Interprofessional Education Collaborative Expert Panel. (2011). *Core competencies for interprofessional collaborative practice: Report of an expert panel*. Interprofessional Education Collaborative Expert Panel.

Interprofessional Education Collaborative Expert Panel. (2016). *Core competencies for interprofessional collaborative practice: 2016 update*. https://ipecollaborative.org/uploads/IPEC-2016-Updated-Core-Competencies-Report__final_release_.PDF

Kahaleh, A. A., Danielson, J., Franson, K. L., Nuffer, W. A., & Umland, E. M. (2015). An interprofessional education panel on development, implementation, and assessment strategies. *American Journal of Pharmaceutical Education, 79*(6), 78. doi:10.5688/ajpe79678 PMID:26430265

King, H. B., Battles, J., Baker, D. P., Alonso, A., Salas, E., Webster, J., Toomey, L., & Salisbury, M. (2008). *TeamSTEPPS™ (Team Strategies and Tools to Enhance Performance and Patient Safety) tools and materials*. https://www.ahrq.gov/downloads/pub/advances2/vol3/advances-king_1.pdf

Kirkpatrick, D. (1967). Evaluation of training. In R. Craig & L. Bittel (Eds.), *Training and development handbook* (pp. 131–167). McGraw-Hill.

Kohn, L. T., Corrigan, J., & Donaldson, M. S. (2000). *To err is human: Building a safety health system*. National Academy Press.

Lutfiyya, M. N., Chang, L. F., McGrath, C., Dana, C., & Lipsky, M. S. (2019). The state of the science of interprofessional collaborative practice: A scoping review of the patient health-related outcomes based literature published between 2010 and 2018. *PLoS One*, *14*(6), e0218578. Advance online publication. doi:10.1371/journal.pone.0218578 PMID:31242239

Mathieu, J. E., Heffner, T. S., Goodwin, G. F., Salas, E., & Cannon-Bowers, J. A. (2000). The influence of shared mental models on team processes and performance. *The Journal of Applied Psychology*, *85*(2), 273–283. doi:10.1037/0021-9010.85.2.273 PMID:10783543

Mitchell, P., Wynia, M., Golden, R., McNellis, B., Okun, S., Webb, C. E., Rohrbach, V., & Von Kohorn, I. (2012). *Core principles and values of effective team-based health care: Discussion Paper*. Institute of Medicine. doi:10.31478/201210c

National Board of Medical Examiners. (2019). *2019-2020 Orientation Guide, COMLEX-USA Level 2-PE*. Retrieved from https://www.nbome.org/wordpress/wp-content/uploads/2017/03/COMLEX-USA_L2PE_Orientation_Guide-website-20192020.pdf

Palaganas, J., Brunette, V., & Winslow, B. (2016). Prelicensure simulation-enhanced interprofessional education: A critical review of the research literature. *Simulation in Healthcare*, *11*(6), 404–418. doi:10.1097/SIH.0000000000000175 PMID:27602706

Peltonen, J., Leino-Kilpi, H., Heikkilä, H., Rautava, P., Tuomela, K., Siekkinen, M., Sulosaari, V., & Stolt, M. (n.d.). Instruments measuring interprofessional collaboration in healthcare – a scoping Review. *Journal of Interprofessional Care*. Advanced online publication. https://doi:10.1080/13561820.2019.1637336

Reeves, S., Boet, S., Zierler, B., & Kitto, S. (2015). Interprofessional education and practice guide no. 3: Evaluating interprofessional education. *Journal of Interprofessional Care*, *29*(4), 305–312. doi:10.3109/13561820.2014.1003637 PMID:25671416

Reeves, S., Suter, E., Goldman, J., Martimianakis, T., Chatalalsingh, C., & Dematteo, D. C. (2007). *A scoping review to identify organizational and education theories relevant for interprofessional practice and education*. Retrieved from http://www.cihc.ca/files/publications/ScopingReview_IP_Theories_Dec07.pdf

Reid, R., Bruce, D., Allstaff, K., & McLernon, D. (2006). Validating the Readiness for Interprofessional Learning Scale (RIPLS) in the postgraduate context: Are health care professionals ready for IPL? *Medical Education*, *40*(5), 415–422. doi:10.1111/j.1365-2929.2006.02442.x PMID:16635120

Rogers, G. D., Thistlethwaite, J. E., Anderson, E. S., Dahlgren, M. A., Grymonpre, R. E., Moran, M., & Samarasekera, D. D. (2016). International consensus statement on the assessment of interprofessional learning outcomes. *Medical Teacher*, *26*, 1–13. PMID:28024436

Salas, E., DiazGranados, D., Klein, C., Burke, C. S., Stagl, K. C., Goodwin, G. F., & Halpin, S. M. (2008). Does team training improve performance? A meta-analysis. *Human Factors*, *50*(6), 903–933. doi:10.1518/001872008X375009 PMID:19292013

Sargeant, J. (2009). Theories to aid in understanding and implementation of interprofessional education. *The Journal of Continuing Education in the Health Professions*, *29*(3), 178–184. doi:10.1002/chp.20033 PMID:19728383

Schot, E., Tummers, L., & Noordegraaf, M. (2019): Working on working together. A systematic review on how healthcare professionals contribute to interprofessional collaboration. *Journal of Interprofessional Care*. Advanced online publication. https://doi:10.1080/13561820.2019.1636007

Suter, E., Goldman, J., Martimianakis, T., Chatalalsingh, C., DeMatteo, D. J., & Reeves, S. (2013). The use of systems and organizational theories in the interprofessional field: Findings from a scoping review. *Journal of Interprofessional Care*, *27*(1), 57–64. doi:10.3109/13561820.2012.739670 PMID:23148862

Thurston, M. M., Chesson, M. M., Harris, E. C., & Ryan, G. J. (2017). Professional stereotypes of interprofessional education naive pharmacy and nursing students. *American Journal of Pharmaceutical Education*, *81*(5), 1–9. PMID:28720912

van Dongen, J. J. J., van Bokhoven, M. A., Daniels, R., van der Weijden, T., Petronella Emonts, W. W. G., & Beurskens, A. (2016). Developing interprofessional plans in chronic care: A scoping review. *BMC Family Practice*, *17*(1), 137. doi:10.118612875-016-0535-7 PMID:27655185

Wilson, K. A., Burke, C. S., Priest, H. A., & Salas, E. (2005). Promoting health care safety through training high reliability teams. *Quality & Safety in Health Care*, *14*(4), 303–309. doi:10.1136/qshc.2004.010090 PMID:16076797

Wooding, E. L., Gale, T. C., & Maynard, V. (2019). Evaluation of teamwork assessment tools for interprofessional simulation: A systematic literature review. *Journal of Interprofessional Care*. Advanced online publication. https://doi:10.1080/13561820.2019.1650730

Zorek, J., & Raehl, C. (2013). Interprofessional education accreditation standards in the USA: A comparative analysis. *Journal of Interprofessional Care, 27*(2), 123–130. doi:10.3109/13561820.2012.718295 PMID:22950791

ENDNOTES

1 Members of the steering committee included: Edmund D. Pellegrino, (Chair) Vice President for Health Affairs, University of Tennessee; Donald C. Brodie, Director, Pharmacy-Related Programs, National Center for Health Services Research & Development; John H. Bryant, Director, School of Public Health and Administrative Medicine, Columbia University; J. Thomas Grayston, Vice President for Health Sciences, University of Washington; James Haughton, Executive Director, Cook County Hospital Corporation Governing Committee; John I. Ingle, Senior Staff Officer, Institute of Medicine; Eleanor C. Lambertsen, Dean, School of Nursing, Cornell University; Lucile P. Leone, San Francisco, CA; J. Warren Perry, Director, Study of Allied Health Education, American Association of Community and Junior Colleges; Rozella M. Schlotfeldt, Professor of Nursing, School of Nursing, Case Western Reserve University; Lawrence C. Weaver, Dean, School of Pharmacy, University of Minnesota; Roger J. Bulger, ex officio, Executive Officer, Institute of Medicine.

2 The following individuals provided extensive and thoughtful responses to the initial questions posed by Provost Ben Cohen. Clinton Adams, Dean College of Osteopathic Medicine; Stephanie Bowlin, Dean College of Allied Health; Tina Meyer, Director Master in Health Sciences; Karen Hanford, Dean College of Graduate Nursing; Diane Lithgow, College of Graduate Nursing; Daniel Robinson, Dean College of Pharmacy; Wallace Murray, Associate Dean Academic Affairs College of Pharmacy; Shirley Johnston, Dean College of Veterinary Medicine; Steve Waldham, College of Veterinary Medicine; Paula Harmer, Office of Institutional Research; Linda Niessen, College of Dental Medicine; Robert Trombly, College of Dental Medicine; Lawrence Harkless, Dean College of Podiatric Medicine; Lester Jones, College of Podiatric Medicine; Willard Bleything, College of Optometry.

3 The Expert Panel members included Susan Mackintosh, D.O., M.P.H. and Daniel Robinson, Pharm.D., F.A.S.H.P, of WesternU as well as Susan M. Meyer,

RPh, Ph.D., Leo E. Rouse, D.D.S., F.A.C.D., Andrew A. Sorensen, Ph.D., M.P.H. Chair, Thomas R. Viggiano, M.D., M.Ed. and Deanna Wathington, M.D., M.P.H., F.A.A.F.P..

4 While the number of students enrolled in IPE grew from 800+ at inception to nearly 1,000 on the Pomona campus, the program has been challenged by a static number of rooms and a limited number of facilitators. Whereas the initial ideal team size was envisioned to be nine students plus one facilitator, teams have had to grow in size in order to accommodate enrollment. The program has experienced growth pains in terms of physical facilities and available faculty to serve as facilitators.

Compilation of References

(2005). Bluml, B Definition of Medication Therapy Management. *Development of Professionwide Consensus J Am Pharm Assoc.*, *45*, 566–572. doi:10.1331/1544345055001274

AAMC. (1999). Learning objectives for medical student education–guidelines for medical schools. *Academic Medicine*, *74*(1), 13–18. doi:10.1097/00001888-199901000-00010 PMID:9934288

AboutUs. (2019, October 22). Retrieved from https://www.caipe.org/about-us

Abu-Rish, E., Kim, S., Choe, L., Varpio, L., Malik, E., White, A. A., Craddick, K., Blondon, K., Robins, L., Nagasawa, P., Thigpen, A., Chen, L., Rich, J., & Zierler, B. (2012). Current trends in interprofessional education of health sciences students: A literature review. *Journal of Interprofessional Care*, *2*(6), 444–445. doi:10.3109/13561820.2012.715604 PMID:22924872

Accreditation Council for Pharmacy Education (ACPE). (2016). *Accreditation standards and key elements for the professional program in Pharmacy leading to the Doctor of Pharmacy degree*. Retrieved from https://www.acpe-accredit.org/pdf/Standards2016FINAL.pdf

Accreditation Review Commission on Education for the Physician Assistant, Inc. (2019). *Accreditation Standards for Physician Assistant Education*. Retrieved from http://www.arc-pa.org/wp-content/uploads/2018/06/Standards-4th-Ed-March-2018.pdf

Ackermann, R. T., & Marrero, D. G. (2007). Adapting the Diabetes Prevention Program lifestyle intervention for delivery in the community: The YMCA model. *The Diabetes Educator*, *33*(1), 74–65. doi:10.1177/0145721706297743 PMID:17272794

Adams, R., Hebert, C. J., McVey, L., & Williams, R. (2016). Implementation of the YMCA Diabetes Prevention Program throughout an Integrated Health System: A Translational Study. *The Permanente Journal*, *20*(4), 82–86. doi:10.7812/TPP/15-241 PMID:27828773

Aebersold, M., Tschannen, D., & Sculli, G. (2013). Improving nursing student's communication skills using crew resource management strategies. *The Journal of Nursing Education*, *52*(3), 125–130. doi:10.3928/01484834-20130205-01 PMID:23380022

Agency for Healthcare Research and Quality (AHRQ). (n.d.). Retrieved December 11, 2019, from https://www.ahrq.gov/

Agency for Healthcare Research and Quality. (2017). *Assessment tools for palliative care. Technical Brief Number 30.* Retrieved from https://effectivehealthcare.ahrq.gov/sites/default/files/pdf/palliative-care-tools_technical-brief-2017.pdf

Agency for Healthcare Research and Quality. (n.d.). *TeamSTEPPS®.* https://www.ahrq.gov/teamstepps/index.html

Aguirre, E., Castellanos, F., Galicia, H., González, A., Fabián, O., Ojeda, C., Sánchez, J., Servin, D., Vargas, R. C., & Vázquez, J. (2012). *Perfil por competencias docentes del profesor de medicina.* Asociación Mexicana de Facultades y Escuelas de Medicina.

AHIMA. (n.d.). *Telehealth and Relaxed HIPAA Enforcement During COVID-19.* Retrieved from https://journal.ahima.org/ahima-special-update-telehealth-and-relaxed-hipaa-enforcement-during-covid-19/

AI Models. (n.d.). Center for Healthcare Strategies Web site: https://www.chcs.org/project/advancing-integrated-models/

Alicke, M. D., & Govorun, O. (2005). The Better-Than-Average Effect. In M. D. Alicke, D. A. Dunning, & J. I. Krueger (Eds.), *Studies in self and identity. The Self in Social Judgment* (pp. 85–106). Psychology Press.

Allport, G. W. (1954). *The nature of prejudice.* AddisonWesley.

Al-Sowygh, Z. H. (2013). Academic distress perceived stress and coping strategies among dental students in Saudi Arabia. *The Saudi Dental Journal, 25*(3), 97–105. doi:10.1016/j.sdentj.2013.05.002 PMID:24179318

American Academy of Pediatrics Section on Ophthalmology. (2009). Joint statement—Learning disabilities, dyslexia, and vision. *Pediatrics, 124*(2), 837–844. doi:10.1542/peds.2009-1445 PMID:19651597

American Diabetes Association. (2015). Standards of Medical Care in Diabetes—2015: Summary of Revisions. *Diabetes Care, 38*(Suppl. 1), S4. doi:10.2337/dc15-S003

American Diabetes Association. (2016). Classification and diagnosis of diabetes. Sec. 2. In Standards of Medical Care in Diabetes. *Diabetes Care, 39*(Suppl. 1), S13–S22. doi:10.2337/dc16-S005 PMID:27555625

American Diabetes Association. (2018). Economic costs of diabetes in the U.S. in 2017. *Diabetes Care, 41*(5), 917–928. doi:10.2337/dci18-0007 PMID:29567642

American Geriatric Society. (2019). *Existing formal geriatric competencies and milestones.* Accessed June 13, 2019 from https://www.americangeriatrics.org/geriatrics-profession/core-competencies

American Institutes for Research. (2010). *TeamSTEPPS Teamwork Perceptions Questionnaire (TPQ).* Manual.

American Medical Association. (2019). *Prevent Diabetes STAT*. Retrieved from http://www.ama-assn.org/sub/prevent-diabetes-stat/

American Optometric Association. (1997). *Vision, learning and dyslexia*. Retrieved from https://cdn.ymaws.com/www.covd.org/resource/resmgr/position_papers/vision-learning-dyslexia_-_j.pdf

American Optometric Association. (1999). *Vision Therapy Information for Health Care and Other Allied Professionals*. Retrieved from https://cdn.ymaws.com/www.covd.org/resource/resmgr/position_papers/vision-therapy_-_jops_aao_&_.pdf

American Optometric Association. (2007). *Optometric Clinical Practice Guideline Care of the Patient with Visual Impairment (Low Vision Rehabilitation)*. Retrieved from https://www.aoa.org/documents/optometrists/CPG-14.pdf

American Optometric Association. (2009). *Definition of optometric vision therapy*. Retrieved from https://www.aoa.org/Documents/CRG/definition-of-optometric-vision-therapy.pdf

American Optometric Association. (2015). *AOA Optometric Clinical Practice Guidelines- Adult Eye Exam*. Retrieved from https://www.aoa.org/optometrists/tools-and-resources/clinical-care-publications/clinical-practice-guidelines

American Optometric Association. (2017). *Evidence-Based Clinical Practice Guideline: Comprehensive Pediatric Eye and Vision Examination*. Retrieved from http://aoa.uberflip.com/i/807465-cpg-pediatric-eye-and-vision-examination/0?m4=

American Optometric Association. (n.d.a). Retrieved from https://www.aoa.org/optometrists/tools-and-resources/vision-rehabilitation/neuro

American Optometric Association. (n.d.b). *Low Vision. American Optometric Association. Realeyes Program*. Retrieved from https://www.aoa.org/the-realeyes-program

American Optometric Association. (n.d.c). *Sports & Performance Vision*. Retrieved from https://www.aoa.org/optometrists/tools-and-resources/sports-and-performance-vision

American Optometric Association. (n.d.d). *What is a Doctor of Optometry?* Retrieved from https://www.aoa.org/about-the-aoa/what-is-a-doctor-of-optometry

Amodio, D., & Ratner, K. (2011). A memory systems model of implicit social cognition. *Current Directions in Psychological Science*, *20*(3), 143–148. doi:10.1177/0963721411408562

Appelbaum, L. G., & Erickson, G. (2018). Sports vision training: A review of the state-of-the-art in digital training techniques. *International Review of Sport and Exercise Psychology*, *11*(1), 160–189. doi:10.1080/1750984X.2016.1266376

Apple. (2010). *Challenge Based Learning: A Classroom Guide*. Apple Inc.

Aravamudhan, R., Vitek, M., & Casser, L. (2015). The Implementation and Assessment of an Interprofessional Education Initiative at Salus University. *Optometric Education*, *40*(3), 11–15.

Association of American Medical Colleges. (2017). *Core entrustable professional activities for entering residency*. https://www.aamc.org/download/484778/data/epa13toolkit.pdf

Association of Schools and Colleges of Optometry. (n.d.). *Interprofessional Education and Collaborative Practice*. Retrieved from https://optometriceducation.org/interprofessional-education/

Aston, S. J., Rheault, W., Arenson, C. F., Tappert, S., Stoeker, J., Orzoff, J., Galitski, H., & Mackintosh, S. (2012). Interprofessional education: A review and analysis of programs from three academic health centers. *Academic Medicine*, *87*(7), 949–955. doi:10.1097/ACM.0b013e3182583374 PMID:22622216

Aston, S., Mackintosh, S., & Orzoff, J. (2010). Interprofessional Education program, Western University of Health Sciences. *Journal of Allied Health*, *39*(Suppl1), e137–e138. PMID:21174033

Aveiro, M. F., Castro, M., Martins, C., Costa, A. D., Castro, J. F., Veronese, M. L., & Almedia, L. E. (2009). Group mentoring for junior Medical students: Perceptions of mentees and mentors. *Revista Brasileira de Educação Médica*, *33*(4), 670–675. doi:10.1590/S0100-55022009000400019

Avorn, J. (1990). The elderly and drug policy: Coming of age. *Health Affairs*, *9*(3), 6–19. doi:10.1377/hlthaff.9.3.6 PMID:2121636

Azer, S. (2008). *Navigating problem-based learning*. Elsevier.

Baggs, J. G., Schmitt, M. H., Mushlin, A. I., Mitchell, P. H., Eldredge, D. H., Oakes, D., & Hutson, A. D. (1999). Association between nurse-physician collaboration and patient outcomes in three intensive care units. *Critical Care Medicine*, *27*(9), 1991–1998. doi:10.1097/00003246-199909000-00045 PMID:10507630

Baker, D. P., Gustafson, S., Beaubien, J., Salas, E., & Barach, P. (2003, October 20). *Medical Teamwork and Patient Safety: The Evidence-Based Relation*. Rockville, MD: Agency for Healthcare Research and Quality. Available from: https://archive.ahrq.gov/research/findings/final-reports/medteam/medteamwork.pdf

Balasubramanian, M., Short, S. D., & Gallagher, J. E. (2018). Dental professionals for a new century: Transforming dentistry through interprofessional education and collaborative practice. *Indian Journal of Dental Research*, *29*(4), 401–403. doi:10.4103/ijdr.IJDR_495_18 PMID:30127184

Barnsteiner, J. H., Disch, J. M., Hall, L., Mayer, D., & Moore, S. M. (2007). Promoting interprofessional education. *Nursing Outlook*, *55*(3), 144–150. doi:10.1016/j.outlook.2007.03.003 PMID:17524802

Barr, H., Gray, R., Helme, M., Low, H., & Reeves, S. (2016). *CAIPE- Interprofessional Education Guidelines: Centre for Advancement of Interprofessional Education*. Available from: https://www.caipe.org/resources/publications/barr-h-grayr-helmem-low-h-reeves-2016-interprofessional-education-guidelines

Barr, H. (2009). Interprofessional education as an emerging concept. In *Interprofessional education: Making it happen*. Palgrave Macmillan. doi:10.1007/978-1-137-08028-8_1

Barr, H. (2014). *Leading the way: Leadership Development for Interprofessional Education and Practice* (D. Forman, M. Jones, & J. E. Thistlethwaite, Eds.). Palgrave.

Barr, H., Koppel, I., Reeves, S., Hammick, M., & Freeth, D. (2005). *Effective interprofessional education: argument, assumption and evidence*. Blackwell. doi:10.1002/9780470776445

Barrows, H., & Tamblin, R. (1980). *Problem based Learning*. Springer Publications.

Barry, C. N., Abraham, K. M., Weaver, K. R., & Bowersox, N. W. (2016). Innovating Team-Based Outpatient Mental health Care in the Veterans Health Administration: Staff-Perceived Benefits and Challenges to Pilot Implementation of the Behavioral health Interdisciplinary Program (BHIP). *Psychological Services*, *13*(2), 148–155. doi:10.1037er0000072 PMID:27148949

Basehore, P. M., Mortensen, L. H., Katsaros, E. P., Linsenmeyer, M., McClain, E. K., Sexton, P. S., & Wadsworth, N. (2017). Entrustable Professional Activities for Entering Residency: Establishing Common Osteopathic Performance Standards in the Transition From Medical School to Residency. *The Journal of the American Osteopathic Association*, *117*(11), 712–718. doi:10.7556/jaoa.2017.137 PMID:29084324

Basehore, P., Soper, E., Getz, R., Graneto, J., Hover, M., Kalousek, K., Katsaros, E., Kaufmann, J., Langenau, E., Linsenmeyer, M., Mehdi, S., Sexton, P., & Told, T. (2016). *Osteopathic Considerations for Core Entrustable Professional Activities (EPAs) for Entering Residency*. American Association of Colleges of Osteopathic Medicine. http://www. aacom.org/docs/default-source/med-ed-presentations/core-epas.pdf ? sfvrsn=20

Bauer, A., Berkley-Patton, J., Bowe-Thompson, C., & Christensen, K. (2018). Predictors and missed opportunities for blood glucose screening among African Americans: Implications for church-based populations. *Journal of Health Disparities Research and Practice*, *12*(2), 4.

Baxi, G., & Palekar, T. (2015). Health science teacher's attitude towards interprofessional education. *National Journal of Integrated Research in Medicine*, *6*(3), 84–87.

Béland, F., Bergman, H., Lebel, P., Clarfield, A.M., Tousignant, P., Contandriopoulos, A.P., & Dallaire, L. (2006). A System of Integrated Care for Older persons with disabilities in Canada: a randomized, controlled trial. *J Gerontol A Biol Sci Med Sci.*, *61*(4), 367–73.

Bell, D. Jr. (2009, July). The Role of Podiatry in Wound Management. *The Journal of the American College of Certified Wound Specialists*, *1*(3), 78–79. doi:10.1016/j.jcws.2009.05.003 PMID:24527119

Benefits of IPE/C. (n.d.). Retrieved from https://education2practice.org/benefits-of-ipec/

Benner, P. (1982). From novice to expert. *The American Journal of Nursing*, *82*(3), 402–409. PMID:6917683

Benor, D. E. (2014). A New Paradigm Is Needed for Medical Education in the Mid-Twenty-First Century and Beyond: Are We Ready? *Rambam Maimonides Medical Journal*, *5*(3), e0018. doi:10.5041/RMMJ.10152 PMID:25120918

Berkley-Patton, J., Bowe Thompson, C., Bauer, A., Berman, M., Bradley-Ewing, A., & ... . (2018a). Using faith community engagement to increase reach and impact of a diabetes/CVD health promotion intervention in African American churches. *Annals of Behavioral Medicine*, *52*(Suppl 1), S2.

Berkley-Patton, J., Bowe Thompson, C., Bradley-Ewing, A., Berman, M., Booker, A., & .... (2018b). Identifying health conditions, priorities, and relevant multilevel health promotion intervention strategies in African American churches: A faith community health needs assessment. *Evaluation and Program Planning*, *31*(67), 19–28. doi:10.1016/j.evalprogplan.2017.10.012 PMID:29156312

Berman, A. M. (1993). Clinical evaluation of the athlete. *Optometry Clinics*, *3*(1), 1–26. PMID:8324319

Bernabei, R., Landi, F., Gambassi, G., Sgadari, A., Zuccala, G., Mor, V., Rubenstein, L. Z., & Carbonin, P. (1998). Randomised trial of impact of model of integrated care and case management for older people living in the community. *BMJ (Clinical Research Ed.)*, *316*(7141), 1348–1351. doi:10.1136/bmj.316.7141.1348 PMID:9563983

Berwick, D. M., Nolan, T. W., & Whittington, J. (2008). The triple aim: Care, health, and cost. *Health Affairs*, *27*(3), 759–769. doi:10.1377/hlthaff.27.3.759 PMID:18474969

Berwick, D., & Finkelstein, J. (2010). Preparing medical students for the continual improvement of health and health care: Abraham Flexner and the New "Public Interest". *Academic Medicine*, *85*, S56–S65. doi:10.1097/ACM.0b013e3181ead779 PMID:20736631

Bhatia, A., Singh, N., & Dhaliwal, U. (2013). Mentoring for first year medical students: Humanising medical education. *Indian Journal of Medical Ethics*, (2). Advance online publication. doi:10.20529/IJME.2013.030 PMID:23697488

Bhugra, D., Till, A., & Sartorius, N. (2013). What is mental health? *The International Journal of Social Psychiatry*, *59*(1), 3–4. doi:10.1177/0020764012463315 PMID:23349505

Bias. (2019). In *Macmillan dictionary*. Retrieved September 10,2019, from https://www.macmillandictionary.com/dictionary/british/biasMacmillan

Bias. (2019). In *Merriam-Webster.com*. Retrieved September 10, 2019, from https://www.merriam-webster.com/dictionary/biasmerriam-webster

Binder, F. V., Nichols, M., Reinehr, S. S., & Malucelli, A. (2017). Challenge Based Learning Applied to Mobile Software Development Teaching. *The 30th IEEE Conference on Software Engineering Education and Training*, 57-64.

Blair, I. V., Ma, J. E., & Lenton, A. P. (2001). Imagining stereotypes away: The moderation of implicit stereotypes through mental imagery. *Journal of Personality and Social Psychology*, *81*(5), 828–841. doi:10.1037/0022-3514.81.5.828 PMID:11708560

Blind, A. F. t. (n.d.). *Blindness and Low Vision*. Retrieved from https://www.afb.org/blindness-and-low-vision

Blowers, A. N., Davis, B., Shenk, D., Kalaw, K., Smith, M., & Jackson, K. (2012). A multidisciplinary approach to detecting and responding to elder mistreatment: Creating a university-community partnership. *American Journal of Criminal Justice*, *37*(2), 276–290. doi:10.100712103-012-9156-4

Blue, A. V., Mitcham, M., Smith, T., Raymond, J., & Greenberg, R. (2010). Changing the future of health professions: Embedding interprofessional education within an academic health center. *Academic Medicine*, *85*(8), 1290–1295. doi:10.1097/ACM.0b013e3181e53e07 PMID:20671454

Bodenheimer, T., & Sinsky, C. (2014). From Tripe to Quadruple Aim: Care of the patient requires care of the provider. *Annal Family Med*, *12*(6), 573-576.

Boltri, J. M., Davis-Smith, M., Okosun, I. S., Seale, J. P., & Foster, B. (2011). Translation of the National Institutes of Health Diabetes Prevention Program in African American churches. *Journal of the National Medical Association*, *103*(3), 194–202. doi:10.1016/S0027-9684(15)30301-1 PMID:21671523

Borsting, E., Mitchell, G. L., Kulp, M. T., Scheiman, M., Amster, D. M., Cotter, S., ... Group, C. S. (2012). Improvement in academic behaviors after successful treatment of convergence insufficiency. *Optometry and Vision Science*, *89*(1), 12–18. doi:10.1097/OPX.0b013e318238ffc3 PMID:22080400

Boult, C., Kane, R. L., Pacala, J. T., & Wagner, E. H. (1999). Innovative healthcare for chronically ill older persons: Results of a national survey. *The American Journal of Managed Care*, *5*, 1162–1172. PMID:10621082

Bourne, R. R. A., Flaxman, S. R., Braithwaite, T., Cicinelli, M. V., Das, A., Jonas, J. B., ... Vision Loss Expert, G. (2017). Magnitude, temporal trends, and projections of the global prevalence of blindness and distance and near vision impairment: A systematic review and meta-analysis. *The Lancet. Global Health*, *5*(9), e888–e897. doi:10.1016/S2214-109X(17)30293-0 PMID:28779882

Bowe Thompson, C., Ruhland Petty, T., Berkley-Patton, J., & Berman, M., C., Booker, A., et al. (2015, November). *Project FIT (Faith Influencing Transformation): The Good, the Bad, and the Ugly of Sunday Morning Health Screenings in African American Churches.* Paper presented at the 143rd Annual Meeting and Scientific Session of the American Public Health Association, Chicago, IL.

Bradley, P. (2006). The history of simulation in medical education and possible future directions. *Medical Education*, *40*(3), 254–262. doi:10.1111/j.1365-2929.2006.02394.x PMID:16483328

Brandt, B., Lutfiyya, M. N., King, J. A., & Chioreso, C. (2014). A scoping review of interprofessional collaborative practice and education using the lens of the Triple Aim. *Journal of Interprofessional Care*, *28*(5), 393–399. doi:10.3109/13561820.2014.906391 PMID:24702046

Brennan, D. S., Balasubramanian, M., & Spencer, A. J. (2015). Trends in dental service provision in Australia: 1983-1984 to 2009-2010. *International Dental Journal*, *65*(1), 39–44. doi:10.1111/idj.12141 PMID:25371293

Bridgeman, M. B., Rusay, M., Afran, J., Yeh, D. S., & Sturgill, M. G. (2018). Impact of an interprofessional medication error workshop on healthcare student perceptions. *Currents in Pharmacy Teaching & Learning*, *10*(7), 975–981. doi:10.1016/j.cptl.2018.04.013 PMID:30236436

Brukner, H. (1999). Giving effective feedback to medical students: A workshop for faculty and house staff. *Medical Teacher*, *21*(2), 161–166. doi:10.1080/01421599979798 PMID:21275731

Brunisholz, K. D., Kim, J., Savitz, L. A., Hashibe, M., Gren, L. H., Hamilton, S., Huynh, K., & Joy, E. A. (2017). A formative evaluation of a diabetes prevention program using the RE-AIM framework in a learning health care system, Utah, 2013-2015. *Preventing Chronic Disease*, *14*(E58), 160556. doi:10.5888/pcd14.160556 PMID:28727546

Buckholtz, R. (2017, September 27). *Looking at new ICD-10-CM Codes for Blindness*. Retrieved from https://www.icd10monitor.com/looking-at-new-icd-10-cm-codes-for-blindness

Budning, A., & El-Defrawy, S. (2016). Interprofessional collaboration in eye health care. *Canadian Journal of Ophthalmology*, *51*(3), 130–132. doi:10.1016/j.jcjo.2016.04.007 PMID:27316255

Buff, S. M., Jenkins, K., Kern, D., Worrall, C., Howell, D., Martin, K., & Blue, A. (2015). Interprofessional service-learning in a community setting: Findings from a pilot study. *Journal of Interprofessional Care*, *29*(2), 159–161. doi:10.3109/13561820.2014.934956 PMID:25003549

Buhse, M., & Della Ratta, C. (2017). Enhancing Interprofessional Education with Team-Based Learning. *Nurse Educator*, *42*(5), 240–244. doi:10.1097/NNE.0000000000000370 PMID:28252549

Buring, S. M., Bhushan, A., Broeseker, A., Conway, S., Duncan-Hewitt, W., Hansen, L., & Westberg, S. (2009). Interprofessional education: Definitions, student competencies, and guidelines for implementation. *American Journal of Pharmaceutical Education*, *73*(4), 59. doi:10.5688/aj730459 PMID:19657492

Byrne, N., & Cohen, R. (1973). Observational study of clinical clerkship activities. *Academic Medicine*, *48*(10), 919–927. doi:10.1097/00001888-197310000-00005 PMID:4728311

CAIPE. (2002). *Defining IPE.* Available at: http://caipe.org.uk/about-us/defining-ipe

Callahan, C. M., Boustani, M. A., Unverzagt, F. W., Austrom, M. G., Damush, T. M., Perkins, A. J., Fultz, B. A., Hui, S. L., Counsell, S. R., & Hendrie, H. C. (2006). Effectiveness of collaborative care for older adults with Alzheimer disease in primary care: A randomized controlled trial. *Journal of the American Medical Association*, *295*(18), 2148–2157. doi:10.1001/jama.295.18.2148 PMID:16684985

Callahan, D. (1998). Managed Care and the Goals of Medicine. *Journal of the American Geriatrics Society*, *46*(3), 385–388. doi:10.1111/j.1532-5415.1998.tb01060.x PMID:9514393

Campbell, J. C., Coben, J. H., McLoughlin, E., Dearwater, S., Nah, G., Glass, N., Lee, D., & Durborow, N. (2001). An Evaluation of a System-change Training Model to Improve Emergency Department Response to Battered Women. *Academic Emergency Medicine*, *8*(2), 131–138. doi:10.1111/j.1553-2712.2001.tb01277.x PMID:11157288

Canadian Interprofessional Health Collaborative. (2010). *A National Interprofessional Competency Framework*. University of British Columbia. Retrieved from http://www.cihc.ca/files/CIHC_IPCompetencies_Feb1210.pdf

Canadian Interprofessional Health Collaborative. (2012). *An inventory of quantitative tools measuring interprofessional education and collaborative practice outcomes*. Retrieved from http://cihc.ca

Capacity. (2019). In *Merriam-Webster.com*. Retrieved September 1, 2019 from https://www.merriam-webster.com/dictionary/capacity

Capella, J., Smith, S., Philp, A., Putnam, T., Gilbert, C., Fry, W., Harvey, E., Wright, A., Henderson, K., Baker, D., Ranson, S., & ReMine, S. (2010). Teamwork training improves the clinical care of trauma patients. *Journal of Surgical Education*, *67*(6), 439–443. doi:10.1016/j.jsurg.2010.06.006 PMID:21156305

Capoccia, K. L., Boudreau, D. M., Blough, D. K., Ellsworth, A. J., Clark, D. R., Stevens, N. G., Katon, W. J., & Sullivan, S. D. (2004). Randomized trial of pharmacist interventions to improve depression care and outcomes in primary care. *American Journal of Health-System Pharmacy*, *61*(4), 364–372. doi:10.1093/ajhp/61.4.364 PMID:15011764

Carels, R. A., Darby, L., Cacciapaglia, H. M., Konrad, K., Coit, C., Harper, J., Kaplar, M. E., Young, K., Baylen, C. A., & Versland, A. (2007). Using motivational interviewing as a supplement to obesity treatment: A stepped-care approach. *Health Psychology*, *26*(3), 369–374. doi:10.1037/0278-6133.26.3.369 PMID:17500624

Carney, P. A., Thayer, E. K., Palmer, R., Galper, A. B., Zierler, B., & Eiff, M. P. (2019). The benefits of interprofessional learning and teamwork in primary care ambulatory training settings. *Journal of Interprofessional Education & Practice*, *15*, 119–126. doi:10.1016/j.xjep.2019.03.011

Centers for Disease Control and Prevention. (1996). *International Classification of Diseases, Ninth Revision, Clinical Modification (ICD-9-CM)*. Retrieved from https://www.cdc.gov/nchs/icd/icd9cm.htm

Centers for Disease Control and Prevention. (2013a). CDC health disparities and inequalities report – United States 2011. Diabetes— United States, 2006 and 2010. *Morbidity and Mortality Weekly Report*, *62*(Suppl 3), 99–104.

Centers for Disease Control and Prevention. (2013b). CDC health disparities and inequalities report – United States 2011. Obesity— United States, 1999–2010. *Morbidity and Mortality Weekly Report*, *62*(Suppl 3), 120–128.

Centers for Disease Control and Prevention. (2017). *National diabetes statistics report: estimates of diabetes and its burden in the United States, 2017*. Atlanta, GA: U.S. Department of Health and Human Services, Centers for Disease Control and Prevention. Retrieved from https://www.cdc.gov/diabetes/data/statistics/statistics-report.html

Centers for Disease Control and Prevention. (2018a). *Screen & Refer Patients to a Lifestyle Change Program*. Retrieved from https://www.cdc.gov/diabetes/prevention/why-refer.html

Centers for Disease Control and Prevention. (2018b). *National Diabetes Prevention Program. Curricula and Handouts*. Retrieved from https://www.cdc.gov/diabetes/prevention/resources/curriculum.html

Centers for Disease Control and Prevention. (n.d.). *Keep an Eye on Your Vision Health*. Retrieved from https://www.cdc.gov/features/healthyvision/index.html

Centers for Disease Control and Prevention. (n.d.). *Public Health Professionals Gateway*. https://www.cdc.gov/publichealthgateway/publichealthservices/essentialhealthservices.html

Centers for Disease Control. (2016). *Health U.S. Chartbook on Long-term Trends Report 2016*, pg. 25. Retrieved from https://www.cdc.gov/nchs/data/hus/hus16.pdf

Centers for Medicare & Medicaid Services Documentation requirements for inpatient rehabilitation (A18990). (n.d.). http://www.wvtra.org/conference/2006/Veritus_IRF.doc

Centre for the Advancement of Interprofessional Education (CAIPE). (1997). Interprofessional education - a definition. *CAIPE Bulletin, 13*, 19. Retrieved from www.caipe.org/resources/publications/archived

Chakrabarti, O. (2019). Telehealth: Emerging evidence on efficiency. *International Review of Economics & Finance, 60*, 257–264. doi:10.1016/j.iref.2018.10.021

Challis, D., Darton, R., Johnson, L., Stone, M., & Traske, K. (1991). An evaluation of an alternative to long-stay hospital care for frail elderly patients: II. Costs and effectiveness. *Age and Ageing, 20*(4), 245–254. doi:10.1093/ageing/20.4.245 PMID:1656718

Chan, C. Y. Z. (2013). Critical thinking and creativity in nursing: Learners' perspectives. *Nurse Education Today, 33*(5), 558–563. doi:10.1016/j.nedt.2012.09.007 PMID:23058105

Charles, G., Bainbridge, L., & Gilbert, J. (2010). The University of British Columbia model of interprofessional education. *Journal of Interprofessional Care, 24*(1), 9–18. doi:10.3109/13561820903294549 PMID:20001544

Chen, A. S., Yau, B., Revere, L., & Swails, J. (2019). Implementation, evaluation, and outcome of TeamSTEPPS in interprofessional education: a scoping review. *Journal of Interprofessional Care*. Advanced online publication. https://doi:10.1080/13561820.2019.1594729

Chen, H. C., van der Broek, W. E. S., & ten Cate, O. (2015). The Case for Use of Entrustable Professional Activities in Undergraduate Medical Education. *Academic Medicine, 90*(4), 431-436. https://www.cdc.gov/onehealth/index.html

Choi, B., & Pak, A. (2007). Multidisciplinarity, interdisciplinarity, and transdisciplinarity in health research, services, education and policy: 2. Promotors, barriers, and strategies of enhancement. *Clinical and Investigative Medicine. Medecine Clinique et Experimentale, 30*(6), E224–E232. doi:10.25011/cim.v30i6.2950 PMID:18053389

Chorazy, M. L., & Klinedinst, K. S. (2019). Learn by doing: A model for incorporating high-impact experiential learning into an undergraduate public health curriculum. *Frontiers in Public Health*, *7*, 31. doi:10.3389/fpubh.2019.00031 PMID:30863743

Christian, L. W., MacIver, S., & Alfieri, M. (2015). Evaluation of Interprofessional Education and Collaboration in Optometry. *Optometric Education*, *40*(3), 16–22.

Clark, A. (2018). What does Alzheiumer's Disease feel like? *The Senior List*. Retrieved from https://www.theseniorlist.com/blog/patented-tool-provides-a-glimpse-into-the-world-of-alzheimers-disease/

Clark, K. M. (2018). Interprofessional education: Making our way out of the silos. *Respiratory Care*, *63*(5), 637–639. doi:10.4187/respcare.06234 PMID:29703797

Coggeshall, L. T. (1966). Planning for medical progress through education. *Journal of the American Medical Association*, *197*(11), 909–912. doi:10.1001/jama.1966.03110110133032 PMID:5952783

Cohen, A. B., Wright, M. S., Cooney, L. Jr, & Fried, T. (2015). Guardianship and end-of-life decision making. *Journal of the American Medical Association. Internal Medicine (Tokyo, Japan)*, *175*(10), 1687–1691.

Cohen, E. V., Hagestuen, R., González-Ramos, G., Cohen, H. W., Bassich, C., Book, E., Bradley, K. P., Carter, J. H., Di Minno, M., Gardner, J., Giroux, M., González, M. J., Holten, S., Joseph, R., Kornegay, D. D., Simpson, P. A., Tomaino, C. M., Vandendolder, R. P., Walde-Douglas, M., ... Morgan, J. C. (2016). Interprofessional education increases knowledge, promotes team building, and changes practice in the care of Parkinson's disease. *Parkinsonism & Related Disorders*, *22*, 21–27. doi:10.1016/j.parkreldis.2015.11.001 PMID:26620547

Cohen, L. C., Dahlen, G., Escobar, A., Fejerskov, O., Johnson, N. W., & Manji, F. (2017). Dentistry in crisis: Time to change. La cascada declaration. *Australian Dental Journal*, *62*(3), 258–260. doi:10.1111/adj.12546 PMID:28793371

Cohen, L. C., Dahlen, G., Escobar, A., Fejerskov, O., Johnson, N. W., & Manji, F. (2017). Why a radical overhaul of dentistry is needed. *Indian Journal of Dental Research*, *28*(5), 471–474. doi:10.4103/ijdr.IJDR_449_17 PMID:29072204

Coleman, K., & Reid, R. (2013). Continuous and team-based healing relationships: improving patient care through teams. In K. E. Phillips & V. Weir (Eds.), *Safety Net Medical Home Initiative Implementation Guide Series* (2nd ed.). Qualis Health and The MacColl Center for Health Care Innovation at the Group Health Research Institute.

Colenbrander, A. (2010). Assessment of functional vision and its rehabilitation. *Acta Ophthalmologica*, *88*(2), 163–173. doi:10.1111/j.1755-3768.2009.01670.x PMID:20039847

College of Optometrists in Vision Development. (n.d.a). *Locate a Doctor*. Retrieved from https://www.covd.org

College of Optometrists in Vision Development. (n.d.b). *Research on Vision Therapy*. Retrieved from https://www.covd.org/page/research

Committee on Improving the Quality of Cancer Care. (2013). *Addressing the Challenges of an Aging Population; Board on Health Care Services*. Washington, DC: National Academies Press. Available from: https://www.ncbi.nlm.nih.gov/books/NBK202149/

Competence. (2019). In *Merriam-Webster.com*. Retrieved September 1, 2019 from https://www.merriam-webster.com/dictionary/competence

Congdon, N., O'Colmain, B., Klaver, C. C., Klein, R., Munoz, B., & Friedman, D. S. (2004). Causes and prevalence of visual impairment among adults in the United States. *Archives of Ophthalmology*, *122*(4), 477–485. doi:10.1001/archopht.122.4.477 PMID:15078664

Cook, A. F., Arora, V. M., Rasinski, K. A., Curlin, F. A., & Yoon, J. D. (2014). The Prevalence of Medical Student Mistreatment and Its Association with Burnout. *Academic Medicine*, *89*(5), 749–754. doi:10.1097/ACM.0000000000000204 PMID:24667503

Cook, D. A. (2005). Models of interprofessional learning in Canada. *Journal of Interprofessional Care*, *19*(sup1), 107–115. doi:10.1080/13561820500082354 PMID:16096149

Coombs, B. (n.d.). *Telehealth visits are booming as doctors and patients embrace distancing amid the coronavirus crisis*. Retrieved from https://www.cnbc.com/2020/04/03/telehealth-visits-could-top-1-billion-in-2020-amid-the-coronavirus-crisis.html

Coster, S., Norman, I., Murrells, T., Kitchen, S., Meerabeau, E., Sooboodoo, E., & d'Avray, L. (2008). Interprofessional attitudes amongst undergraduate students in the health professions: A longitudinal questionnaire survey. *International Journal of Nursing Studies*, *45*(11), 1667–1681. doi:10.1016/j.ijnurstu.2008.02.008 PMID:18423644

Courtenay, M., Nancarrow, S., & Dawson, D. (2013). Interprofessional teamwork in the trauma setting: A scoping review. *Human Resources for Health*, *11*(1), 57. doi:10.1186/1478-4491-11-57 PMID:24188523

Craddock, D., O'Halloran, C., Borthwick, A., & McPherson, K. (2006). Interprofessional education in health and social care: Fashion or informed practice. *Learning in Health and Social Care*, *5*(4), 220–242. doi:10.1111/j.1473-6861.2006.00135.x

Curran, V. R., Sharpe, D., & Forristall, J. (2007). Attitudes of health sciences students towards interprofessional teamwork and education. *Medical Education*, *41*(9), 892–896. doi:10.1111/j.1365-2923.2007.02823.x PMID:17696982

Dacey, M., Kennedy, M., Polak, R., & Phillips, E. (2014). Physical activity counseling in medical school education: A systematic review. *Medical Education Online*, *19*(1), 24325. doi:10.3402/meo.v19.24325 PMID:25062944

Dall, T. M., Mann, S. E., Zhang, S., Quick, W. W., Seifert, R. F., Martin, J., Huang, E. A., & Zhang, S. (2009). Distinguishing the economic costs associated with type 1 and type 2 diabetes. *Population Health Management*, *12*(2), 103–110. doi:10.1089/pop.2009.12203 PMID:19361253

Dall, T. M., Roary, M., Yang, W., Zhang, S., Chen, Y. J., & .... (2011). Health care use and costs for participants in a diabetes disease management program, United States, 2007-2008. *Preventing Chronic Disease*, *8*(3), A53. PMID:21477493

D'Amour, D., Ferrada-Videla, M., San Martin Rodriguez, L., & Beaulieu, M. (2005). The conceptual basis for interprofessional collaboration: Core concepts and theoretical frameworks. *Journal of Interprofessional Care, 19*(sup1), 116-131.

Dargahi, H., Shirazi, M., & Yazdanparast, S. A. (2012). Interprofessional learning: The attitudes of medical, nursing and pharmacy students to shared learning at Tehran University of Medical Sciences. *Thrita J Med Sci*, *1*(2), 44–48. doi:10.5812/thrita.5203

Davis-Smith, M. (2007). Implementing a diabetes prevention program in a rural African-American church. *Journal of the National Medical Association*, *99*, 440–446. PMID:17444435

De Bono, E. (2016). *Six Thinking Hats*. Penguin UK.

DeCaporale-Ryan, L. N., Ahmed-Sarwar, N., Upham, R., Mahler, K., & Lashway, K. (2017). Reducing Hospital Readmission Through Team-Based Primary Care: A 7-Week Pilot Study Integrating Behavioral health and Pharmacy. *Families, Systems & Health*, *35*(2), 217–226. doi:10.1037/fsh0000269 PMID:28617022

Deslauriers, L., McCarty, L. S., Miller, K., Callaghan, K., & Kestin, G. (2019). Measuring actual learning versus the feeling of learning in response to being actively engaged in the classroom. *Proceedings of the National Academy of Sciences*. 10.1073/pnas.1821936116

Diabetes Prevention Program Research Group. (2002). Reduction in the incidence of Type 2 diabetes with lifestyle intervention or metformin. *The New England Journal of Medicine*, *346*(6), 393–403. doi:10.1056/NEJMoa012512 PMID:11832527

Diabetes Prevention Program Research Group. (2004). Achieving weight and activity goals among Diabetes Prevention Program Lifestyle participants. *Obesity Research*, *12*(9), 1426–1434. doi:10.1038/oby.2004.179 PMID:15483207

Dickter, D. N., Stielstra, S., & Lineberry, M. (2015). Interrater reliability of standardized actors versus nonactors in a simulation based assessment of interprofessional collaboration. *Simulation in Healthcare*, *10*(4), 249–255. doi:10.1097/SIH.0000000000000094 PMID:26098494

Dickter, D. N., Stielstra, S., Mackintosh, S., Garner, S., Finocchio, V. A., & Aston, S. J. (2013). Development of the Ambulatory Team Observed Structured Clinical Evaluation (ATOSCE). *Medical Science Educator*, *23*(S3, 3S), 554–558. doi:10.1007/BF03341676

Dodani, S., & Fields, J. Z. (2010). Implementation of the Fit Body and Soul, a church-based life style program for diabetes prevention in high risk African Americans: A feasibility study. *The Diabetes Educator*, *36*(3), 465–472. doi:10.1177/0145721710366756 PMID:20508263

Donahue, S. P., & Nixon, C. N., Section on Opthamology, A. A. o. P., Committee on, P., Ambulatory Medicine, A. A. o. P., American Academy of, O., . . . American Association of Certified, O. (2016). Visual System Assessment in Infants, Children, and Young Adults by Pediatricians. *Pediatrics, 137*(1), 28–30. doi:10.1542/peds.2015-3596 PMID:29756730

Dowd, L., & Smith, J. P. (2015). Incorporating Interprofessional Education into a VA Optometric Residency. *Optometric Education, 40*(3), 38–41.

Downes, M. A., Healy, P., Page, C. B., Bryant, J. L., & Isbister, G. K. (2009). Structured team approach to the agitated patient in the emergency department. *Emergency Medicine Australasia, 21*, 196–202. PMID:19527279

Dubuc, N., Dubois, M., Raîche, M., Gueye, N. R., & Hébert, R. (2011). Meeting the home-care needs of disabled older persons living in the community: Does integrated services delivery make a difference? *BMC Geriatrics, 11*(1), 67. doi:10.1186/1471-2318-11-67 PMID:22029878

Dyrbye, L. N., Thomas, M. R., Massie, F. S., Power, D. V., Eacker, A., Harper, W., Durning, S., Moutier, C., Szydlo, D. W., Novotny, P. J., Sloan, J. A., & Shanafelt, T. D. (2008). Burnout and Suicidal Ideation among U.S. Medical Students. *Annals of Internal Medicine, 149*(5), 334. doi:10.7326/0003-4819-149-5-200809020-00008 PMID:18765703

Eaglehouse, Y. L., Venditti, E. M., Kramer, M. K., Arena, V. C., Vanderwood, K. K., Rockette-Wagner, B., & Kriska, A. M. (2017). Factors related to lifestyle goal achievement in a diabetes prevention program dissemination study. *Translational Behavioral Medicine, 7*(4), 873–880. doi:10.100713142-017-0494-0 PMID:28397158

Eckel, F.M. (2014). Pharmacy Workforce Center's 2014 National Pharmacist Workforce Survey. *Pharmacy Times.*

Educating primary care teams for the future: family medicine and physician assistant interprofessional education. (2012). *The Journal of Physician Assistant Education: The Official Journal Of The Physician Assistant Education Association, 23*(3), 33–41. Retrieved from http://search.ebscohost.com.proxy.library.umkc.edu/login.aspx?direct=true&db=cmedm&AN=23072069&site=eds-live&scope=site

Edwards, S., Molina, P. E., McDonough, K. H., Mercante, D. E., & Gunaldo, T. P. (2018). The potential of interprofessional education to translate physiology curricula effectively into future team-based healthcare. *Advances in Physiology Education, 42*(2), 354–359. doi:10.1152/advan.00183.2017 PMID:29761708

Eliot, K., Carlson, J., Breitbach, A., Gockel-Blessing, E., & Kienstra, K. (2013, Fall). From buy-in to integration: Melding an interprofessional initiative into academic programs in the health professions. *Journal of Allied Health, 42*(3), e67–e73. PMID:24013253

El-Jawahri, A., Greer, J. A., Pirl, W. F., Park, E. R., Jackson, V. A., Back, A. L., Kamdar, M., Jacobsen, J., Chittenden, E. H., Rinaldi, S. P., Gallagher, E. R., Eusebio, J. R., Fishman, S., VanDusen, H., Li, Z., Muzikansky, A., & Temel, J. S. (2017). Effects of Early Integrated Palliative Care on Caregivers of Patients with Lung and Gastrointestinal Cancer: A Randomized Clinical Trial. *The Oncologist*, *22*(12), 1528–1534. doi:10.1634/theoncologist.2017-0227 PMID:28894017

Eng, C., Pedulla, J., Eleazer, G. P., McCann, R., & Fox, N. (1997). Program of All-inclusive Care for the Elderly (PACE): An innovative model of integrated geriatric care and financing [see comments]. *Journal of the American Geriatrics Society*, *45*(2), 223–232. doi:10.1111/j.1532-5415.1997.tb04513.x PMID:9033525

Eraña Rojas, I. E., López Cabrera, M. V., Ríos, E., & Membrillo-Hernández, J. (2019). A challenge-based learning experience in forensic medicine. *Journal of Forensic and Legal Medicine*, *68*, 101873. doi:10.1016/j.jflm.2019.101873 PMID:31627125

Evans, S., Ward, C., Shaw, N., Walker, A., Knight, T., & Sutherland-Smith, W. (n.d.). Interprofessional education and practice guide No. 10: Developing, supporting and sustaining a team of facilitators in online interprofessional education. *Journal of Interprofessional Care, 31*, 1-7. Advanced online publication. https://doi:10.1080/13561820.2019.1632817

Fagin, C. M. (1992). Collaboration between nurses and physicians: No longer a choice. *Academic Medicine*, *67*(5), 295–303. doi:10.1097/00001888-199205000-00002 PMID:1575859

Fernandopulle, R., Ferris, T., Epstein, A., McNeil, B., Newhouse, J., Pisano, G., & Blumenthal, D. (2003). A research agenda for bridging the "quality chasm". *Health Affairs (Project Hope)*, *22*(2), 178–190. doi:10.1377/hlthaff.22.2.178 PMID:12674420

Ferrell, B., Sun, V., Hurria, A., Cristea, M., Raz, D. J., Kim, J. Y., Reckamp, K., Williams, A. C., Borneman, T., Uman, G., & Koczywas, M. (2015). Interdisciplinary Palliative Care for Patients With Lung Cancer. *Journal of Pain and Symptom Management*, *50*(6), 758–767. doi:10.1016/j.jpainsymman.2015.07.005 PMID:26296261

Finley, P. R., Crismon, M. L., & Rush, A. J. (2003). Evaluating the Impact of Pharmacists in Mental Health: A Systematic Review. *Pharmacotherapy*, *23*(12), 1634–1644. doi:10.1592/phco.23.15.1634.31952 PMID:14695043

Finley, P. R., Rens, H. R., Pont, J. T., Gess, S. L., Louie, C., Bull, S. A., Lee, J. Y., & Bero, L. A. (2003). Impact of a Collaborative Care Model on Depression in a Primary Care Setting: A Randomized Controlled Trial. *Pharmacotherapy*, *23*(9), 1175–1185. doi:10.1592/phco.23.10.1175.32760 PMID:14524649

Fisher, N. (2018). The history of hospice: A different kind of health care. *Forbes*. Retrieved from https://www.forbes.com/sites/nicolefisher/2018/06/22/the-history-of-hospice-a-different-kind-of-health-care/#7a072e70660c

Fishman Hellerstein, L. B. I. F. (1999). Collaboration Between Occupational Therapists and Optometrists. *Journal of Behavioral Optometry*, *10*, 147–152.

FitzGerald, C., & Hurst, S. (2017). Implicit bias in healthcare professionals: A systematic review. *BMC Medical Ethics*, *18*(1), 19. doi:10.118612910-017-0179-8 PMID:28249596

Flexner, A. (1910). *Medical Education in the United States and Canada*. A Report to the Carnegie Foundation for the Advancement of Teaching. Bulletin No. 4. Boston: Updyke.

Flynn, T., Carraccio, C., & Cleary, L. (2014). *Core Entrustable Professional Activities for Entering Residency: Curriculum Developers*. Association of American Medical Colleges. https:// members.aamc.org/eweb/upload/Core%20 EPA%20Curriculum%20Dev%20Guide.pdf

Folkman, S., & Lazarus, R. S. (1980). An Analysis of Coping in a Middle-Aged Community Sample. *Journal of Health and Social Behavior*, *21*(3), 219–239. doi:10.2307/2136617 PMID:7410799

Folkman, S., Lazarus, R. S., Dunkel-Schetter, C., DeLongis, A., & Gruen, R. J. (1986). Dynamics of a Stressful Encounter: Cognitive Appraisal, Coping, and Encounter Outcomes. *Journal of Personality and Social Psychology*, *50*(5), 992–1003. doi:10.1037/0022-3514.50.5.992 PMID:3712234

Forbes. (2017). Mexicanos, los más estresados del mundo por su trabajo. *Forbes México*. Retrieved from https://www.forbes.com.mx/mexicanos-los-mas-estresados-del-mundo-por-su-trabajo/

Forciea, M. A. (2014). Geriatric Medicine: History of a young specialty. *American Medical Association Journal of Ethics*, *16*(5), 385–389. PMID:24847710

Fornari, A., Murray, T., Menzin, A., Woo, V., Clifton, M., Lombardi, M., & Shelov, S. (2014). Mentoring program design and implementation in new medical schools. *Medical Education Online*, *19*(1), 24570. doi:10.3402/meo.v19.24570 PMID:24962112

Francis, J., & Abraham, S. (2014). Clinical pharmacists: Bridging the gap between patients and physicians. *Saudi Pharmaceutical Journal*, *22*(6), 600–602. doi:10.1016/j.jsps.2014.02.011 PMID:25561874

Frank, J. R., Snell, L., & Sherbino, J. (2015). *CanMEDS 2015: Physician Competency Framework*. Royal College of Physicians of Canada.

Fransworth, T. J., Seikel, J. A., Hudock, D., & Holst, J. (2015). History and Development of Interprofessional Education. *Journal of Phonetics and Audiology*, *1*(101). Advance online publication. doi:10.4172/2471-9455.1000101

Freeth, D., Hammick, M., Reeves, S., Koppel, I., & Barr, H. (2007). A critical review of evaluations of interprofessional education. King's College, London: Higher Education Academy.

Freeth, D., Hammick, M., Reeves, S., Koppel, I., & Barr, H. (2005). *Effective interprofessional education: Development, delivery & evaluation*. Blackwell Publishing. doi:10.1002/9780470776438

Frei, E., Stamm, M., & Buddeberg-Fischer, B. (2010). Mentoring programs for medical students – a review of the PubMed literature 2000 – 2008. *BMC Medical Education*, *10*(32), 1–14. PMID:20433727

Frenk, J., Chen, L., Bhutta, Z.A., Cohen, J., Crisp, N., Evans, T., . . . Zurayk, H. (2010). Health professionals for a new century: Transforming education to strengthen health systems in an interdependent world. *Lancet, 376*(9756), 1923-58. DOI:(10)61854-5 doi:10.1016/S0140-6736

Friederike-Grabel, B. (2017). *The relationship between wellbeing and academic achievement A systematic review* (Master's thesis).

Friedrichsen, S., Martinez, T. S., Hostetler, J., & Tang, J. M. W. (2014). Innovations in interprofessional education: Collaborative practice skills. *California Dental Association Journal, 42*(9), 629–635. PMID:25265729

Frost, J. S., Hammer, D. P., Nunez, L. M., Adams, J. L., Chesluk, B., Grus, C., Harvison, N., McGuinn, K., Mortensen, L., Nishimoto, J. H., Palatta, A., Richmond, M., Ross, E. J., Tegzes, J., Ruffin, A. L., & Bentley, J. P. (2019, January 2). The intersection of professionalism and interprofessional care: Development and initial testing of the interprofessional professionalism assessment (IPA). *Journal of Interprofessional Care, 33*(1), 102–115. doi:10.1080/13561820.2018.1515733 PMID:30247940

Fulmer, T., & Gaines, M. (2014). Partnering with Patient, Families and Communities to Link Interprofessional Practice and Education. *Proceeding of a conference sponsored by the Josiah Macy Jr. Foundation in April 2014.* New York: Josiah Macy Jr. Foundation.

Gaba, D. M. (2004). The future vision of simulation in health care. *Quality & Safety in Health Care, 13*(1), 2–10. doi:10.1136/qshc.2004.009878 PMID:15465951

Gagliardi, A., Dobrow, M., & Wright, F. (2001). How can we improve cancer care? A review of interprofessional collaboration models and their use in clinical management. *Surgical Oncology, 20*(3), 146–154. doi:10.1016/j.suronc.2011.06.004 PMID:21763127

Gale, N. K., Heath, G., Cameron, E., Rashid, S., & Redwood, S. (2013). Using the framework method for the analysis of qualitative data in multi-disciplinary health research. *BMC Medical Research Methodology, 13*(1), 117. Advance online publication. doi:10.1186/1471-2288-13-117 PMID:24047204

Gao, Y., Chen, L., Yang, S. N., Wang, H., Yao, J., Dai, Q., & Chang, S. (2015). Contributions of Visuo-oculomotor Abilities to Interceptive Skills in Sports. *Optometry and Vision Science, 92*(6), 679–689. doi:10.1097/OPX.0000000000000599 PMID:25930979

Garbee, D. D., Paige, J. T., Bonanno, L. S., Rusnak, V. V., Barrier, K. M., Kozmenko, L. S., ... Nelson, T. K. (2013). Effectiveness of teamwork and communication education using an interprofessional high-fidelity human patient simulation critical care code. *Journal of Nursing Education and Practice, 3*(3), 1–12. doi:10.5430/jnep.v3n3p1

Garmel, G. M. (2004). Mentoring Medical Students in Academic Emergency Medicine. *Academic Emergency Medicine, 11*(12), 1351–1357. doi:10.1197/j.aem.2004.06.013 PMID:15576528

Gary-Webb, T. L., Walker, E. A., Realmuto, L., Kamler, A., Lukin, J., Tyson, W., Carrasquillo, O., & Weiss, L. (2018). Translation of the National Diabetes Prevention Program to engage men in disadvantaged neighborhoods in New York City: A description of Power Up for Health. *American Journal of Men's Health, 12*(4), 998–1006. doi:10.1177/1557988318758788 PMID:29540131

Gazelle, G., Liebschutz, J., & Riess, H. (2014). Physician Burnout. Coaching a Way Out. *Journal of General Internal Medicine, 30*(4), 508–513. doi:10.100711606-014-3144-y PMID:25527340

Genn, J. M. (2001). AMEE Medical Education Guide No. 23 (Part 2): Curriculum, environment, climate, quality and change in medical education – a unifying perspective. *Medical Teacher, 23*(5), 445–454. PMID:12098364

Gibu, M., Clark, J., & Gold, J. (2018). Mental health pharmacists as interim prescribers. *Ment Health Clin, 7*(3), 111–115. doi:10.9740/mhc.2017.05.111 PMID:29955508

Gilbert, J. V., Yan, J., & Hoffman, S. J. (2010). A WHO Report: Framework for action on interprofessional education and collaborative practices. *Journal of Allied Health, 39*, 196–197. PMID:21174039

Givler, A., & Maani-Fogelman, P. A. (2019). The importance of cultural competence in pain and palliative care. *StatPearls, 5*(13). Retrieved from https://www.ncbi.nlm.nih.gov/books/NBK493154/

Goldstone, L. W., DiPaula, B. A., Caballero, J., Park, S., Price, C., & Sister, M. (2015). Improving medication-related outcomes for patients with psychiatric and neurologic disorders: Value of psychiatric pharmacists as part of the health care team. *MHC, 5*(1), 1–23. doi:10.9740/mhc.2015.01.001

Gorrindo, P., Alon, P., & Ladner, T. (2014). Medical students as health educators at a student-run free clinic: Improving the clinical outcomes of diabetic patients. *Academic Medicine, 89*(4), 625–631. doi:10.1097/ACM.0000000000000164 PMID:24556762

Granet, D. B., Gomi, C. F., Ventura, R., & Miller-Scholte, A. (2005). The relationship between convergence insufficiency and ADHD. *Strabismus, 13*(4), 163–168. doi:10.1080/09273970500455436 PMID:16361187

Green, B., & Johnson, C. (2015). Interprofessional collaboration in research, education, and clinical practice: Working together for a better future. *The Journal of Chiropractic Education, 29*(1), 1–10. doi:10.7899/JCE-14-36 PMID:25594446

Green, J. (2019). *See Change Clearly: Leveraging Adversity to Sharpen Your Vision and Build Resilient Teams*. Lioncrest Publishing.

Greiner, A., & Knebel, E. (2003). Health professions education: A bridge to quality. Washington, DC: National Academies Press.

Gunaldo, T. P., Brisolara, K. F., Davis, A. H., & Moore, R. (2017). Aligning interprofessional education collaborative sub-competencies to a progression of learning. *Journal of Interprofessional Care, 31*(3), 394–396. doi:10.1080/13561820.2017.1285273 PMID:28272902

Gunn-Tove, M. (2015). A culturally sensitive approach to elderly care. *The Journal of Gerontology and Geriatric Research, 4*(241). Retrieved from https://www.omicsonline.org/open-access/a-culturallysensitive-approach-to-elderly-care-2167-7182-1000241.php?aid=64251

Haglund, M. E. M., aan het Rot, M., Cooper, N. S., Nestadt, P. S., Muller, D., Southwick, S. M., & Charney, D. S. (2009). Resilience in the Third Year of Medical School: A Prospective Study of the Associations Between Stressful Events Occurring During Clinical Rotations and Student Well-Being. *Academic Medicine, 84*(2), 258–268. doi:10.1097/ACM.0b013e31819381b1 PMID:19174682

Hale, L. S., & DiLollo, A. (2016). Immersive Interprofessional Education Using an Evidence-Based Practice Course. *The Journal of Physician Assistant Education: the Official Journal of the Physician Assistant Education Association, 27*(3), 117–125. doi:10.1097/JPA.0000000000000083 PMID:27548762

Hall, L. W., & Zierler, B. K. (2015). Interprofessional Education and Practice Guide No. 1: Developing faculty to effectively facilitate interprofessional education. *Journal of Interprofessional Care, 29*(1), 1, 3–7. doi:10.3109/13561820.2014.937483 PMID:25019466

Hall, P. (2005). Interprofessional teamwork: Professional cultures as barriers. *Journal of Interprofessional Care, 19*(sup1), 188–196. doi:10.1080/13561820500081745 PMID:16096155

Hammick, M., Freeth, D., Koppel, I., Reeves, S., & Barr, H. (2007). A best evidence systematic review of interprofessional education: BEME guide no. 9. *Medical Teacher, 29*(8), 735–751. doi:10.1080/01421590701682576 PMID:18236271

Harden, R. M. (1998). AMEE guide No. 12: Multiprofessional education: Part 1- effective multiprofessional education: a three-dimensional perspective. *Medical Teacher, 20*(5), 402–408. doi:10.1080/01421599880472

Harden, R. M., & Laidlaw, J. M. (2017). *Essential skills for a medical teacher*. Elsevier.

Harden, R. M., & Lilley, P. (2018). *The eight roles of the medical teacher*. Elsevier.

Harper, J. C. (2019). IPEC's core competency 2 roles and responsibilities: What more do we need to implement these? *Journal of Nursing Education and Practice, 9*(7).

Hartmann, E. E., Block, S. S., & Wallace, D. K. (2015). Vision and eye health in children 36 to <72 months: Proposed data system. *Optometry and Vision Science, 92*(1), 24–30. doi:10.1097/OPX.0000000000000445 PMID:25562478

Hattie, J., & Timperley, H. (2007). The Power of Feedback. *Review of Educational Research, 77*(1), 81–112. doi:10.3102/003465430298487

Havyer, R. D., Nelson, D. R., Wingo, M. T., Comfre, N. I., Halvorsen, A. J., McDonalds, F. S., & Reed, D. A. (2016). Addressing the Interprofessional Collaboration Competencies of the Association of American Medical Colleges: A Systematic Review of Assessment Instruments in Undergraduate Medical Education. *Academic Medicine, 91*(6), 865–888. doi:10.1097/ACM.0000000000001053 PMID:26703415

Hayden, J. K., Smiley, R. A., & Gross, L. (2014). Simulation in Nursing Education: Current Regulations and Practices. *Journal of Nursing Regulation, 5*(2), 25–30. doi:10.1016/S2155-8256(15)30084-3

Health Professions Accreditors Collaborative. (2019). *Guidance on developing quality interprofessional education for the health professions*. Health Professions Accreditors Collaborative.

Hean, S., Craddock, D., Hammick, M., & Hammick, M. (2012). Theoretical insights into interprofessional education: AMEE Guide No. 62. *Medical Teacher, 34*(2), e78–e101. doi:10.3109/0142159X.2012.650740 PMID:22289015

Hébert, R., Raiche, M., Dubois, M. F., Gueye, N. R., Dubuc, N., & Tousignant, M. (2010). Impact of PRISMA, a coordination-type integrated service delivery system for frail older people in Quebec (Canada): A quasi-experimental study. *The Journals of Gerontology. Series B, Psychological Sciences and Social Sciences, 65B*(1), 107–118. doi:10.1093/geronb/gbp027 PMID:19414866

Hedge, S., Gajre, M. P., Shah, H., & Soares, N. S. (2016). Interprofessional Education and practice in an Indian setting. *J Taibah Univ Med Sci, 12*(3), 265–267. doi:10.1016/j.jtumed.2016.08.005 PMID:31435249

Hendrick, A. M., & Maria, V. (2015). Diabetic Retinopathy. *Primary Care Clinical Office Practice, 42*(3), 451–464. doi:10.1016/j.pop.2015.05.005 PMID:26319349

Henry & Hardin. (2006, Oct. 1). The Contact Hypothesis Revisited: Status Bias in the Reduction of Implicit Prejudice in the United States and Lebanon. *Psychological Science*.

Hesketh, E. A., & Laidlaw, J. M. (2002). Developing the teaching instinct, 1: Feedback. *Medical Teacher, 24*(3), 243–248. PMID:12098410

Hodge, A. N., & Marshal, A. P. (2007). Violence and aggression in the emergency department: A critical care perspective. *Australian Critical Care, 20*(2), 61–67. doi:10.1016/j.aucc.2007.03.001 PMID:17568534

Hodge, C., Chan, C., Zantos, S., Kokkinakis, J., Stapleton, F., & Sutton, G. (2015). Therapeutic treatment of keratoconus: A survey of local optometric practice criteria. *Clinical & Experimental Optometry, 98*(4), 312–318. doi:10.1111/cxo.12233 PMID:26104590

Hoffman, J., Pham, D.Q., & Robinson, D. (2014). Interprofessional education: The road to interprofessional practice. *California Pharmacist*, 42-44.

Hoffman, J., & Redman-Bentley, D. (2012). Comparison of faculty and student attitudes toward teamwork and collaboration in interprofessional education. *Journal of Interprofessional Care, 26*(1), 66–68. doi:10.3109/13561820.2011.602441 PMID:22233371

Hogg, M. A. (2018). Social identity theory. In P. J. Burke (Ed.), *Contemporary social psychological theories* (pp. 112–138). Stanford University Press.

Hojat, M., Vergare, M., Isenberg, G., Cohen, M., & Spandorfer, J. (2015). Underlying construct of empathy, optimism, and burnout in medical students. *International Journal of Medical Education, 6*, 12–16. doi:10.5116/ijme.54c3.60cd PMID:25633650

Ho, K., Jarvis-Selinger, S., Borduas, F., Frank, B., Hall, P., Handfield-Jones, R., Hardwick, D. F., Lockyer, J., Sinclair, D., Lauscher, H. N., Ferdinands, L., MacLeod, A., Robitaille, M.-A., & Rouleau, M. (2008). Making interprofessional education work: The strategic roles of the academy. *Academic Medicine, 83*(10), 934–940. doi:10.1097/ACM.0b013e3181850a75 PMID:18820523

Hooker, R. S., Cawley, J. F., & Everett, C. M. (2017). *Physician Assistants: Policy and practice* (4th ed.). F. A. Davis Company.

Hoppe, E. (1992). Evaluating the laws defining blindness. *Journal of the American Optometric Association, 63*(6), 390–394. PMID:1634739

Hoppe, K., Williams, M., Thomas, N., Zella, J., Drewry, A., Kim, K., Havighurst, T., & Johnson, H. (2019). Telehealth with remote blood pressure monitoring for postpartum hypertension: A prospective single-cohort feasibility study. *Pregnancy Hypertension, 15*, 171–176. doi:10.1016/j.preghy.2018.12.007 PMID:30825917

Hosny, S., Kamel, M. H., El-Wazir, Y., & Gilbert, J. (2013). Integrating interprofessional education in community-based learning activities: Case study. *Medical Teacher, 35*(sup1), S68–S73. doi:10.3109/0142159X.2013.765550 PMID:23581899

Hshieh, T., Inouye, T., & Inouye, S. (2014). Delirium. In Current Diagnosis and Treatment: Geriatrics (2nd ed.). Academic Press.

Huffman, M., Bowe Thompson, C., Lister, S., Johnson, N., Ervie, K., & … . (Manuscript submitted for publication). Can health professional students help fight the diabetes epidemic? A report on an interprofessional service-learning opportunity in African American churches. *Journal of Interprofessional Care.*

Hughes, A. M., Gregory, M. E., Joseph, D. L., Sonesh, S. C., Marlow, S. L., Lacerenza, C. N., Benishek, L. E., King, H. B., & Salas, E. (2016). Saving lives: A meta-analysis of team training in healthcare. *The Journal of Applied Psychology, 101*(9), 1266–1304. doi:10.1037/apl0000120 PMID:27599089

Hummels, J., & de Leede, J. (2000). Teamwork and morality: Comparing lean production and socio-technology. *Journal of Business Ethics, 26*(1), 75–88. doi:10.1023/A:1006242516664

Illingworth, P., & Chelvanayagam, S. (2007). Benefits of interprofessional education in health care. *British Journal of Nursing (Mark Allen Publishing), 16*(2), 121–124. doi:10.12968/bjon.2007.16.2.22773 PMID:17353824

InfantSEE. (n.d.a). Retrieved from https://www.infantsee.org/

InfantSEE. (n.d.b)About InfantSEE. Retrieved from https://www.infantsee.org/about-us.xml

InfantSEE. (n.d.c). *InfantSEE. Ways to help infant vision development.* Retrieved from https://www.infantsee.org/parents-center/ways-to-help-infant-vision-development.xml

Institute for Healthcare Improvement. (n.d.). *The IHI Triple Aim.* Retrieved from http://www.ihi.org:80/Engage/Initiatives/TripleAim/Pages/default.aspx

Institute of Medicine (US) Committee on Quality of Health Care in America. (2000). *To Err is Human: Building a Safer Health System* (L. T. Kohn, J. M. Corrigan, & M. S. Donaldson, Eds.). Retrieved from https://www.ncbi.nlm.nih.gov/books/NBK225182/

Institute of Medicine and National Research Council. (1999). *Ensuring quality cancer care.* National Academy Press.

Institute of Medicine Committee on the Health Professions Education Summit. (2003). Health Professions Education: A Bridge to Quality. National Academy Press.

Institute of Medicine. (1972). *Educating for the health team: Report of the conference on the interrelationships of educational programs for health professional.* Washington, DC: National Academy of Sciences. Available through http://books.google.com

Institute of Medicine. (1978). *A Manpower Policy for Primary Health Care: Report of a Study.* The National Academies Press., doi:10.17226/9932

Institute of Medicine. (2001). Crossing the quality chasm. National Academies Press.

Institute of Medicine. (2001). *Crossing the quality chasm: A new health system for the 21st Century*. National Academy Press.

Institute of Medicine. (2001). *Crossing the Quality Chasm: A New Health System for the 21st Century*. The National Academies Press. doi:10.17226/10027

Institute of Medicine. (2003). *Health Professions Education: A Bridge to Quality*. The National Academies Press. doi:10.17226/10681

Institute of Medicine. (2015). *Measuring the Impact of Interprofessional Education on Collaborative Practice and Patient Outcomes*. The National Academies Press., doi:10.17226/21726

International Sports Vision Association. (n.d.). *Dynamic Visual Skills for Sports*. Retrieved from https://www.sportsvision.pro

Interprofessional Education Collaborative Expert Panel. (2011). *Core competencies for interprofessional collaborative practice: Report of an expert panel*. Interprofessional Education Collaborative.

Interprofessional Education Collaborative Expert Panel. (2011). *Core competencies for interprofessional collaborative practice: report of an expert panel*. Retrieved from www.umassmed.edu/.../collaborativepractice

Interprofessional Education Collaborative Expert Panel. (2016). *Core competencies for interprofessional collaborative practice: 2016 update.* https://ipecollaborative.org/uploads/IPEC-2016-Updated-Core-Competencies-Report__final_release_.PDF

Interprofessional Education Collaborative Mission and Vision. (n.d.). https://www.ipecollaborative.org/vision---mission.html

Interprofessional Education Collaborative. (2016). *Core Competencies for Interprofessional Collaborative Practice: 2016 Update.* http://bit.ly/2zLEARR

Interprofessional Education Collaborative. (2016). *Core competencies for interprofessional collaborative practice: 2016 update.* Interprofessional Education Collaborative.

Interprofessional Education Collaborative. (2016). *Core competencies for interprofessional collaborative practice: 2016 update.* Washington, DC: Interprofessional Education Collaborative. (https://www.ipecollaborative.org/membership.html

Interprofessional Education Collaborative. (2016). *Core competencies for interprofessional collaborative practice: Report of Expert Panel 2016 update.* Washington, DC: Interprofessional Education Collaborative. Retrieved 11-4-2019 from: https://ipecollaborative.org/uploads/IPEC-Core-Competencies.pdf

Jacka, F. (2017). Nutritional Psychiatry: Where to Next? *EBioMedicine*, *17*, 24–29. doi:10.1016/j.ebiom.2017.02.020 PMID:28242200

Jackson, D., Sibson, R., & Riebe, L. (2014). Undergraduate perceptions of the development of team-working skills. *Education + Training*, *56*(1), 7–20. doi:10.1108/ET-01-2013-0002

Jaiswal, S., Asper, L., Long, J., Lee, A., Harrison, K., & Golebiowski, B. (2019). Ocular and visual discomfort associated with smartphones, tablets and computers: What we do and do not know. *Clinical & Experimental Optometry*, *102*(5), 463–477. doi:10.1111/cxo.12851 PMID:30663136

Jaleel, A., Rahman, M. A., & Huda, N. (2001). Problem-based learning in biochemistry at Ziauddin Medical University, Karachi, Pakistan. *Biochemistry and Molecular Biology Education*, *29*(2), 80–84. doi:10.1016/S1470-8175(01)00021-2

Janis, I. L. (1972). *Victims of Groupthink: A Psychological Study of Foreign-Policy Decisions and Fiascoes.* Houghton Mifflin.

Jiang, L., Manson, S. M., Dill, E. J., Beals, J., Johnson, A., Huang, H., Acton, K. J., & Roubideaux, Y. (2015). Participant and site characteristics related to participant retention in a diabetes prevention translational project. *Prevention science. The Official Journal of the Society for Prevention Research*, *16*(1), 41–52. doi:10.100711121-013-0451-1 PMID:24384689

Johnson, D. W., Johnson, R. T., & Smith, K. A. (2014). Cooperative Learning: Improving University Instruction By Basing Practice On Validated Theory. *Journal on Excellence in University Teaching*, *25*(4), 1–26.

Johnson, L. F., Smith, R. S., Smythe, J. T., & Varon, R. K. (2009). *Challenge-Based Learning: An Approach for Our Time*. The New Media Consortium.

Johnsons, L., & Brown, S. (2011). *Challenge Based Learning: The Report from the Implementation Project*. The New Media Consortium.

Jordon, J. (2005). *Mentorship and Preceptorship. Teaching Learners in Clinical Practice*. School of Health Studies.

Kahaleh, A. A., Danielson, J., Franson, K. L., Nuffer, W. A., & Umland, E. M. (2015). An interprofessional education panel on development, implementation, and assessment strategies. *American Journal of Pharmaceutical Education, 79*(6), 78. doi:10.5688/ajpe79678 PMID:26430265

Kaltman, S., & Tankersley, A. (2019). Teaching motivational interviewing to medical students: A systematic review. *Academic Medicine*. Advance online publication. doi:10.1097/ACM.0000000000003011 PMID:31577585

Kandiah, D. (2017). Perception of educational value in clinical rotations by medical students. *Advances in Medical Education and Practice, 8*, 149–162. doi:10.2147/AMEP.S129183 PMID:28223855

Kayingo, G., Kidd, V. D., Gilani, O., & Warner, M. L. (2015). Primary Care Teams, Composition, Roles, and Satisfaction of PA Students During Primary Care Rotations. *The Journal of Physician Assistant Education: the Official Journal of the Physician Assistant Education Association, 26*(2), 88–93. doi:10.1097/JPA.0000000000000022 PMID:26211031

Keijsers, C.J.P.W., Dreher, R., Tanner, S., Forde-Johnston, C., Thompson, S. (2016). Interprofessional education in geriatric medicine. *Elsevier Masson SAS*. doi:10.1016/j.eurger.2016.01.011

Kelly, D. P. (2013). Interdisciplinary collaborative future for developmental-behavioral pediatrics: Barriers and opportunities. *Journal of Developmental and Behavioral Pediatrics, 34*(7), 523–528. doi:10.1097/DBP.0b013e31829d1f44 PMID:24042083

Kemp, S., Hu, W., Bishop, J., Forrest, K., Hudson, J. N., Wilson, I., Teodorczuk, A., Rogers, G. D., & Wearn, A. (2019). Medical student wellbeing – a consensus statement from Australia and New Zealand. *BMC Medical Education, 69*(19). Advance online publication. doi:10.118612909-019-1505-2 PMID:30832630

Kesten, K. S. (2011). Role-play using SBAR technique to improve observed communication skills in senior nursing students. *The Journal of Nursing Education, 50*(2), 79–87. doi:10.3928/01484834-20101230-02 PMID:21210611

King, H. B., Battles, J., Baker, D. P., Alonso, A., Salas, E., Webster, J., Toomey, L., & Salisbury, M. (2008). *TeamSTEPPS™ (Team Strategies and Tools to Enhance Performance and Patient Safety) tools and materials*. https://www.ahrq.gov/downloads/pub/advances2/vol3/advances-king_1.pdf

Kirkpatrick, D. (1967). Evaluation of training. In R. Craig & L. Bittel (Eds.), *Training and development handbook* (pp. 131–167). McGraw-Hill.

KJ, J., & HC, C. (n.d.). *Teamwork Training*. Retrieved from https://www.psnet.ahrq.gov/primer/teamwork-training

Kohll, D. (2010). *Multiple Medication Dilemmas*. Retrieved from http://www.dorlandhealth.com

Koh, M., Hum, A. Y. M., Khoo, H. S., Ho, A. H. Y., Chong, P. H., Ong, J., ... Yong, W. C. (2019). Burnout And Resilience after a Decade in Palliative Care (BARD) (2019). What "Survivors" have to teach us. A Qualitative Study of Palliative Care Clinicians with more than 10 years of experience. *Journal of Pain and Symptom Management*. PMID:31465787

Kohn, L. T., Corrigan, J. M., & Donaldson, M. S. (Eds.). (2000). To Err is Human: Building a Safer Health System. National Academy Press.

Kohn, L. T., Corrigan, J. M., & Donaldson, M. S. (2000). *To Err is Human: Building a Safer Health System*. National Academy Press. Available at http://www.nap.edu/books/0309068371/html

Kohn, L. T., Corrigan, J. M., & Donaldson, M. S. (2000). *To Err is Human: Building a Safer Health System. Washington*. National Academies Press.

Kohn, L. T., Corrigan, J., & Donaldson, M. S. (2000). *To err is human: Building a safety health system*. National Academy Press.

Kraft, S., Wise, H. H., Jacques, P. F., & Burik, J. K. (2013). Discharge Planning Simulation: Training the Interprofessional Team for the Future Workplace. *Journal of Allied Health, 42*(3), 175–181.

Krein, S. L., Klamerus, M. L., Vijan, S., Lee, J. L., Fitzgerald, J. T., Pawlow, A., Reeves, P., & Hayward, R. A. (2004). Case management for patients with poorly controlled diabetes: A randomized trial. *The American Journal of Medicine, 116*(11), 732–739. doi:10.1016/j.amjmed.2003.11.028 PMID:15144909

Krumholtz, I. (2004). Educating the educators: Increasing grade-school teachers' ability to detect vision problems. *Optometry (St. Louis, Mo.), 75*(7), 445–451. doi:10.1016/S1529-1839(04)70159-1 PMID:15296377

Kumanyika, S. K., Whitt-Glover, M. C., & Haire-Joshu, D. (2014). What works for obesity prevention and treatment in black Americans? Research directions. *Obesity Reviews, 15*, 204–212. doi:10.1111/obr.12213 PMID:25196414

Kusnoor, A. V., & Stelljes, L. A. (2016). Interprofessional learning through shadowing: Insights and lessons learned. *Medical Teacher, 38*(12), 1278–1284. doi:10.1080/0142159X.2016.1230186 PMID:27647042

Lachs, M., & Pillemer, K. (2015). Elder Abuse. *The New England Journal of Medicine, 373*(2), 1947–1955. doi:10.1056/NEJMra1404688 PMID:26559573

Lack, D. (2010). Another joint statement regarding learning disabilities, dyslexia, and vision—A rebuttal. *Optometry (St. Louis, Mo.), 81*(10), 533–543. doi:10.1016/j.optm.2009.11.007 PMID:20728412

Lalis, T., Anson, J., & Greenfield, D. (2014). Barriers and enablers that influence sustainable interprofessional education: A literature review. *Journal of Interprofessional Care*, *8*(4), 305–310. doi:10.3109/13561820.2014.895977 PMID:24625198

Landi, F., Gambassi, G., Pola, R., Tabaccanti, S., Cavinato, T., Carbonin, P., & Bernabei, R. (1999). Impact of integrated home care services on hospital use. *Journal of the American Geriatrics Society*, *47*(12), 1430–1434. doi:10.1111/j.1532-5415.1999.tb01562.x PMID:10591237

Langhorne, P., & Dennis, M. S. (2004). Stroke units: The next 10 years. *Lancet*, *363*(9412), 834–835. doi:10.1016/S0140-6736(04)15771-1 PMID:15031023

Langton, H. (2009). *Interprofessional education in higher education institutions: Models, pedagogies and realities*. Palgrave Macmillan. Retrieved from www.worldcat.org/title/interprofessional

Lapkin, S., Levett-Jones, T., & Gilligan, C. (2011). The effectiveness of interprofessional education in university-based health professional programs: A systematic review. *Joanna Briggs Institute Library of Systematic Reviews*, *9*(46), 1917–1970. doi:10.11124/jbisrir-2011-103 PMID:27820537

Lasher, S. K. (2015). *IDOC: Interpreting Data from the Oyler Clinic Thesis*. Academic Press.

Lavretsky, H. (2010). Spirituality and aging. *Medscape. Aging Health*, *6*(6), 749–769. doi:10.2217/ahe.10.70

Lawrenson, J. G., Hull, C. C., & Downie, L. E. (2017). The effect of blue-light blocking spectacle lenses on visual performance, macular health and the sleep-wake cycle: A systematic review of the literature. *Ophthalmic & Physiological Optics*, *37*(6), 644–654. doi:10.1111/opo.12406 PMID:29044670

Lee, A. M. I. (n.d.). *Individuals With Disabilities Education Act (IDEA): What You Need to Know*. Retrieved from https://www.understood.org/en/school-learning/your-childs-rights/basics-about-childs-rights/individuals-with-disabilities-education-act-idea-what-you-need-to-know

Lewis, H. (2006). *Excellence Without a Soul: How a Great University Forgot Education*. Public Affairs.

Liaison Committee on Medical Education. (2019). *Functions and Structure of a Medical School. Standards for Accreditation of Medical Education Programs Leading to the MD Degree*. Association of American Medical Colleges and American Medical.

Lie, D. A., Forest, C. P., Walsh, A., Banzali, Y., & Lohenry, K. (2016). What and how do students learn in an interprofessional student-run clinic? An educational framework for team-based care. *Medical Education Online*, *21*(1), 31900. doi:10.3402/meo.v21.31900 PMID:27499364

Lie, D. A., Walsh, A., Segal-Gidan, F., Banzali, Y., & Lohenry, K. (2013). Physician Assistant Students' Views Regarding Interprofessional Education: A Focus Group Study. *The Journal of Physician Assistant Education: the Official Journal of the Physician Assistant Education Association*, *24*(1), 35–41. Advance online publication. doi:10.1097/01367895-201324010-00005 PMID:23858824

Lingard, L. (2013). Rethinking competence in the context of teamwork. In B. D. Hodges & L. Lingard (Eds.), *The Question of Competence: Reconsidering Medical Education in the Twenty-First Century* (pp. 14–41). ILR Press.

Lin, J., Thompson, T. J., Cheng, Y. J., Zhuo, X., Zhang, P., Gregg, E., & Rolka, D. B. (2018). Projection of the future diabetes burden in the United States through 2060. *Population Health Metrics, 16*(1), 9. doi:10.118612963-018-0166-4 PMID:29903012

Linsenmeyer, M., Wimsatt, L., Speicher, M., Powers, P., Miller, S., & Katsaros, E. (2018). Assessment Considerations for Core Entrustable Professional Activities for Entering Residency. *J Am Osteopath Assoc., 118*(4), 243-251. Doi:10.7556/jaoa.2018.049

Li, R., Qu, S., Zhang, P., Chattopadhyay, S., Gregg, E. W., Albright, A., Hopkins, D., & Pronk, N. P. (2015). Economic evaluation of combined diet and physical activity promotion rograms to prevent type 2 diabetes among persons at increased risk: A systematic review for the Community Preventive Services Task Force. *Annals of Internal Medicine, 163*(6), 452–460. doi:10.7326/M15-0469 PMID:26167962

Locke, A., & Kamo, N. (2016). Utilizing clinical pharmacists to improve delivery of evidence-based care for depression and anxiety in primary care. *BMJ Quality Improvement Reports, 5*(1), 1–5. doi:10.1136/bmjquality.u211816.w4748 PMID:27493753

Long, D. D., & Rosen, I. (2017). Social Work and Optometry: Interprofessional Practice Revisited. *Health & Social Work, 42*(2), 117–120. doi:10.1093/hsw/hlx002 PMID:28339798

Long, J., & Helland, M. (2012). A multidisciplinary approach to solving computer related vision problems. *Ophthalmic & Physiological Optics, 32*(5), 429–435. doi:10.1111/j.1475-1313.2012.00911.x PMID:22540950

López Cabrera, M. V., Hernandez-Rangel, E., Mejía, G. P., & Cerano, J. L. (2019). Factors that enable the adoption of educational technology in medical schools. *Educación Médica, 20*(1), 3–9.

López Cabrera, M. V., & Valdez, J. E. (2019). Organizational philosophy and planning: the keys to the adoption of educational technology. In *Maria Clausen, A Closer Look at Educational Technology*. NOVA Science Publishers.

López, M.V., & Valdez-García, J.E. (2019). Virtual reality in residents training. *Annals of Eye Science*. doi:10.21037/aes.2019.08.01

Lutfiyya, M. N., Chang, L. F., McGrath, C., Dana, C., & Lipsky, M. S. (2019). The state of the science of interprofessional collaborative practice: A scoping review of the patient health-related outcomes based literature published between 2010 and 2018. *PLoS One, 14*(6), e0218578. Advance online publication. doi:10.1371/journal.pone.0218578 PMID:31242239

Maeno, T., Haruta, J., Takayashiki, A., Yoshimoto, H., Goto, R., & Maeno, T. (2019). Interprofessional education in medical schools in Japan. *PLoS One, 14*(1), e0210912. doi:10.1371/journal.pone.0210912 PMID:30653563

Maestre, J. M., & Rudolph, J. W. (2015). Theories and styles of debriefing:the good judgment method as a tool for formative assessment in healthcare. *Revista Espanola de Cardiologia, 68*, 282–287. doi:10.1016/j.recesp.2014.05.018 PMID:25239179

Mahdi, R., Sukarman, S. S., & Chan, M. K. Y. (2015). Fostering creativity through innovation engagement in science and technology education: Case study of Unversiti Teknologi MARA students. *Procedia: Social and Behavioral Sciences, 167*, 256–260. doi:10.1016/j.sbspro.2014.12.671

Mahler, C., Berger, S., & Reeves, S. (2015). The Readiness for Interprofessional Learning Scale (RIPLS): A problematic evaluative scale for the interprofessional field. *Journal of Interprofessional Care, 29*(4), 289–291. doi:10.3109/13561820.2015.1059652 PMID:26176984

Makary, M. A., Sexton, J. B., Freischlag, J. A., Holzmueller, C. G., Millman, E. A., Rowen, L., & Pronovost, P. J. (2006). Operating room teamwork among physicians and nurses: Teamwork in the eye of the beholder. *Journal of the American College of Surgeons, 202*(5), 746–752. doi:10.1016/j.jamcollsurg.2006.01.017 PMID:16648014

Mann, K. V., Mcfetridge-Durdle, J., Martin-Misener, R., Clovis, J., Rowe, R., Beanlands, H., & Sarria, M. (2009). Interprofessional education for students of the health professions: The "Seamless Care" model. *Journal of Interprofessional Care, 23*(3), 224–233. doi:10.1080/13561820802697735 PMID:19387906

Marsh-Tootle, W. L., Russ, S. A., & Repka, M. X. (2015). Vision and eye health in children 36 to <72 months: Proposed data definitions. *Optometry and Vision Science, 92*(1), 17–23. doi:10.1097/OPX.0000000000000444 PMID:25562477

Martin, J. S., Ummenhofer, W., Manser, T., & Spirig, R. (2010). Interprofessional collaboration among nurses and physicians: Making a difference in patient outcome. *Swiss Medical Weekly, 140*, w13062. doi:10.4414mw.2010.13062 PMID:20458647

Maternal and Child Health Bureau. (n.d.). Retrieved from https://mchb.hrsa.gov/

Mathieu, J. E., Heffner, T. S., Goodwin, G. F., Salas, E., & Cannon-Bowers, J. A. (2000). The influence of shared mental models on team processes and performance. *The Journal of Applied Psychology, 85*(2), 273–283. doi:10.1037/0021-9010.85.2.273 PMID:10783543

Maxwell, J. (2013). *Qualitative research design*. SAGE Publications.

Mcalister, F., Stewart, S., Ferrua, S., & Mcmurray, J. (2004). Multidisciplinary strategies for the management of heart failure patients at high risk for admissionA systematic review of randomized trials. *Journal of the American College of Cardiology, 44*(4), 810–819. doi:10.1016/S0735-1097(04)01123-4 PMID:15312864

McBride, J. M., & Drake, R. L. (2015). Student perceptions of an interprofessional educational experience: The importance of goal articulation. *Anatomical Sciences Education, 8*(4), 381–385. doi:10.1002/ase.1547 PMID:26040781

McCray. (2008). Resident physician burnout: Is there hope? *Family Medicine, 40*(9), 626–632. https://www.ncbi.nlm.nih.gov/pubmed/18830837 PMID:18830837

McCulloch, A. (2009). The student as co-producer: Learning from public administration about the student-university relationship. *Studies in Higher Education, 34*(2), 171–183. doi:10.1080/03075070802562857

McLaughlin, K., Veale, P., McIlwrick, J., de Groot, J., & Wright, B. (2013). A practical approach to mentoring students with repeated performance deficiencies. *BMC Medical Education, 13*(1), 56. Advance online publication. doi:10.1186/1472-6920-13-56 PMID:23597111

McLeod, S. A. (2019, Oct 24). Social identity theory. *Simply Psychology*. https://www.simplypsychology.org/social-identity-theory.html

McLeod, A., & Bush, S. (2015). Pilot Assessment of Teaching Anterior Segment Evaluation to Develop Interprofessional Education Programs. *Optometric Education, 40*(3), 42–47.

Medicine. (2011). *Team-Based Care and the Learning Culture*. National Academies Press.

Mishra, A., Krishna, G. S., Alla, S., Kurian, T. D., Kurian, J., Ramesh, M., & Kishor, M. (2017). Impact of Pharmacist-Psychiatrist Collaborative Patient Education on Medication Adherence and Quality of Life (QOL) of Bipolar Affective Disorder (BPAD) Patients. *Frontiers in Pharmacology, 8*(722), 722. doi:10.3389/fphar.2017.00722 PMID:29066976

Mitchell, P., Wynia, M., Golden, R., McNellis, R., Okun, S., Webb, C. E., Rohrbach, V., & Von Korhorn, I. (2012). *Core principles and values of effective team-based health care*. Institute of Medicine. doi:10.31478/201210c

Mohammadi, S. F., Aghazade Amiri, M., Naderifar, H., Rakhshi, E., Vakilian, B., Ashrafi, E., & Behesht-Nejad, A. H. (2016). Vision Examination Protocol for Archery Athletes Along With an Introduction to Sports Vision. *Asian Journal of Sports Medicine, 7*(1), e26591. doi:10.5812/asjsm.26591 PMID:27217923

Montero, L., Triviño, X., Dois, A., Sirhan, M., & Leiva, L. (2017). Percepción de los académicos del rol docente del médico. *Investigación en Educación Médica, 6*(23), 198–205. doi:10.1016/j.riem.2017.01.001

Morano, C. L. (2017). *Perspectives on interprofessional education and practice*. NASW Press.

Morey, J. C., Simon, R., Jay, G. D., Wears, R. L., Salisbury, M., Dukes, K. A., & Berns, S. D. (2002). Error reduction and performance improvement in the emergency department through formal teamwork training: Evaluation results of the MedTeams project. *Health Services Research, 37*(6), 1553–1581. doi:10.1111/1475-6773.01104 PMID:12546286

Moss, M., Good, V. S., Gozal, D., Kleinpell, R., & Sessler, C. N. (2016). An Official Critical Care Societies Collaborative Statement: Burnout Syndrome in Critical Care Health Care Professionals: A Call for Action. *American Journal of Critical Care, 25*(4), 368–376. doi:10.4037/ajcc2016133 PMID:27369038

Mueller, C., Schur, C., & O'Connell, J. (1997). Prescription drug spending: The impact of age and chronic disease status. *American Journal of Public Health, 87*(10), 1626–1629. doi:10.2105/AJPH.87.10.1626 PMID:9357343

Muñoz, F., Medina, A., Carrasco, D., Pérez, C., & Ortiz, L. (2016). Burnout en estudiantes de Odontología y su relación con sus características sociodemográficas y antecedentes académicos. *Educación Médica Superior*, *30*(2). http://www.ems.sld.cu/index.php/ems/article/view/762/375

Murphy, J. (2013 November 15). *Current Trends in Comanagement*. Retrieved from https://www.reviewofoptometry.com/article/current-trends-in-comanagement-44930

National Academies of Practice. (n.d.). *14 Health Professions Joining Together*. Retrieved from https://napractice.org/About-NAP/Academies/Optometry%20accessed%20on%208/16/19

National Association of School Nurses. (2017). *Vision and eye health*. Retrieved from https://www.nasn.org/nasn-resources/practice-topics/vision-health

National Board of Medical Examiners. (2019). *2019-2020 Orientation Guide, COMLEX-USA Level 2-PE*. Retrieved from https://www.nbome.org/wordpress/wp-content/uploads/2017/03/COMLEX-USA_L2PE_Orientation_Guide-website-20192020.pdf

National Eye Health Education Program. (n.d.). *Vision Rehabilitation: Helping People with Low Vision*. Retrieved from https://nei.nih.gov/sites/default/files/nehep-pdfs/Low_Vision_Fact_Sheet_v3.pdf

National, P. T. A. (2005). *Position Statement - Elements of Comprehensive Health Programs*. Retrieved from https://www.pta.org/home/advocacy/ptas-positions/Individual-Position-Statements/Position-Statement-Elements-of-Comprehensive-Health-Programs

Navarro, A. E., Gassoumis, Z. D., & Wilber, K. H. (2013). Holding abusers accountable: An elder abuse forensic center increases criminal prosecution of financial exploitation. *The Gerontologist*, *53*(2), 303–312. doi:10.1093/geront/gns075 PMID:22589024

Naylor, C., Griffiths, R., & Fernandez, R. (2004). Does a multidisciplinary total parenteral nutrition team improve patient outcomes? A systematic review. *Journal of Parenteral and Enteral Nutrition*, *28*(4), 251–258. doi:10.1177/0148607104028004251 PMID:15291407

Nehmad, L., Reynolds, S. A., & Anderson-Worts, P. (2015). Interprofessional Education on a Mission. *Optometric Education*, *40*(3), 51–54.

Nelson, S., Turnbull, J., Bainbridge, L., Caufield, T., Hudon, G., Kendel, D., & Sketris, I. (2014). *Optimizing Scopes of Practice: New Models for a New Health Care System: Report of the Expert Panel Appointed by the Canadian Academy of Health Sciences*. Canadian Academy of Health Sciences. Retrieved from www.cahs-acss.ca/completed-projects

Nelson, S., White, C. F., Hodges, B. D., & Tassone, M. (2017). Interprofessional team training at the prelicensure level: A review of the literature. *Academic Medicine*, *92*(5), 709–716. doi:10.1097/ACM.0000000000001435 PMID:27782914

Nexus, I. P. E. (n.d.). *National Center for Interprofessional Practice and Education. Picker Institutes Eight Principles of Effective Patient Care*. https://nexusipe.org/informing/resource-center/picker-institute's-eight-principles-patient-centered-care

Nhim, K., Gruss, S. M., Porterfield, D. S., Jacobs, S., Elkins, W., Luman, E. T., Van Aacken, S., Schumacher, P., & Albright, A. (2019). Using a RE-AIM framework to identify promising practices in National Diabetes Prevention Program implementation. *Implementation Science; IS*, *14*(1), 81. doi:10.118613012-019-0928-9 PMID:31412894

Nisbet, G., Lee, A., Kumar, K., Thistlethwaite, J., & Dunston, R. (2011). *Inter- professional Health Education: A Literature Review. Overview of international and Australian developments in interprofessional health education (IPE).* Retrieved from www.health.wa.gov.au/wactn/docs/IPEAUSlitreview2011

Noonan, C. D., Scow, S., Sheagley, B. A., & Bunn, J. (2018). Shifting Perspectives on Pain Management after an Interprofessional International Service Learning Experience: A Qualitative Assessment of Pilot Data. *Journal of Interprofessional Care*, *32*(5), 645–647. https://doi-org.proxy.library.umkc.edu/10.1080/13561820.2018.1471053. doi:10.1080/13561820.2018.1471053 PMID:29741408

Obeso, V., Brown, D., Aiyer, M., Barron, B., Bull, J., Carter, T., Emery, M., Gillespie, C., Hormann, M., Hyderi, A., Lupi, C., Schwartz, M. L., Uthman, M., Vasilevskis, E. E., Yingling, S., & Phillipi, C. (Eds.). (2017). For Core EPAs for Entering Residency Pilot Program. Toolkits for the 13 Core Entrustable Professional Activities for Entering Residency. Washington, DC: Association of American Medical Colleges. aamc.org/initiatives/coreepas/publicationsandpresentations

Office of Minority Health. (2016). *Diabetes and African Americans.* Retrieved from http://minorityhealth.hhs.gov/omh/browse.aspx?lvl=4&lvlID=18

Olivares, S.L., Adame, E., Treviño, J., López Cabrera, M.V., & Turrubiates, M. (2019). *Action Learning: Challenges that impact employability skills.* Higher Education, Skills, and Work-Based Learning; Ahead-of-print.

Olivares, S. L., López Cabrera, M. V., & Valdez-García, J. E. (2018). Aprendizaje basado en retos: Una experiencia de innovación para enfrentar problemas de salud pública. *Educación Médica*, *19*, 230–237. doi:10.1016/j.edumed.2017.10.001

Olivares, S. L., & Valdez, J. E. (2017). *Aprendizaje Centrado en el Paciente.* Editorial Médica Panamericana.

Olupeliyawa, A., Balasooriya, C., Hughes, C., & O'Sullivan, O. (2014). Educational impact of an assessment of medical students' collaboration in health care teams. *Medical Education*, *48*(2), 146–156. doi:10.1111/medu.12318 PMID:24528397

OneSight. (n.d.). *Vision Center at Oyler School.* Retrieved from https://www.cincinnati-oh.gov/health/assets/File/Oyler%20Vision%20Center.pdf

Optimal Team Practice. (n.d.). *Learn More About OTP.* Retrieved December 11, 2019, from AAPA website: https://www.aapa.org/advocacy-central/optimal-team-practice/

Optometric Extension Program Foundation. (n.d.). *Shop OEPF.* Retrieved from https://www.oepf.org/

Osteopathic Core Competencies for Medical Students. (2012). *American Association of Colleges of Osteopathic Medicine*. https://www.aacom.org/docs/default-source/core-competencies/corecompetencyreport2012.pdf?sfvrsn=4

Oxford Dictionary. (2019). *Definition of mentor noun*. Retrieved from: https://www.oxfordlearnersdictionaries.com/us/definition/english/mentor?q=mentor

Oxford English Dictionary. (n.d.). *art, n. 1*. Oxford University Press.

Ozkan, H., Degirmenci, B., Musal, B., Itil, O., Akalın, E., Kilinç, O., Ozkan, S., & Alici, E. (2006). Task-based learning program for clinical years of medical education. *Education for Health*, *19*(1), 32–42. doi:10.1080/13576280500534826 PMID:16531300

Palaganas, J., Brunette, V., & Winslow, B. (2016). Prelicensure simulation-enhanced interprofessional education: A critical review of the research literature. *Simulation in Healthcare*, *11*(6), 404–418. doi:10.1097/SIH.0000000000000175 PMID:27602706

Palatta, A., Cook, B. J., Anderson, E. L., & Valachovic, R. W. (2015). 20 Years Beyond the Crossroads: The Path to Interprofessional Education at U.S. Dental Schools. *Journal of Dental Education*, *79*(8), 982–996. PMID:26466391

Palmer, R., & Stilp, C. (2017). Learning by Doing: The MD-PA Interprofessional Education Rural Rotation. *Rural and Remote Health*, *17*(1). Advance online publication. doi:10.22605/RRH4167 PMID:28328232

Parsell, G., & Bligh, J. (1999). The development of a questionnaire to assess the readiness for health care students for interprofessional learning (RIPLS). *Medical Education*, *33*(2), 95–100. doi:10.1046/j.1365-2923.1999.00298.x PMID:10211258

Patel, R.S., Bachu, R., Adikey, A., Malik, M., & Shah, M. (2018). Factors related to physician burnout and its consequences: a review. *Behav Sci, 8*(11), 98.

Patel, P. B., & Vinson, D. R. (2005). Team assignment system: Expediting emergency department care. *Annals of Emergency Medicine*, *46*(6), 499–506. doi:10.1016/j.annemergmed.2005.06.012 PMID:16308063

Peltonen, J., Leino-Kilpi, H., Heikkilä, H., Rautava, P., Tuomela, K., Siekkinen, M., Sulosaari, V., & Stolt, M. (n.d.). Instruments measuring interprofessional collaboration in healthcare – a scoping Review. *Journal of Interprofessional Care*. Advanced online publication. https://doi:10.1080/13561820.2019.1637336

Pérez, C., Parra, P., Fasce, E., Ortiz, L., Bastías, N., & Bustamante, C. (2012). Estructura factorial y confiabilidad del inventario de burnout de Maslach en universitarios chilenos. *Revista Argentina de Clínica Psicológica*, *21*(3), 255–263.

Pew Research Center. (2015). *America's Changing Religious Landscape*. Retrieved from https://www.pewforum.org/files/2015/05/RLS-05-08-full-report.pdf

Phillips, W. R., & Keys, T. (2018). Interprofessional Primary Care Course Curriculum and Evaluation. *Family Medicine*, *50*(3), 217–222. doi:10.22454/FamMed.2018.998057 PMID:29537465

Physician Assistant Education Association. (2019). *Core Competencies for New Physician Assistant Graduates*. Retrieved from https://paealearning.org/wp-content/uploads/2018/10/Core-Competencies-for-New-PA-Graduates_FINAL_061918.pdf

Pippitt, K., Moloney-Johns, A., Jalilibahabadi, S., & Gren, L. H. (2015). Collaboration Versus Competition: An Interprofessional Education Experience. *Family Medicine*, *47*(4). PMID:25853601

Piras, A., Lobietti, R., & Squatrito, S. (2010). A study of saccadic eye movement dynamics in volleyball: Comparison between athletes and non-athletes. *The Journal of Sports Medicine and Physical Fitness*, *50*(1), 99–108. PMID:20308980

Poltavski, D., & Biberdorf, D. (2015). The role of visual perception measures used in sports vision programmes in predicting actual game performance in Division I collegiate hockey players. *Journal of Sports Sciences*, *33*(6), 597–608. doi:10.1080/02640414.2014.951952 PMID:25142869

Porter, C., & Zupek, J. (2020). Use of Telehealth Experiences To Facilitate Interprofessional Education. *American Journal of Health-System Pharmacy*, *17*. doi:10.1093/ajhp/zxaa033 PMID:32179887

Prades, J., Remue, E., van Hoof, E., & Borras, J. (2015). Is it worth reorganizing cancer services on the basis of multidisciplinary teams (MDTs)? A systematic review of the objectives and organization of MDTs and their impact on patient outcomes. *Health Policy (Amsterdam)*, *119*(4), 464–474. doi:10.1016/j.healthpol.2014.09.006 PMID:25271171

Progressive Education. (n.d.). In *Wikipedia*. Available from: https://en.wikipedia.org/wiki/Progressive_education.

Qin, Z., Johnson, D. W., & Johnson, R. T. (1995). Cooperative Versus Competitive Efforts and Problem Solving. *Review of Educational Research*, *65*(2), 129–143. doi:10.3102/00346543065002129

Rao, C., Darshan, B., Das, N., Rajan, V., Bhogun, M., & Gupta, A. (2012). Practice of Physical Activity among Future Doctors: A Cross Sectional Analysis. *International Journal of Preventive Medicine*, *3*(5), 365–369. PMID:22708033

Rathfon, E., & Jones, G. (2011). *Family Physicians and Physician Assistants: Team-Based Family Medicine. A Joint Policy Statement of the American Academy of Family Physicians and American Academy of Physician Assistants*. Retrieved from: https://www.aafp.org/about/policies/all/fp-pa.html

Rea, K. E., Rao, P., Hill, E., Saylor, K. M., & Cousino, M. K. (2018). Families' Experiences With Pediatric Family-Centered Rounds: A Systematic. *La Revue de Pediatrie*, *141*(3), 2–13. doi:10.1542/peds.2017-1883 PMID:29437931

Reeves, S., Suter, E., Goldman, J., Martimianakis, T., Chatalalsingh, C., & Dematteo, D. C. (2007). *A scoping review to identify organizational and education theories relevant for interprofessional practice and education.* Retrieved from http://www.cihc.ca/files/publications/ScopingReview_IP_Theories_Dec07.pdf

Reeves, S. (2016). Why we need interprofessional education to improve the delivery of safe and effective care. *Interface (Botucatu), 20*(56), 185–197. doi:10.1590/1807-57622014.0092

Reeves, S. A., Denault, D., Huntington, J. T., Ogrinc, G., Southard, D. R., & Vebell, R. (2017). Learning to Overcome Hierarchical Pressures to Achieve Safer Patient Care: An Interprofessional Simulation for Nursing, Medical, and Physician Assistant Students. *Nurse Educator, 42*, S27–S31. doi:10.1097/NNE.0000000000000427 PMID:28832459

Reeves, S., Boet, S., Zierler, B., & Kitto, S. (2015). Interprofessional education and practice guide no. 3: Evaluating interprofessional education. *Journal of Interprofessional Care, 29*(4), 305–312. doi:10.3109/13561820.2014.1003637 PMID:25671416

Reeves, S., Fletcher, S., Barr, H., Birch, I., Boet, S., Davies, N., McFadyen, A., Rivera, J., & Kitto, S. (2016). A BEME systematic review of the effects of interprofessional education: BEME Guide No. 39. *Medical Teacher, 38*(7), 656–668. doi:10.3109/0142159X.2016.1173663 PMID:27146438

Reeves, S., Lewin, S., Espin, S., & Zwarenstein, M. (2010). *A Conceptual Framework for Interprofessional Teamwork.* John Wiley and Sons. Interprofessional Teamwork for Health and Social Care. doi:10.1002/9781444325027.ch4

Reeves, S., Pelone, F., Harrison, R., Goldman, J., & Zwarenstein, M. (2017). Interprofessional collaboration to improve professional practice and healthcare outcomes. *Cochrane Database of Systematic Reviews.* Advance online publication. doi:10.1002/14651858.CD000072.pub3 PMID:28639262

Reeves, S., Perrier, L., Goldman, J., Freeth, D., & Zarenstein, M. (2013). Interprofessional education: Effects on professional practice and healthcare outcomes (update). *Cochrane Database of Systematic Reviews*, (3), CD00213. doi:10.1002/14651858.CD002213.pub3 PMID:23543515

Reid, R., Bruce, D., Allstaff, K., & McLernon, D. (2006). Validating the Readiness for Interprofessional Learning Scale (RIPLS) in the postgraduate context: Are health care professionals ready for IPL? *Medical Education, 40*(5), 415–422. doi:10.1111/j.1365-2929.2006.02442.x PMID:16635120

Reinberg, S. (2017). High blood pressure may not be all bad in elderly. *WebMD.* Retrieved from https://www.webmd.com/hypertension-high-blood-pressure/news/20170117/high-blood-pressure-elderly-dementia#1

Remick, K. (2018). *Eyes On Track; Ages 4-Adult: A manual to improve vision processing.* Academic Press.

Remmen, R., Derese, A., Scherpbier, A., Denekens, J., Hermann, I., Van der Vleuten, C., Royen, P. V., & Bossaert, L. (2002). Can medical schools rely on clerkships to train students in basic clinical skills? *Medical Education, 33*(8), 600–605. Advance online publication. doi:10.1046/j.1365-2923.1999.00467.x PMID:10447847

Report of the Graduate Medical Education National Advisory Committee to the Secretary, Department of Health and Human Services electronic resource. (1981). Hyattsville, MD: U.S. Dept. of Health and Human Services, Public Health Service, Health Resources Administration, Office of Graduate Medical Education; For sale by the Supt. of Docs., G.P.O. Retrieved from http://search.ebscohost.com.proxy.library.umkc.edu/login.aspx?direct=true&db=edsgpr&AN=edsgpr.ocn690419361&site=eds-live&scope=site

Rich, M. W., Beckham, V., Wittenberg, C., Leven, C. L., Freedland, K. E., & Carney, R. M. (1995). A multidisciplinary intervention to prevent the readmission of elderly patients with congestive heart failure. *The New England Journal of Medicine, 333*(18), 1190–1195. doi:10.1056/NEJM199511023331806 PMID:7565975

Rintoul, Y., Wynaden, D., & McGowan, S. (2009). Managing aggression in the emergency department: Promoting an interdisciplinary approach. *International Emergency Nursing, 17*(2), 122–127. doi:10.1016/j.ienj.2008.11.005 PMID:19341998

Rizzo, V. M., Burnes, D., & Chalfy, A. (2015). A systematic evaluation of a multidisciplinary social work-lawyer elder mistreatment intervention model. *Journal of Elder Abuse & Neglect, 27*(1), 1–18. doi:10.1080/08946566.2013.792104 PMID:24965802

Robben, S., Perry, M., van Nieuwenhuijzen, L., van Achterberg, T., Rikkert, M. O., Schers, H., Heinen, M., & Melis, R. (2012). Impact of interprofessional education on collaboration attitudes, skills, and behavior among primary care professionals. *The Journal of Continuing Education in the Health Professions, 32*(3), 196–204. doi:10.1002/chp.21145 PMID:23008082

Roch-Levecq, A. C., Brody, B. L., Thomas, R. G., & Brown, S. I. (2008). Ametropia, preschoolers' cognitive abilities, and effects of spectacle correction. *Archives of Ophthalmology, 126*(2), 252–258. doi:10.1001/archophthalmol.2007.36 PMID:18268218

Rodriguez, E., Srivastava, A., & Landau, M. (2018). Increasing Screening Follow-Up for Vulnerable Children: A Partnership with School Nurses. *International Journal of Environmental Research and Public Health, 15*(8), 1572. Advance online publication. doi:10.3390/ijerph15081572 PMID:30044383

Rogers, G. D., Thistlethwaite, J. E., Anderson, E. S., Dahlgren, M. A., Grymonpre, R. E., Moran, M., & Samarasekera, D. D. (2016). International consensus statement on the assessment of interprofessional learning outcomes. *Medical Teacher, 26*, 1–13. PMID:28024436

Roland, D. (2015). But I told you she was ill! The role of families in preventing avoidable harm in children. *BMJ Quality & Safety, 24*(3), 186–187. doi:10.1136/bmjqs-2015-003950 PMID:25628427

Rollason, V., & Vogt, N. (2003). Reduction of Polypharmacy in the Elderly. *Drugs & Aging, 20*(11), 817–832. doi:10.2165/00002512-200320110-00003 PMID:12964888

Rosen, K. R. (2008). The history of medical simulation. *Journal of Critical Care*, *23*(2), 157–166. doi:10.1016/j.jcrc.2007.12.004 PMID:18538206

Rosenstein, A. H., & O'Daniel, M. (2005). Disruptive behavior and clinical outcomes: Perceptions of nurses and physicians. *The American Journal of Nursing*, *105*(1), 54–64. doi:10.1097/00000446-200501000-00025 PMID:15659998

Rummans, T. A., Clark, M. M., Sloan, J. A., Frost, M. H., Bostwick, J. M., Atherton, P. J., Johnson, M. E., Gamble, G., Richardson, J., Brown, P., Martensen, J., Miller, J., Piderman, K., Huschka, M., Girardi, J., & Hanson, J. (2006). Impacting quality of life for patients with advanced cancer with a structured multidisciplinary intervention: A randomized controlled trial. *Journal of Clinical Oncology*, *24*(4), 635–642. doi:10.1200/JCO.2006.06.209 PMID:16446335

Ryan, D. J., O'Sullivan, F., & Jackson, S. H. D. (2016). Clinical pharmacology: Prescribing medicines for older patients. *Medicine*, *44*(7), 433–437. doi:10.1016/j.mpmed.2016.04.005

Salas, E., DiazGranados, D., Klein, C., Burke, C. S., Stagl, K. C., Goodwin, G. F., & Halpin, S. M. (2008). Does team training improve performance? A meta-analysis. *Human Factors*, *50*(6), 903–933. doi:10.1518/001872008X375009 PMID:19292013

Sambunjak, D., Straus, S. E., & Marusic, A. (2006). Mentoring in Academic Medicine A Systematic Review. *Journal of the American Medical Association*, *296*(9), 1103–1115. doi:10.1001/jama.296.9.1103 PMID:16954490

Sanchez-Diaz, P. C., Ann Parker, R. A., Valdes, M. S., Ramirez, M. N., Narayanan, S., Dominguez, D. G., & Jones, M. E. (2015). Shaping Student Attitudes Toward Healthcare Teams Through a Hybrid and an Online Interprofessional Education Course: Results from a Pilot Study. *Optometric Education*, *40*(3), 23–30.

Sarcevic, A. (n.d.). *Understanding teamwork in trauma resuscitation through analysis of team errors* (Dissertation). Rutgers University. Available at: https://pdfs.semanticscholar.org/f29e/2fc608d82a7c9dfd0550670c7b56c05f4ac7.pdf

Sargeant, J. (2009). Theories to aid in understanding and implementation of interprofessional education. *The Journal of Continuing Education in the Health Professions*, *29*(3), 178–184. doi:10.1002/chp.20033 PMID:19728383

Sattin, R. W., Williams, L. B., Dias, J., Garvin, J. T., Marion, L., Joshua, T. V., Kriska, A., Kramer, M. K., & Venkat Narayan, K. M. (2016). Community trial of a faith-based lifestyle intervention to prevent diabetes among African-Americans. *Journal of Community Health*, *41*(1), 87–96. doi:10.100710900-015-0071-8 PMID:26215167

Schapmire, T. J., Head, B. A., Nash, W. A., Yankeelov, P. A., Furman, C. D., Wright, R. B., Gopalraj, R., Gordon, B., Black, K. P., Jones, C., Hall-Faul, M., & Faul, A. C. (2018). Overcoming barriers to interprofessional education in gerontology: The Interprofessional Curriculum for the Care of Older Adults. *Advances in Medical Education and Practice*, *9*, 109–118. doi:10.2147/AMEP.S149863 PMID:29497345

Scheele, F., Teunissen, P., Luijk, S. V., Heineman, E., Fluit, L., Mulder, H., Meininger, A., Wijnen-Meijer, M., Glass, G., Sluiter, H., & Hummel, T. (2008). Introducing competency-based postgraduate medical education in the Netherlands. *Medical Teacher, 30*(3), 248–253. doi:10.1080/01421590801993022 PMID:18484450

Schernhammer, E. (2005). Taking Their Own Lives — The High Rate of Physician Suicide. *The New England Journal of Medicine, 352*(24), 2473–2476. doi:10.1056/NEJMp058014 PMID:15958803

Schmitt, M., Blue, A., Aschenbrener, C., & Viggiano, T. (2011). Core Competencies for Interprofessional Collaborative Practice: Reforming Health Care by Transforming Health Professionals' Education. *Academic Medicine, 86*(11), 1351. doi:10.1097/ACM.0b013e3182308e39 PMID:22030650

Schot, E., Tummers, L., & Noordegraaf, M. (2019): Working on working together. A systematic review on how healthcare professionals contribute to interprofessional collaboration. *Journal of Interprofessional Care*. Advanced online publication. https://doi:10.1080/13561820.2019.1636007

Segal-Gidan, F., Walsh, A., Lie, D., Fung, C. C., & Lohenry, K. (2014). Knowledge and Attitude Change in Physician Assistant Students After an Interprofessional Geriatric Care Experience: A Mixed Methods Study. *The Journal of Physician Assistant Education: the Official Journal of the Physician Assistant Education Association, 25*(2), 25–30. doi:10.1097/01367895-201425020-00006 PMID:25016910

Segura, N.A., Eraña, I.E., Luna-de-la-Garza, M.V., Castorena-Ibarra, J., López Cabrera, M.V. (2019). *Analysis of anxiety on early clinical encounters: Experiences using clinical simulation in undergraduate students*. Educación Médica. Transformar la educación para fortalecer los sistemas de salud.

Segura-Azuara, N. A., Valencia, J. L., & López Cabrera, M. V. (2018). Desarrollo del pensamiento crítico mediante simulación de alta fidelidad con estudiantes de medicina. In Ed Med, 7(28), 55-64.

Seif, G., Coker-Bolt, P., Kraft, S., Gonsalves, W., Simpson, K., & Johnson, E. (2014). The development of clinical reasoning and interprofessional behaviors: Service-learning at a student run free clinic. *Journal of Interprofessional Care, 28*(6), 559–564. doi:10.3109/13561820.2014.921899 PMID:24865993

Shah, K., & Villareal, D. T. (2017). Obesity. In H. M. Fillit, K. Rockwood, & J. Young (Eds.), *Brocklehurst's Textbook of Geriatric Medicine* (8th ed.). Elsevier.

Shoemaker, M. J., Platko, C. M., Cleghorn, S. M., & Booth, A. (2014). Virtual patient care: An interprofessional education approach for physician assistant, physical therapy and occupational therapy students. *Journal of Interprofessional Care, 28*(4), 365–367. doi:10.3109/13561820.2014.891978 PMID:24593330

Shrader, S., Kern, D., Zoller, J., & Blue, A. (2013). Interprofessional Teamwork Skills as Predictors of Clinical Outcomes in a Simulated Healthcare Setting. *Journal of Allied Health, 42*(1), e1-6.

Shumer, R. (1994). Community-based learning: Humanizing education. *Journal of Adolescence, 17*(4), 357–367. doi:10.1006/jado.1994.1032

Sibyl, S., Bennadi, D., Kshetrimayum, N., & Reddy, C.V.K. (2018). Readiness for interprofessional learning among dental undergraduate students: An institutional study. *J Indian Assoc Public Health Dent, 16*(4), 328-32. Doi:10.4103/jiaphd.jiaphd_59_18

Simmons, B., Egan-Lee, E., Wagner, S. J., Esdaile, M., Baker, L., & Reeves, S. (2011). Assessment of interprofessional learning: The design of an interprofessional objective structured clinical examination (iOSCE) approach. *Journal of Interprofessional Care, 25*(1), 73–74. doi:10.3109/13561820.2010.483746 PMID:20645683

Singer, S. J., Falwell, A., Gaba, D. M., Meterko, M., Rosen, A., Hartmann, C. W., & Baker, L. (2009). Identifying organizational cultures that promote patient safety. *Health Care Management Review, 34*(4), 300–311. doi:10.1097/HMR.0b013e3181afc10c PMID:19858915

Singh, U. (n.d.). *Department of Geriatrics*. Retrieved from https://www.healthplanofnevada.com

Singh, P. M., Kaur, M., & Trikha, A. (2012). Virtual reality in anesthesia "simulation.". *Anesthesia, Essays and Researches, 6*(2), 134–139. doi:10.4103/0259-1162.108289 PMID:25885605

Smith CB, Phillips T, Smith TJ. (2017). Using the New ASCO Clinical Practice Guideline for Palliative Care Concurrent With Oncology Care Using the TEAM Approach. *Am Soc Clin Oncol Educ B.*, (37), 714-723. doi:10.1200/EDBK_175474

Smithburger, P. L., Kane-Gill, S. L., Kloet, M. A., Lohr, B., & Seybert, A. L. (2013). Advancing interprofessional education through the use of high fidelity human patient simulators. *Pharmacy Practice, 11*(2), 61–65. doi:10.4321/S1886-36552013000200001 PMID:24155851

Smith, E. R., & DeCoster, J. (2000). Dual-process models in social and cognitive psychology: Conceptual integration and links to underlying memory systems. *Personality and Social Psychology Review, 4*(2), 108–131. doi:10.1207/S15327957PSPR0402_01

Smith, S., Shochet, R., Keeley, M., Fleming, A., & Moynahan, K. (2014). The Growth of Learning Communities in Undergraduate Medical Education. *Academic Medicine, 89*(6), 928–933. doi:10.1097/ACM.0000000000000239 PMID:24871245

Soares, N. S., Gajre, M. P., & Manglani, M. V. (2016). Building developmental- behavioral pediatrics in low-middle income countries through international collaboration. *Journal of Developmental and Behavioral Pediatrics, 37*(6), 508–510. doi:10.1097/DBP.0000000000000306 PMID:27366958

Solomon, P. (2011). Student perspectives on patient educators as facilitators of interprofessional education. *Medical Teacher, 33*(10), 851–853. doi:10.3109/0142159X.2010.530703 PMID:21942483

Sommers, L. S., Marton, K. I., Barbaccia, J. C., & Randolph, J. (2000). Physician, nurse, and social worker collaboration in primary care for chronically ill seniors. *Archives of Internal Medicine, 160*(12), 1825–1833. doi:10.1001/archinte.160.12.1825 PMID:10871977

Sonney, J., Willgerodt, M., Lindhorst, T., & Brock, D. (2018, January). Elizabeth: Typical or Troubled Teen? A Training Case for Health Professionals to Recognize and Report Child Maltreatment. *MedEdPORTAL : The Journal of Teaching and Learning Resources*, *14*(1), mep_2374-8265.10712. Advance online publication. doi:10.15766/mep_2374-8265.10712 PMID:30800912

South Dakota School of Mines and Technology Student Activities and Leadership Center. (n.d.). *Understanding Group Process*. Retrieved from https://www.sdsmt.edu/uploadedFiles/Content/Campus_Life/Student_Activities/Organizations/Understanding%20Group%20Process.pdf

Stanika, N., & Peter, L. (2018). Community, strategic partner of the educational organization in the 21st Century. *International Conference of Knowledge-based Organization*, *24*, 416-420.

Stefanidis, D., Sevdalis, N., Paige, J., Zevin, B., Aggarwal, R., Grantcharov, T., & Jones, D. (2015). Simulation in Surgery. *Annals of Surgery*, *261*(5), 846–853. doi:10.1097/SLA.0000000000000826 PMID:25243562

Steineman, S., Berg, B., Skinner, A., Ditulio, A., Anzelon, K., Teráda, K., ... Speck, C. (2011). In situ, multidisciplinary, simulation-based teamwork training improves early trauma care. *Journal of Surgical Education*, *68*(6), 472–2. doi:10.1016/j.jsurg.2011.05.009 PMID:22000533

Stelmack, J. A., Tang, X. C., Wei, Y., Wilcox, D. T., Morand, T., Brahm, K., ... Group, L. I. S. (2017). Outcomes of the Veterans Affairs Low Vision Intervention Trial II (LOVIT II): A Randomized Clinical Trial. *JAMA Ophthalmology*, *135*(2), 96–104. doi:10.1001/jamaophthalmol.2016.4742 PMID:27978569

Stets, J.E., & Burke, P.J. (2000). Identity Theory and Social Identity Theory. *Social Psychology Quarterly*, *63*(3), 224-237. http://links.jstor.org/sici?sici=0190-2725%28200009%2963%3A3%3C224%3AITASIT%3E2.0.CO%3B2-V

Stewart, R. M., Myers, J. G., Dent, D. L., Ermis, P., Gray, G. A., Villarreal, R., Blow, O., Woods, B., McFarland, M., Garavaglia, J., Root, H. D., & Pruitt, B. A. Jr. (2003). Seven hundred fifty-three consecutive deaths in a level I trauma center: The argument for injury prevention. *The Journal of Trauma Injury Infection and Critical Care*, *54*(1), 66–71. doi:10.1097/00005373-200301000-00009 PMID:12544901

Stocker, M., Burmester, M., & Allen, M. (2014). Optimization of simulated team training through the application of learning theories: A debate for a conceptual framework. *BMC Medical Education*, *14*(1), 69–78. doi:10.1186/1472-6920-14-69 PMID:24694243

Strasser, D. C., Falconer, J. A., Stevens, A. B., Uomoto, J. M., Herrin, J., Bowen, S. E., & Burridge, A. B. (2008). Team training and stroke rehabilitation outcomes: A cluster randomized trial. *Archives of Physical Medicine and Rehabilitation*, *89*(1), 10–15. doi:10.1016/j.apmr.2007.08.127 PMID:18164324

Straus, S., Chatur, F., & Taylor, M. (2009). Issures in the Mentor-Mentee relationship in academic medicine: A qualitative study. *Academic Medicine*, *84*(1), 135–139. doi:10.1097/ACM.0b013e31819301ab PMID:19116493

Stuart Foundation. (2002). Creating, Implementing, and Sustaining Interprofessional Education (Vol. 3). San Francisco, CA: Author.

Sullivan, K., Charrette, A., Massey, C., Bartlett, D., Walker, C., Bond, I., & Fong, J. J. (2015). Interprofessional education with a community fall prevention event. *Journal of Interprofessional Care, 29*(4), 374–376. doi:10.3109/13561820.2014.969834 PMID:25317499

Surowiecki, J. (2005). *The wisdom of crowds: Why the many are smarter than the few*. Abacus.

Suter, E., Goldman, J., Martimianakis, T., Chatalalsingh, C., DeMatteo, D. J., & Reeves, S. (2013). The use of systems and organizational theories in the interprofessional field: Findings from a scoping review. *Journal of Interprofessional Care, 27*(1), 57–64. doi:10.3109/13561820.2012.739670 PMID:23148862

Symonds, I., Cullen, L., & Fraser, D. (2003). Evaluation of a formative interprofessional team objective structured clinical examination (ITOSCE): A method of shared learning in maternity education. *Medical Teacher, 25*(1), 38–41. doi:10.1080/0142159021000061404 PMID:14741857

Tackett, S., Wright, S., Colbert-Getz, J., & Shochet, R. (2018). Associations between learning community engagement and burnout, quality of life, and empathy among medical students. *International Journal of Medical Education, 9*(1), 316–322. doi:10.5116/ijme.5bef.e834 PMID:30504524

Taherian, K., & Shekarchian, M. (2008). Mentoring for doctors. Do its benefits outweigh its disadvantages? *Medical Teacher, 30*(4), e95–e99. doi:10.1080/01421590801929968 PMID:18569651

Taplin, S. H., Weaver, S., Salas, E., Chollette, V., Edwards, H. M., Bruinooge, S. S., & Kosty, M. P. (2015). Reviewing cancer care team effectiveness. *Journal of Oncology Practice / American Society of Clinical Oncology, 11*(3), 239–246. doi:10.1200/JOP.2014.003350 PMID:25873056

Taylor, R. J., Chatters, L. M., & Levin, J. (2004). *Religion in the lives of African Americans: social, psychological, and health perspectives*. Sage.

Teaster, P. B., Nerenberg, L., & Stansbury, K. L. (2003). A national look at elder abuse multidisciplinary teams. *Journal of Elder Abuse & Neglect, 15*(3-4), 91–107. doi:10.1300/J084v15n03_06

Tejos, R., Chahuán, J., Uslar, T., Inzunza, M., Villagrán, I., Riquelme, V., Padilla, O., Pizarro, M., Corvetto, M., Varas, J., & Riquelme, A. (2018). Simulated training program in abdominal paracentesis for undergraduate medical students. *Gastroenterologia y Hepatologia, 42*(4), 239–247. doi:10.1016/j.gastrohep.2018.10.001 PMID:30471721

Temel, J. S. (2010). Early palliative care for patients with metastatic non-small-cell lung cancer. *The New England Journal of Medicine*.

The Role of the Physical Therapist in National Health Care Reform. (n.d.). *APTA's Health Care*. https://www.apta.org/uploadedFiles/APTAorg/Advocacy/Federal/Health_Care_Reform/APTA_Position/RoleofPTinHealthCareReform.pdf

The WHO Framework for Action. (2010). The WHO Framework for Action. *Journal of Interprofessional Care, 24*(5), 475–478. doi:10.3109/13561820.2010.504134 PMID:20718593

Thomas, P. A., Kern, D. E., Hughes, M. T., & Chen, B. Y. (2016). *Curriculum development for medical education: a six-step approach.* Johns Hopkins University Press.

Thompson, B. M., Bratzler, D. W., Fisher, M. J., Torres, A., Faculty, E., & Sparks, R. A. (2016). Working together: Using a unique approach to evaluate an interactive and clinic-based longitudinal interprofessional education experience with 13 professions. *Journal of Interprofessional Care, 30*(6), 754–761. doi:10.1080/13561820.2016.1227962 PMID:27797628

Thorell, M., Fridorff-Jens, P. K., Lassen, P., Lange, T., & Kayser, L. (2015). Transforming students into digital academics: A challenge at both the individual and the institutional level. *BMC Medical Education, 15*(1), 48. doi:10.118612909-015-0330-5 PMID:25890174

Thurston, M. M., Chesson, M. M., Harris, E. C., & Ryan, G. J. (2017). Professional stereotypes of interprofessional education naive pharmacy and nursing students. *American Journal of Pharmaceutical Education, 81*(5). Advance online publication. doi:10.5688/ajpe81584 PMID:28720912

Tietze, M., Woods, S., Brown, G., & Brown, S. (n.d.). *Telehealth: Delivering on Interprofessional, Analytic and Patient Safety/Quality With Community Based Partnerships.* Retrieved from https://community.ania.org/HigherLogic/System/

Timeline. (n.d.a). Retrieved December 11, 2019, from Institute for Healthcare Improvement website: http://www.ihi.org/about/Documents/IHI_Timeline_2018.pdf

Timeline. (n.d.b). Retrieved December 11, 2019, from Physician Assistant History Society website: https://pahx.org/timeline/

Tinnetti, M. E., Williams, T. F., & Mayewski, R. (1986). Fall Risk Assessment for elderly patients based on number of chronic disabilities. *The American Journal of Medicine, 80*(3), 429–434. doi:10.1016/0002 9343(86)90717-5 PMID:3953620

Tourigny, A., Durand, P.J., Bonin, L., Hébert, R., & Rochette, L. (2004). Quasi-experimental Study of the Effectiveness of an Integrated Service Delivery Network for the Frail Elderly. *Canadian Journal on Aging/La Revue canadienne du vieillissement, 23*(3), 231-246.

Trivedi, D., Goodman, C., Gage, H., Baron, N., Scheibl, F., Iliffe, S., Manthorpe, J., Bunn, F., & Drennan, V. (2013). The effectiveness of interprofessional working for older people living in the commuity: A systematic review. *Health & Social Care in the Community, 21*(2), 113–128. doi:10.1111/j.1365-2524.2012.01067.x PMID:22891915

Tsai, J., Cheng, M., Tsai, H., Hung, H., & Chen, Y. (2019). Acceptance and resistance of telehealth: The perspective of dual-factor concepts in technology adoption. *International Journal of Information Management, 49*, 34–44. doi:10.1016/j.ijinfomgt.2019.03.003

Turk, M. A., & Nitu-Maquise, A. D. (2015). Rehabilitation team functioning. *Physical Medicine & Rehabilitation Knowledge.* https://now.aapmr.org/rehabilitation-team-functioning/

U.S. Department of Education. (n.d.). *IDEA Individuals with Disabilities Education Act*. Retrieved from https://sites.ed.gov/idea/

U.S. Preventive Services Task Force. (2011). U.*S. Preventive Services Task Force Issues Final Recommendation Statement for Vision Screening in Children Ages 1 to 5*. Retrieved from https://www.uspreventiveservicestaskforce.org/Announcements/News/Item/us-preventive-services-task-force-issues-final-recommendation-statement-for-vision-screening-in-children-ages-1-to-5

United States Census Bureau. (2017). *Population Projections*. Retrieved from https://www.census.gov/programs-surveys/popproj.html

United States Census Bureau. (2018). Older people projected to outnumber children for the first time in US history. *Newsroom*. Release number CB18-41. Retrieved from https://www.census.gov/newsroom/press-releases/2018/cb18-41-population-projections.html on September 18, 2019.

Valdez-García, J. E. (2004). Brevísima Historia de la Educación Médica. *Avances*, *1*(3), 37–38.

Valdez-García, J. E., & Uscanga, V. M. (2006). Nuevos campos clínicos en la educación médica: Análisis comparativo campos clínicos hospitalario y ambulatorio. *Avances*, *9*, 33–40.

van Dongen, J. J. J., van Bokhoven, M. A., Daniels, R., van der Weijden, T., Petronella Emonts, W. W. G., & Beurskens, A. (2016). Developing interprofessional plans in chronic care: A scoping review. *BMC Family Practice*, *17*(1), 137. doi:10.118612875-016-0535-7 PMID:27655185

Villanueva, T., Núñez Tapia, R. M, Syr Salas Perea, R., & Rodríguez-Orozco, A. R. (2007). The undergraduate medical internship and the clinical competences: Mexico in the Latin American context. *Educación Médica Superior, 21*(4). Retrieved from http://scielo.sld.cu/scielo.php?script=sci_arttext&pid=S0864-21412007000400005&lng=es&tlng=en

Vision & Mission. (n.d.). Retrieved from IPEC Interprofessional Education Collaborative website: http://ipecollaborative.org/vision---mission.html

Von Korff, M., Gruman, J., Schaefer, J., Curry, S. J., & Wagner, E. H. (1997). Collaborative management of chronic illness: Essential elements. *Annals of Internal Medicine*, *127*(12), 1097–1102. doi:10.7326/0003-4819-127-12-199712150-00008 PMID:9412313

Walders, N., Kercsmar, C., Schluchter, M., Redline, S., Kirchner, H. L., & Drotar, D. (2006). An interdisciplinary intervention for undertreated pediatric asthma. *Chest*, *129*(2), 292–299. doi:10.1378/chest.129.2.292 PMID:16478844

Walsh, K. (2013). *Oxford Textbook of Medical Education*. Oxford University Press. doi:10.1093/med/9780199652679.001.0001

Walston, J. D. (2016). Common clinical sequelae of aging. In L. Goldman & A. Schafer (Eds.), *Goldman-Cecil Medicine* (25th ed.). Elsevier Saunders.

Walter, H. J., Vernacchio, L., Trudell, E. K., Bromberg, J., Goodman, E., Barton, J., Young, G. J., DeMaso, D. R., & Focht, G. (2019). Five-Year Outcomes of Behavioral Health Integration in Pediatric Primary Care. *Pediatrics*, *144*(1), e20183243. doi:10.1542/peds.2018-3243 PMID:31186366

Wang, R., Shi, N., Bai, J., Zheng, Y., & Zhao, Y. (2015). Implementation and evaluation of an interprofessional simulation-based education program for undergraduate nursing students in operating room nursing education: A randomized controlled trial. *BMC Medical Education*, *15*(1), 115. doi:10.118612909-015-0400-8 PMID:26155839

Weinstein, R., Krupinski, E., & Doarn, C. (2018). Clinical Examination Component of Telemedicine, Telehealth, mHealth, and Connected Health Medical Practices. *The Medical Clinics of North America*, *102*(3), 533–544. doi:10.1016/j.mcna.2018.01.002 PMID:29650074

Weller, J., Boyd, M., & Cumin, D. (2014). Teams, tribes, and patient safety: Overcoming barriers to effective teamwork in healthcare. *Postgraduate Medical Journal*, *90*(1061), 149–154. doi:10.1136/postgradmedj-2012-131168 PMID:24398594

Wenger, E. (2002). *Comunidades de práctica*. Paidós.

West, C., Graham, L., Palmer, R. T., Miller, M. F., Thayer, E. K., Stuber, M. L., Awdishu, L., Umoren, R. A., Wamsley, M. A., Nelson, E. A., Joo, P. A., Tysinger, J. W., George, P., & Carney, P. A. (2016). Implementation of interprofessional education (IPE) in 16 U.S. medical schools: Common practices, barriers and facilitators. *J Interprofessional Educ Pract Online*, *4*, 41–49. doi:10.1016/j.xjep.2016.05.002 PMID:28184380

West, S. K., Rubin, G. S., Broman, A. T., Munoz, B., Bandeen-Roche, K., & Turano, K. (2002). How does visual impairment affect performance on tasks of everyday life? The SEE Project. Salisbury Eye Evaluation. *Archives of Ophthalmology*, *120*(6), 774–780. doi:10.1001/archopht.120.6.774 PMID:12049583

Whitcomb, M. E. (2009). Commentary: Flexner redux 2010: Graduate medical education in the United States. *Academic Medicine*, *84*(11), 1476–1478. doi:10.1097/ACM.0b013e3181bb25db PMID:19858793

WHO Study Group on Multiprofessional Education of Health Personnel. (Ed.). (1988). *Learning together to work together for health: Report of a WHO Study Group on Multiprofessional Education of Health Personnel: the team approach*. World Health Organization.

Wilkinson, M. J., Manoogian, E., Zadourian, A., Lo, H., Fakhouri, S., Shoghi, A., Wang, X., Fleischer, J. G., Navlakha, S., Panda, S., & Taub, P. R. (2020). Ten-hour time-restricted eating reduces weight, blood pressure, and atherogenic lipids in patients with metabolic syndrome. *Cell Metabolism*, *31*(1), 1–13. doi:10.1016/j.cmet.2019.11.004 PMID:31813824

Willis, J. (1996). A flexible framework for task-based learning An overview of a task-based framework for language teaching. *Oxford Prabhu*, *1987*, 52–62.

Wilson, K. A., Burke, C. S., Priest, H. A., & Salas, E. (2005). Promoting health care safety through training high reliability teams. *Quality & Safety in Health Care, 14*(4), 303–309. doi:10.1136/qshc.2004.010090 PMID:16076797

Wimmers, P., Schmidt, H., & Splinter, T. A. (2006). Influence of clerkship experiences on clinical competence. *Medical Education, 40*(5), 450–458. Advance online publication. doi:10.1111/j.1365-2929.2006.02447.x PMID:16635125

Wockland, E. (n.d.). *Is There A Difference Between Telemedicine and Telehealth?* Retrieved from https://mhealthintelligence.com/features/is-there-a-difference-between-telemedicine-and-telehealth

Wolf, L., Delao, A., & Perhats, C. (2014). Nothing Changes, Nobody Cares: Understanding the Experience of Emergency Nurses Physically or Verbally Assaulted While Providing Care. *Journal of Emergency Nursing, 40*. . doi:10.1016/j.jen.2013.11.006:1-6

Wong, A., Wing, L., Weiss, B., & Gang, M. (2015). Coordinating a team response to behavioral emergencies in the emergency department: A simulation-enhanced interprofessional curriculum. *The Western Journal of Emergency Medicine, 16*(6), 859–865. doi:10.5811/westjem.2015.8.26220 PMID:26594279

Wooding, E. L., Gale, T. C., & Maynard, V. (2019). Evaluation of teamwork assessment tools for interprofessional simulation: A systematic literature review. *Journal of Interprofessional Care*. Advanced online publication. https://doi:10.1080/13561820.2019.1650730

World Health Organization (WHO). (2010). *Framework for action on interprofessional education & collaborative practice*. WHO.

World Health Organization. (1973). *Continuing Education for Physicians. Report of a WHO (World Health Organization) Expert Committee.* Technical Report Series No. 534.

World Health Organization. (1973). Continuing education for physicians. Report of a WHO expert committee. *World Health Organization Technical Report Series, 534*, 1–32. eric.ed.gov/?id=ED102917 PMID:4204010

World Health Organization. (1988). Learning together to work together for health. Report of a WHO study group on multiprofessional education of health personnel: The team approach. *World Health Organization Technical Report Series, 769*, 1–72. https://apps.who.int/iris/handle/10665/37411 PMID:3140499

World Health Organization. (2006). *Rapid Scaling Up of Health Workforce Production. World Health Assembly. WHA59.23.* Retrieved from https://www.who.int/workforcealliance/knowledge/resources/wha_scalingup/en

World Health Organization. (2010). Framework for action on interprofessional education and collaborative practice. Health Professions Network Nursing and Midwifery Office within the Department of Human Resources for Health.

World Health Organization. (2010). *Framework for Action on Interprofessional Education and Collaborative Practice*. Retrieved from https://www.who.int/hrh/resources/framework_action/en/

World Health Organization. (2010). *Framework for Action on Interprofessional Education and Collaborative Practice*. Retrieved from www.who.int/hrh/resources/framework_action

World Health Organization. (2010). *Framework for action on interprofessional education and collaborative practice*. Retrieved from: https://apps.who.int/iris/bitstream/10665/70185/1/WHO_HRH_HPN_10.3_eng.pdf?ua=1

World Health Organization. (2010). *Framework for action on interprofessional education and collaborative practice*. WHO.

World Health Organization. (2013). *Transforming and scaling up health professional's education and training: World health organization guidelines*. Retrieved from www.who.int/hrh/resources/transf_scaling_hpet/en

World Health Organization. (2015). *The impact of myopia and high myopia*. Retrieved from https://www.who.int/blindness/causes/MyopiaReportforWeb.pdf

World Health Organization. (2016). *Declaration of Alma-Ata: Adopted at the International Conference on Primary Health Care, Alma-Ata, USSR*. Retrieved from www.who.int/publications/almaata_declaration_en.pdf

World Health Organization. (2018 October 11). *Blindness and vision impairment*. Retrieved from https://www.who.int/news-room/fact-sheets/detail/blindness-and-visual-impairment

World Health Organization. (2018). *Abuse Fact Sheet*. Retrieved from https://www.who.int/news-room/fact-sheets/detail/elder-abuse

World Health Organization. (2019). *Dementia Fact Sheet*. Retrieved from https://www.who.int/news-room/fact-sheets/detail/dementia

World Health Organization. (2019). *Preventing suicide: A global perspective*. Retrieved from https://apps.who.int/iris/bitstream/handle/10665/131056/9789241564878_eng.pdf;jsessionid=0E95072A30E5F3DF4DB15AE4CEA79C33?sequence=8

World Health Organization. (n.d.). *Global Health Observatory data*. Retrieved from https://www.who.int/gho/goe/telehealth/en/

Wright, A. A., & Katz, I. T. (2018). Beyond Burnout—Redesigning Care to Restore Meaning and Sanity for Physicians. *The New England Journal of Medicine*, *378*(4), 309–311. doi:10.1056/NEJMp1716845 PMID:29365301

Yadav, N. K., & Ciuffreda, K. J. (2014). Effect of binasal occlusion (BNO) and base-in prisms on the visual-evoked potential (VEP) in mild traumatic brain injury (mTBI). *Brain Injury: [BI]*, *28*(12), 1568–1580. doi:10.3109/02699052.2014.939718 PMID:25058498

Yang, Z., Zhou, Y., Chung, J. W. Y., Tang, Q., Jiang, L., & Wong, T. K. S. (2018). Challenge Based Learning nurtures creative thinking: An evaluative study. *Nurse Education Today*, *71*, 40–47. doi:10.1016/j.nedt.2018.09.004 PMID:30223169

Yeu, E., Donnenfeld, E., & Chang, D. H. (2018 February 21). *Five secrets to success with co-management*. Retrieved from https://www.ophthalmologytimes.com/article/five-secrets-success-co-management

Yon, Y., Mikton, C. R., Gassoumis, Z. D., & Wilber, K. H. (2017). Elder abuse prevalence in community settings: A systematic review and meta-analysis. *The Lancet. Global Health*, *5*(2), e147–e156. Advance online publication. doi:10.1016/S2214-109X(17)30006-2 PMID:28104184

You, P., Malik, N., Scott, G., & Fung, K. (2017). Current state of interprofessional educaiton in Canadian medical schools: Findings from a national survey. *Journal of Interprofessional Care*, *31*(5), 670–672. doi:10.1080/13561820.2017.1315060 PMID:28481135

Yumori, J. W., Dickter, D. N., Napier-Dovorany, K., Wren, V. Q., Tegzes, J. H., & Stielstra, S. (2015). Optometry Students' Knowledge-Based Performance within Interprofessional Education Courses. *Optometric Education*, *40*(3), 31–36.

Zhan, C., Sangl, J., Bierman, A. S., Miller, M. R., Friedman, B., Wickizer, S. W., & Meyer, G. S. (2001). Potentially inappropriate medication use in the community-dwelling elderly. Findings from the 1996 medical expenditure panel survey. *Journal of the American Medical Association*, *286*(22), 2823–2829. doi:10.1001/jama.286.22.2823 PMID:11735757

Zhou, H. Y. (2012). The present situation of curriculum system and transformation of nursing education in China. *J. Qilu Nurs*, *18*(15), 39–40.

Zimmerman, A. B., Lust, K. L., & Bullimore, M. A. (2011). Visual acuity and contrast sensitivity testing for sports vision. *Eye & Contact Lens*, *37*(3), 153–159. doi:10.1097/ICL.0b013e31820d12f4 PMID:21378574

Ziv, A., Wople, P. R., Small, S. D., & Glick, S. (2003). Simulation-based medical education: An ethical imperative. *Academic Medicine*, *78*(8), 783–788. doi:10.1097/00001888-200308000-00006 PMID:12915366

Zoon, H. F. A., deGraf, C., & Boesveldt, S. (2016). Food odours direct specific appetite. *Foods*, *5*(1). Retrieved from https://www.ncbi.nlm.nih.gov/pmc/articles/PMC5224573/

Zorek, J., & Raehl, C. (2013). Interprofessional education accreditation standards in the USA: A comparative analysis. *Journal of Interprofessional Care*, *27*(2), 123–130. doi:10.3109/13561820.2012.718295 PMID:22950791

About the Contributors

Steven D. Waldman, MD, JD, serves as Vice Dean and Chair of the Department Medical Humanities and Bioethics at the University of Missouri-Kansas City School of Medicine. He holds joint academic appointments as Professor of Anesthesiology and Professor of Medical Humanities and Bioethics. The author of 43 textbooks and numerous academic articles on the specialty of interventional pain management, physical diagnosis ultrasound, and medical education, Dr. Waldman also continues his clinical work as an interventional pain management physician as well as an active member of the medical staff at Truman Medical Center.

Stephanie Bowlin is the Founding Chief of Office of Mission Integration at Western University of Health Sciences (WesternU) and is an Associate Professor of Physician Assistant Education. She graduated from the University of La Verne in 1998 with an EdD in Organizational Leadership and earned a Physician Assistant Certificate from Charles R. Drew University of Medicine and Science in 1984 and specializes in pediatrics. She joined the PA Faculty in 1990 at WesternU and served as the Dean of the College of Health Sciences from 1998 to 2019. The college houses a Master's in Science in Health Sciences, Master's in PA Studies and a Doctorate in Physical Therapy. In her current role as Founding Chief of Mission Integration, Dr. Bowlin is responsible for building a culture of cross-departmental integration at the University, ensuring collaborations and unified strategic planning among educational, service and research enterprises. She leads educational departments and services that include Interprofessional Education, faculty development, community engagement, and leadership assessment, and development.

* * *

Manisha Arora received her MD in Anesthesia & Critical Care from University of Delhi-India in 2008. She completed her Senior Residency from University of Delhi-India. In 2013 she was hired as Attending Consultant in Department of Anesthesiology and Pain Management at Rajiv Gandhi Cancer Institute & Research

Centre Delhi-India. Currently she is working as Consultant Pain Physician at Delhi Pain Management Centre Delhi-India. She has a keen interest in spreading awareness about chronic pain and is involved in various research projects on chronic pain.

Julie Wright Banderas earned her PharmD degree at the University of Nebraska Medical Center College of Pharmacy in 1990. She has a longstanding teaching and leadership record of accomplishment at the University of Missouri-Kansas City School of Medicine. She is a tenured professor and Chair for the Department of Graduate Health Professions in Medicine. She has expertise in teaching clinical pharmacology, responsible conduct of research, and concepts of evidence-based medicine, patient safety, and quality improvement. HIV treatment and prevention are the focus of her research and community service efforts.

Christi Bartlett is an Assistant Professor in Palliative Care at The University of Kansas School of Medicine. She completed medical school at the University of Kansas, as well as her Internal Medicine residency and Hospice and Palliative Care fellowship. She is certified by the American Board of Internal Medicine and the American Board of Hospice and Palliative Medicine. Her practice involves hospital-based Palliative Care as well as inpatient hospice care. She is active in medical school and residency education as well as the Palliative Care fellowship program.

Jannette Berkley-Patton, Ph.D., is a professor in the University of Missouri-Kansas City School of Medicine Biomedical and Health Informatics Department. She is also the director of the Community Health Research Group, the director of the UMKC Health Equity Institute, and adjunct faculty in the Department of Psychology at the University of Missouri-Kansas City. Her expertise is in using community-engaged approaches to test and disseminate evidence-based health screening and linkage to care interventions focused on diabetes, heart disease, HIV/STDs/hepatitis c virus, and mental health in community settings. She engages students, community-health-academic partnerships, and ethnic minority populations in addressing health disparities using novel scalable and sustainable methods. She was recently honored with induction into the KU Women's Hall of Fame, awarded the University of Missouri System Cross-Cultural Community Engagement Presidential Award, and appointed as a University of Missouri System Presidential Engagement Fellow.

Carole Bowe Thompson is Project Director for two NIH-funded grants: a) an NIMHD-R24 grant pilot testing a multilevel intervention using a community-based participatory research approach to educate and provide screening, prevention, linkage to care for diabetes/heart disease/stroke in 6 African American churches, b) an NIMH-R01 grant focusing on increasing access to HIV screening, prevention, and linkage to care in 14 African American churches. She contributed largely to a faith-based capacity building grant funded by NMHD (R34) as Co-Project Director of the Heartland Health Network (HHN). HHN established a model partnership network between academic health researchers, the African American faith-based community, and community-based health service organizations to address health disparities in African American communities. She has over 25 years of experience working with health, community, and faith-based organizations where she held numerous leadership roles that focused on project conceptualization and development, coordinating study activities with collaborative partners, creating training programs for research team members and staff members at partnering organizations, managing data collection activities and reports, manualizing study procedures/activities, and supervising research staff on large-scale health promotion interventions in underserved. Ms. Bowe Thompson has also contributed as an author to the conceptualization and preparation of manuscripts from several church-bases studies and have presented findings in over 20 conference presentations.

Brian Burghardt is an assistant professor at the UMKC School of Medicine. He graduated from the Medical College of Wisconsin in 2006. He graduated from the Children's Mercy Pediatrics residency program in 2009 and joined the faculty there, where he serves as a board-certified general pediatrician. He has served as the Associate Director of medical student education there from 2014 to present. He has been the faculty advisor for the UMKC Pediatric Interest Group since 2014. He serves as the attending physician for multiple resident continuity clinics. He holds a special interest in adolescent medicine and mental health.

D. Joshua Cameron, PhD, completed a PhD in Neuroscience at the University of Utah School of Medicine in 2007 and a postdoctoral fellowship in Cellular and Molecular Biology at Harvard University in 2010. He is currently an associate professor of optometry at the Western University of Health Sciences, Pomona, CA.

Raúl René Cantú Hernández is a junior physician, medical education researcher at Tec de Monterrey's School of Medicine and currently a high school biology professor at Prepa Tec.

Ida Chung is a pediatric optometrist in Pomona, CA at WesternU Health Eye Care Institute. She graduated from the SUNY College of Optometry in 1993 and completed her residency in pediatrics and binocular vision at Pennsylvania College of Optometry in 1994. She obtained her fellowship from the College of Optometrists in Vision Development in 1996, and became a fellow of the American Academy of

Optometry in 2001. She is the Associate Dean of Academic Affairs and associate professor of optometry at Western University of Health Sciences College of Optometry.

Valerie Chuy is a third year medical student at the University of Missouri-Kansas City School of Medicine. She is an Admission Ambassador, co-creator of Sojourner Health Clinic's Help a Life Organization, and chair of the university's Camp Cardiac.

David Dickter is the Director of Interprofessional Education (IPE) Research and Strategic Assessment at Western University of Health Sciences. He leads the development and implementation of assessment programs to evaluate IPE programming, including the design of assessment tools and establishment of systems to evaluate the results of various stages, activities, and phases the program. In addition, he manages the development, implementation and evaluation of various university strategic planning activities. Prior to joining WesternU, Dr. Dickter served as an internal and external consultant on assessment and program evaluation projects for over 15 years, including the development of competency assessments; research design; statistical analysis; and program evaluation. He has held internal and external consulting roles in education (Ohio State University, University of Pennsylvania), non-profit organizations (e.g., Educational Testing Services) and corporations (e.g., AT&T). Publications in peer-reviewed journals include the Journal of Applied Psychology and the Journal of Organizational Behavior. Dr. Dickter earned his Ph.D. in Industrial/Organizational Psychology from Ohio State University.

Stefanie Ellison is the associate dean for Learning Initiatives at the UMKC School of Medicine and a Professor of Emergency Medicine at Truman Medical Center. She graduated from the University of Nebraska Medical Center College of Medicine in 1997. She graduated from TMC/UMKC Emergency Medicine residency program in June 2000 and joined the faculty at Truman Medical Center. She is board certified in Emergency Medicine and is a core faculty for the Emergency Medicine residency at Truman Medical Center. She served as the Associate Dean and Chair for the Council on Curriculum at the UMKC School of Medicine from 2000-2017 and was a member of the UMKC SOM Council on Curriculum for over ten years. She served as the Emergency Medicine Clerkship director from 2004-2015. She is an active member of the UMKC Interprofessional Education (IPE) Steering Committee and the Co-convener of the UMKC Health Science IPE Curriculum and Assessment Working Group since 2011.

Irma Elisa Eraña Rojas is Medicine Undergraduate Program Director and Associate Professor at the School of Medicine of Tecnológico de Monterrey, Northern Region. Pathologist at the San José Hospital TecSalud in Monterrey. Fellow at the

Foundation for Advancement of International Medical Education (FAIMER). Judge in the QS Stars Re-imagine Education Awards and in the Novus Educational Innovation Fund. Won the Inspiring Professor Award in 2013 and is member of the faculty that created the Virtual Pathology Laboratory project, which was chosen for the Novus 2013 fund for educational innovation and obtained second place in the International innovation event in education called QS Stars Re-imagine Education Awards in 2015. In the same event in 2017 was selected as shortlisted with the Forensic Science immersion lab project. Obtained the distinction of Microsoft Innovative Educator Expert since 2015 to current date.

Katherine G. Ervie graduated from the Butler University Physician Assistant program in 1998, later obtaining her Masters in Physician Assistant Studies from the University of Nebraska Medical Center in 2003. Katherine worked as a PA primarily in the area of orthopedic surgery before becoming the founding program director of the University of Missouri-Kansas City Physician Assistant Program in 2012. Katherine has a teaching and research interest in interprofessional education, patient safety, service learning, and diversity and inclusion, all of which she has strived to incorporate into the PA program curriculum and learning community.

Izhar Faisal received his MD in Anaesthesiology from Dr. Ram Manohar Lohia Avadh University-India in 2014. He further gained experience by working as Senior Resident from February 2015 to September 2018 at prestigious Govind Ballabh Pant Institute of Postgraduate Medical Education and Research New Delhi-India. Advancing his career in Pain management he completed fellowship in Pain management from Aesculap Academy-Germany. In 2019 he was hired as Attending Consultant in Department of Anesthesiology and Pain Management by Medeor Hospital New Delhi-India. Currently he is working as Attending Consultant in Department of Anesthesiology and Pain Management Medeor Hospital New Delhi-India. Always being on top of his professional career he has many scientific awards to his name including RSACP'S Padmakant Research Award. He has presented his scientific work at various State and National Congresses and has several publications to his name. His area of interest includes chronic pain management and regenerative medicine. He is part of various research projects in Anesthesiology and Pain management.

Saqib Hassan, BA, is a medical student at the University of Missouri Kansas City in Kansas City, MO. He anticipates graduating in May 2021 and as planning to go into a residency program for Anesthesiology. Before graduating, he hopes to help improve interprofessional curriculum to foster a better working environment for all professionals working in healthcare.

Elizabeth Hoppe, OD, MPH, DrPH, is the Founding Dean of the College of Optometry at Western University of Health Sciences.

Emmanuel Katsaros is a graduate of Midwestern University Chicago College of Osteopathic Medicine. He completed his internal medicine residency and rheumatology fellowship at Loma Linda University Medical Center, where he also became the program director of rheumatology fellowship program. He currently is the Chair of Internal Medicine Department at Western University of Health Sciences/College of Osteopathic Medicine of the Pacific and was a member of the American Association for Colleges of Osteopathic Medicine (AACOM) EPA steering Committee, which published a guide for EPA development for undergraduate medical education.

Mildred López Cabrera MSc, PhD, is currently the Director of Educational Innovation at the School of Medicine and Health Sciences at Tecnológico de Monterrey. She is a Fellow of FAIMER Institute (Foundation for Advancement of International Medical Education and Research) in Latin America FRILA and the Pontificia Universidad Católica de Chile. She is an Associate Fellow of AMEE (Association for Medical Education in Europe).

Susan Mackintosh is a graduate of the Western University of Health Sciences, College of Osteopathic Medicine of the Pacific. She completed her Family Medicine residency at Kaiser -Fontana. She is currently the Associate Dean of Multiprofessional Collaboration and College Affairs for the College of Osteopathic Medicine of the Pacific. Dr. Mackintosh was the founding Director for Interprofessional Education at Western University of Health Sciences and additionally was one of the original contributors to the 2011 Core Competencies for Interprofessional Collaborative Practice.

Tine Meyer graduated with the charter PA class from the College of Osteopathic Medicine of the Pacific in 1992. She earned a master's degree from Western University in Health Professions Education in 2005, and the Doctor of Health Sciences from Nova Southeastern University in 2009 where she studied global health delivery systems. Dr. Meyer maintains continuous NCCPA certification since 1992. Her clinical practice included internal and family medicine, hospitalist, long-term care and hospice. Dr. Meyer teaches topics in clinical medicine, public health, education, curriculum design, and program development throughout WesternU. Dr. Meyer served as the Governor's Appointee to the California Medical Board in 2003-2008, Co-Chair of the Diversity Committee of the California Academy of Physician Assistant and served as President of the Western University Alumni Association.

Abigail Montserrat Molina Rodriguez is a Junior Physician, graduated from Instituto Tecnológico y de Estudios Superiores de Monterrey's. During her student years, she co-founded and coordinated as part of the directive board the student group "RREM" which helped to impart RCP courses to the medical and non-medical community, she was honored as a fellow teacher to impart Histology Lab to first year medical students for 2 years, she also helped coordinate MediTEC for 2 years, a clinic run by students for employees and alumni, and she was involved in the implementation of cultural diffusion events in her Medical School. At the end of 2018 and beginning of 2019 she completed an international clinical rotation in Pediatrics and General Surgery in Hospital Reina Sofia in Navarra, Spain and a clinical rotation in Pediatric Oncology and Pediatric Surgery in Hospital Niño de Jesús in Madrid, Spain. During her Social Service Year which she continues, she was honored to be the medical student in charge of the clinical area of the social non-profit organization "Fundación TecSalud" in where she seeks, presents, develops and continues the patient treatment along different clinical experts from General Surgery, Ophtalmology and Cardiology to Neurosurgery to treat over 350 patients a year.

Judith Ovalle-Abuabara is the Clerkship Director for the Psychiatry Department at UMKC School of Medicine, Child and Adolescent Psychiatrist at Truman Medical Center OP Clinic and Faculty member of Greater Kansas City Psychoanalytic Institute (GKCPI). She graduated from The School of Medicine at the Universidad Nacional de Colombia in 1988 and received her degree as a Psychiatrist at El Rosario, University in Bogota, Colombia in 1994 as well as completed her training as a Psychoanalyst at the Sociedad Colombiana de Psychoanalysis in Colombia, getting the International certification as a Psychoanalyst by the International Psychoanalytic Association (IPA) in 2002. She was Director and Psychiatrist of Kennedy Behavioral Health Day Treatment Center for Children and Adolescents which was a psychoanalytic oriented pilot program in Bogota from 1994 to 2002 and also was an Assistant Professor for Psychiatry and Pediatric residents as well as she directed the Child and Adolescent Course for Medical Students at El Rosario University from 1995 to 2003. She graduated from Mizzou-University of Missouri-Columbia Psychiatry residency program in June 2009 and graduated from Child Psychiatry Fellowship also from Mizzou in June 2011. She served as a General and Child and Adolescent Psychiatrist at Pathways Community Behavioral Health Care from 2011 to June 2015 providing mental health services to remote and underserved areas in Missouri, through tele-psychiatry. She is Board Certified in Psychiatry and is a core faculty for the UMKC Psychiatry Residency Program at Truman Medical Center (TMC) since July 2015, where she coordinates the Psychodynamic Psychotherapy Training Program and Track for the Psychiatry Residents. She also has been serving as a psychiatrist for the Hispanic Community at Mattie Rhodes Center, through Truman Medical Center, since November 2016.

Christine T. Pham is an Assistant Professor at Western University of Health Sciences, College of Optometry. She received the Doctorate of Optometry from Western University of Health Sciences, College of Optometry in 2013 and completed a residency in primary eye care and geriatrics at the Edith Nourse Rogers Memorial Veteran in 2014. Her interests are managing and co-managing variety of ocular diseases including macular degeneration, glaucoma, and diabetic retinopathy. Dr. Pham joined Western University of Health Sciences, College of Optometry as faculty in 2015. She became a fellow of the American Academy of Optometry in 2017.

Nurry Pirani MD, FACP, is the Associate Dean and Chair for the Council on Curriculum and an Assistant Professor of Internal Medicine at the University of Missouri - Kansas City School of Medicine. She graduated from the UMKC Internal Medicine residency program in 2011. She served as the Associate Program Director for the Internal Medicine residency from 2013-2017. She practices Internal Medicine at Truman Medical Center and serves as a Docent/Mentor at the UMKC School of Medicine.

Manuel Emiliano Quiroga Garza is a Junior Physician graduated from Instituto Tecnológico y de Estudios Superiores de Monterrey's Class of 2019. Throughout his student years, he helped coordinate MediTEC, a student-run clinic for Campus alumni and employees. In 2015, he was involved in the logistics and implementation of cultural diffusion events in his Medical School. During his Social Service Year, he was honored to be the student in charge of the Learning Communities program for medical students and professors. In this year, he grew professionally by contributing to the expansion of the project to other Health Science spheres and engaging in the development of a Well-Being and Mentorship program for students in Clinical Clerkships. In the year 2011, he was a delegate for the World Health Organization in the UNAUSAMUN Conference in New York. He studied the violin for 13 years and was an active member of the State Symphony Orchestra for 8 years.

Marcella Riley, MD, is a recent graduate of the University of Missouri - Kansas City. She will begin her residency in Obstetrics and Gynecology at Orlando Health, Orlando Florida in July 2020. She has an interest in serving underserved patient populations.

Daniel Robinson, PharmD, FASHP, is the Dean of the College of Pharmacy at Western University of Health Sciences (WesternU). His research and practice interests include drug policy, international pharmacy education, interprofessional education and practice, and political advocacy that support that delivery of pharmaceutical care in all practice settings. Dr. Robinson has over 30 years of experience as a licensed pharmacist and health care educator and over 20 years in academic and health care administration. He has served the American Association of Colleges of Pharmacy on the Professional Affairs Committee, National Patient Safety Task Force, Council of Deans (secretary), Interprofessional Practice Core Competencies Expert Panel, Task Force on Health Care Reform's Impact on Pharmacy Education, MedEdPORTAL-IPEC Advisory Committee, Institutional Research and Assessment Committee, the Academic Leadership Fellows Program as Dean Facilitator and Dean Mentor. He also served on the Board of Directors for the Center for Community Health Education Research and Service, the Board of Directors for the California Pharmacists Association Foundation and the Dean's Advisory Council for the National Community Pharmacists Association. He is past national president of the Rho Chi Pharmacy Honor Society. Dr. Robinson's previous full-time faculty appointments have included University of Nebraska, Department of Clinical Pharmacy; University of Southern California (USC) as Chair of the Department of Pharmacy; Northeastern University as Dean, School of Pharmacy; and Associate Dean, Bouve College of Health Sciences. He established thirteen international academic exchange agreements in nine countries and he co-founded the California Center for Pharmaceutical Care.

Valerie Ruehter is a Clinical Assistant Professor and the Director of Experiential Learning at the University of Missouri Kansas City (UMKC) School of Pharmacy. Dr. Ruehter received her Bachelor of Science in Pharmacy and Doctor of Pharmacy degrees from UMKC. Dr. Ruehter is Board Certified in Psychiatric Pharmacy Practice & Administration (BCPP) and served as a Clinical Psychiatric Pharmacist at Western Missouri Mental Health Center in Kansas City, Missouri from 1993 until 2006. During this time, she held Adjunct faculty appointments with UMKC and the University of Kansas School of Pharmacy serving as a clinical preceptor for senior rotation students. Additionally, she was the Director of the ASHP accredited Psychiatric Pharmacy Practice & Administration Residency Program at Western Missouri Mental Health Center from 1998-2006. Dr. Ruehter coordinates all Introductory and Advanced Pharmacy Practice Experiences in the curriculum at the School of Pharmacy. She is committed to excellence in Experiential Programs and preceptor development for the School of Pharmacy. She is also Co-Convener for the UMKC Health Science Interprofessional Education (IPE) Curriculum and Assessment Working Group and a member of the UMKC IPE Steering Committee.

Saima Salam received her MS in Obstetrics & Gynecology from University of Kashmir-India in 2016. In 2016 she joined as Senior Resident in the Department of Obstetrics & Gynecology Government Medical College at University of Kashmir-India. In 2017 she was hired as Senior Resident in the Department of Obstetrics & Gynecology by University College of Medical Sciences at University of Delhi-India. Currently she is working as Senior Resident in the Department of Obstetrics & Gynecology Government Medical College at University of Kashmir-India. She is actively involved in research activities and has several publications to her name.

Dee Schilling is a tenured Professor at Western University of Health Sciences in Pomona, California where she serves as Interim Dean of the College of Health Sciences. She received her BS in Education from Kent State University, physical therapy degree from Emory, MS in Rehabilitation Medicine from the University of Washington, and a collaborative PhD in Special Education and Rehabilitation Medicine, from the University of Washington. Dee has over 40 years of clinical experience with the majority in pediatrics within the school-based and community settings, as well as serving as Rehabilitation Research Program Specialist at the Cleveland Clinic where she was responsible for the facilitation, coordination and management of Physical Therapists, Occupational Therapists, Orthotists and Prosthetists engaging in multi-disciplinary clinical research and academic trials. Dee has multiple lines of inquiry including educational instruction and assessment, leadership, interprofessional education, behavior and autism. She has presented and published across disciplines, nationally and internationally regarding interprofessional practice, leadership, defining benchmarks for academic excellence and assessment. She is noted for her research and expertise in autism in the areas of sensory strategies for academic success, positive behavior support, and influence of sensorimotor development on function and behavior. She has served as a textbook contributor and editor as well as a reviewer for multiple journals including the Physical Therapy Journal, Journal of Autism and Developmental Disorders, and International Journal of Educational Research. Dee's expertise in behavior and learning, as well as assessment and curricular mapping are rooted in both her undergraduate and graduate degrees in education. She has served school districts k-12 as both an educator and physical therapist. She has served as an external reviewer and curriculum consultant across a variety of disciplines at both the undergraduate and graduate education level including programs such as Kinesiology, Physician Assistant, Health Sciences, Optometry, and Veterinary Medicine. At Western University of Health Sciences, she has served on the University Outcomes Assessment Committee, Strategic Planning Committee, and the IPE Curriculum and Implementation Committees and as Chair of the Institutional Review Board. Dee is a member of APTA's Education, Research, Pediatrics, and Health Policy Administration Sections. She is an active member of the National Interprofessional Education Consortium, serving as Vice Chair, a Fellow in the National Academies of Practice serving as Director at Large – Physical Therapy and a LAMP Institute for Leadership in Physical Therapy faculty member.

Kelley L. Sharp is an emergency room nurse at Hartford Hospital. Kelley received her Bachelor of Science Degree in Nursing from the University of Kansas. She is a Master's Degree candidate in Biomedical Science Research at Ohio State University. Special interests include eldercare bioethics, opioids, perinatal pain management, and interprofessional education. She is currently a first year medical student at the Frank Netter Quinnipiac School of Medicine in Connecticut.

Corey W. Waldman is an ophthalmologist in San Antonio, Texas at UT Health San Antonio. He specializes in cataract and glaucoma surgery. He graduated with honors from University Of Missouri, Kansas City, School Of Medicine in 2012, completed his residency at Sinai Hospital in 2016, and his fellowship in glaucoma at Boston University in 2017. He is Board Certified in ophthalmology and serves as an assistant professor of ophthalmology and as the associate residency program director at UT Health San Antonio as well as the director of medical student education.

Reid Waldman is a dermatology resident at the University of Connecticut. He was born and raised in Leawood, Kansas and stayed in the Kansas City Metro for college and medical school, graduating AOA from the University of Missouri-Kansas City School of Medicine 6 Year BA/MD combined program at the age of 23. After medical school, he completed his intern year at Cedars-Sinai Medical Center in Los Angeles, California. He is an avid writer and researcher. His primary research interest is health services research. He enjoys analyzing data from large national medical record databases to answer pressing clinical issues in dermatology.

Debra Wekesa is a medical student at the University of Missouri- Kansas City. She anticipates graduating in May 2021 and will go on to a residency program in Internal Medicine. She has an interest in academic medicine, working with underserved populations, and increasing diversity in healthcare and diversity and inclusion education in healthcare.

Naveen Yadav is an Assistant Professor at the Western University of Health Sciences College of Optometry. Dr. Yadav received a Bachelor of Science degree with honors in Optometry from the All India Institute of Medical Sciences, a Masters in Vision Science from the University of Waterloo, and a Ph.D. in Vision Science from SUNY, College of Optometry. He has a clinical research interest in the areas of acquired brain injury, clinical electrophysiology, visual perception, pediatric vision, and special need population. His ongoing clinical research project is to assess visual attention objectively in younger children with attention deficit. He is actively involved in reviewing grants and manuscripts in the areas of traumatic brain injury (TBI), clinical electrophysiology, and visual perception. His teaching interest includes visual neurophysiology, visual perception, binocular vision, eye movements, and acquired brain injury.

Kara Zweerink is a medical student at the University of Missouri-Kansas City. She anticipates graduating in May 2021 and plans to complete a residency in Dermatology. As well as practicing as a clinician, Kara is interested in playing a role in educating residents and medical students in her future.

Index

F

G

H

I

L

M

N

O

P

Q

R

S

T

V

W

www.ingramcontent.com/pod-product-compliance
Lightning Source LLC
LaVergne TN
LVHW060005031026
849161LV00025B/1489